FOURTH EDITION

Bipolar Disorder

A Guide for You & Your Loved Ones

FRANCIS MARK MONDIMORE, MD

JOHNS HOPKINS UNIVERSITY PRESS

Baltimore

Note to the Reader: This book is not meant to substitute for medical care, and treatment should not be based solely on its contents. Instead, treatment must be developed in a dialogue between the individual and his or her physician. This book has been written to help with that dialogue.

Drug dosage: The author and publisher have made reasonable efforts to determine that the selection of drugs discussed in this text conform to the practices of the general medical community. The medications described do not necessarily have specific approval by the US Food and Drug Administration for use in the diseases for which they are recommended. In view of ongoing research, changes in governmental regulation, and the constant flow of information relating to drug therapy and drug reactions, the reader is urged to check the package insert of each drug for any change in indications and dosage and for warnings and precautions. This is particularly important when the recommended agent is a new and/or infrequently used drug.

© 1999, 2006, 2014, 2020 Francis Mark Mondimore
All rights reserved. Published 2020
Printed in the United States of America on acid-free paper
9 8 7 6 5 4 3 2 1

Johns Hopkins University Press
2715 North Charles Street
Baltimore, Maryland 21218-4363
www.press.jhu.edu

Library of Congress Cataloging-in-Publication Data

Names: Mondimore, Francis Mark, 1953– author.
Title: Bipolar disorder : a guide for you and your loved ones / Francis Mark
    Mondimore, MD.
Description: Fourth edition. | Baltimore : Johns Hopkins University Press, 2020.
    | Series: A Johns Hopkins Press health book | Includes bibliographical
    references and index.
Identifiers: LCCN 2019059864 | ISBN 9781421439051 (hardcover ; alk. paper)
    | ISBN 9781421439068 (paperback ; alk. paper) | ISBN 9781421439075 (ebook)
Subjects: MESH: Bipolar Disorder | Popular Work
Classification: LCC RC516 | NLM WM 171.7 | DDC 616.89/5—dc23
LC record available at https://lccn.loc.gov/2019059864

A catalog record for this book is available from the British Library.

Special discounts are available for bulk purchases of this book. For more information, please contact Special Sales at specialsales@press.jhu.edu.

Johns Hopkins University Press uses environmentally friendly book materials, including recycled text paper that is composed of at least 30 percent post-consumer waste, whenever possible.

Contents

Preface

About 2 percent of the population suffers from some form of bipolar disorder. If one includes the milder forms of the illness known as *soft* bipolar conditions, that number rises to nearly 5 percent.[1]

Winston Churchill, George Frederic Handel, Lord Byron, Virginia Woolf, Edgar Allan Poe, Napoleon Bonaparte, and Vincent van Gogh are only a few of the politicians, writers, artists, and musicians who, despite having bipolar disorder, left a mark of greatness upon the world.[2] In our own time, musical sensation Mariah Carey, *Star Wars* actress Carrie Fisher, and television anchor and journalist Jane Pauley have acknowledged being diagnosed with bipolar disorder.[3] The list could go on and on.

Most persons who are affected by this illness, however, are just ordinary people who want nothing more than to get back to their everyday lives after they or their family members have been diagnosed with it. This book is written for them.

We psychiatrists have at times become a little complacent about this disease. When lithium became widely available in the United States in the mid-1970s, many psychiatrists thought the battle to control the illness had been won. Indeed, lithium was—and still is—a miracle drug for many people who suffer from what was then known as manic depression. More recent studies indicate that a substantial proportion of patients—according to some studies, as many as half—have a relapse of their illness despite taking lithium. But even as we become more aware of the sobering facts about the difficulty of successfully treating bipolar disorder, an explosion of developments in science and medicine holds great promise for those affected by the disease. In this new edition, I shall relate this good news.

Clinical research has shown again and again that many relapses of bipolar disorder occur not because of medication failure but rather because patients stop taking medication and drop out of treatment. Perhaps they don't understand that relapse and repetition of illness episodes are the hallmark of the disease, that *abruptly* stopping medication has been shown to be especially risky, that medication side effects can often be treated or controlled, and that new medications are becoming available all the time. I hope this book helps those who face difficult treatment decisions to make well-informed and intelligent choices.

A survey of patients with bipolar disorder and other mood disorders, carried out by the National Depressive and Manic-Depressive Association (now, the Depression and Bipolar Support Alliance) in the early 1990s, found that 36 percent of those who responded to the questionnaire had not sought professional treatment until more than *ten years* after their symptoms had begun. Of the bipolar patients in this study, 73 percent had received at least one incorrect diagnosis before being identified as having bipolar disorder—often many years after first seeking help. The average respondent had seen 3.3 physicians before being correctly diagnosed.[4] Another study, done in 2017, showed only a small improvement in the length of time it took persons with bipolar disorder to get into treatment: the number of years had only dropped to just under six.[5]

Why is this illness so difficult to identify correctly? One reason is that the easily diagnosed most severe form of the illness, called bipolar I disorder, is only one of the several forms this chameleon disorder can take—and bipolar I, in fact, is probably less common than the milder forms, in which symptoms of mild depression and subtle "mood swings" may be the only manifestations. We are realizing that many patients with these milder forms of the disorder benefit from treatment with mood-stabilizing medications, too. But they can do so only if they seek treatment and are correctly diagnosed. We shall see why many patients who have a bipolar disorder are told they have "only depression" or a "personality disorder," and we shall also see the consequences of these and other diagnostic errors.

Like any other serious illness, bipolar disorder affects not only the person who suffers from the disease but family, friends, and colleagues as well. Family support is crucial to the effective management of symptoms. The disrupted relationships and interpersonal conflicts that the symptoms of the illness can cause make bipolar disorder all the more difficult and complicated to treat. Information and understanding are definitely part of the treatment for this disease, and this book was written not only for the patient but for the patient's family and friends as well.

Bipolar disorder can be a fatal disease. Although the figures vary among studies, 10 to 15 percent of persons with bipolar disorder die from suicide,[6] while nearly a third make suicide attempts.[7] These are preventable deaths, because very effective treatments for this illness exist. So, yes, I hope that the information this book provides about the treatment of bipolar disorder will save lives.

Many thanks to all who have contributed to this new edition.

I want to especially thank all of the editors and staff at the Johns Hopkins University Press, who have been a pleasure to work with, as always. Special thanks to my editors, Joe Rusko and Juliana McCarthy.

Thanks to Carrie Watterson for her expert copyediting as well as her suggestions for improvements to the content of the manuscript that have made this a better book, and also to Juliet Wilkerson for helping me navigate some thorny stigma issues.

Thanks to Jenna Macfarlane for her handsome illustrations and her patience in dealing with a sometimes persnickety author.

Writers' spouses deserve special gratitude, and mine is no exception. Thank you, Greg, for your patience, your support and encouragement as well as some sound editorial advice.

PART I

What Is
Bipolar Disorder?

A professor of mine once told me, "When you can't figure out *what* the patient has, he or she probably has bipolar disorder." I remember thinking at the time that this was one of the most foolish things I had ever heard a Johns Hopkins faculty member say. But over the years I have come to realize that he was right.

Bipolar disorder is the chameleon of psychiatric disorders, changing its symptoms from one patient to the next and from one episode of illness to the next even in the same patient. It is a phantom that can sneak up on its victim, cloaked in the darkness of melancholy, but then disappear for years at a time—only to return in the resplendent but fiery robes of mania. Although both depression and mania had been described over two millennia previously by Greek and Persian physicians—several of whom thought the conditions were linked in some way—it wasn't until the early part of the twentieth century that a German psychiatrist, Emil Kraepelin, convincingly presented the idea that these opposite conditions were two sides of one pathological coin, the two profiles of a Janus-faced disease that he called manic-depressive insanity.

Why did it take more than two thousand years for someone to solve a puzzle having only two pieces? Because, as my professor knew, there are so many more than two pieces to this mysterious disorder. The depressed phase can be merely gloomy or profoundly despairing, torpid and lethargic, or agitated and churning. The manic phase can be no more than an enthusiastic glow, or it can be an exultant, transcendental fervor, frenzied panic, or delirious, crashing, raving psychosis. Sometimes opposite moods seem to be combined, as inseparable as smoke and fire, mood states that have been given names like *depressive mania*, *manic stupor*, *agitated depression*, and more recently and more simply, *mixed states*. The tendency of the illness to hibernate—for symptoms to spontaneously disappear for years, even decades, at a time—adds to the confusion, perplexing the diagnostician and lulling the patient into dangerous complacency regarding the need for treatment.

In this first part of the book, there are four chapters examining the symptoms, the syndromes, and the diagnosis of bipolar disorder. In chapter 1, "Normal and Abnormal Mood," we review the many symptoms of bipolar disorder, collected into three main clusters: *mania*, *depression*, and the *mixed mood states*. I have not minimized the severity of the symptoms in this chapter; I present all the possible symptoms of the illness, many of them frightening and terrible. But it is important to remember, first, that not every person with bipolar disorder develops all the possible symptoms and, second, that modern treatments usually prevent the development of the worst of them, many of which are now rarely seen even by psychiatrists.

The different forms the disorder can take is the subject of chapter 2, "The Categories of Bipolar Disorder." The diagnosis of bipolar disorder is complex, and there is still some disagreement about how the different symptom clusters are related to one another. Are there several different diseases of mood with different causes? Is there a group of disorders that share common features *and* common causes? Are these illness forms essentially the *same* disorder differing only in details of expression? Do these different forms remain the same over time in each patient, or can one form develop into another? The answers to some of these questions remain unknown. Nevertheless, there are several forms of the illness that can be reliably identified and separated from one another. Identifying one or another of these forms allows for predictions about the course of the illness over time and about the type of treatment that has the best chance of being effective.

Chapter 3, "Bipolar Disorder and the *DSM-5*," reviews the official classification system for the illness that is currently used by the American Psychiatric Association (and by many psychiatrists throughout the world). This chapter might be considered optional reading and will probably be of more interest to students and professionals concerned with the details of illness classification and diagnostic categories.

In chapter 4, "The Mood Disease," I show how psychiatrists came to realize that bipolar disorder is indeed a disease. For decades, persons afflicted with mood disorders were often given the covert message by their physicians that they themselves were to blame for their symptoms. Depression and other mood symptoms were blamed on emotional immaturity or "maladjustment" rather than being recognized as expressions of disordered functioning of the brain. It was only with the discovery of effective pharmaceuticals that psychiatry realized that bipolar disorder is indeed a disease—as real as diabetes or hyperthyroidism.

CHAPTER 1

Normal and Abnormal Mood

Bipolar disorder is a *mood* disorder, one of several emotional disorders whose main symptom is a problem with a person's mood. The first step in understanding the illness, then, is to understand what we mean by the word *mood*. Perhaps more to the point, I want to talk about what psychiatrists mean by the word. The dictionary isn't much help here; it defines *mood* simply as "a conscious state of mind or predominant feeling."[1] "Predominant feeling" begins to capture the idea, but mood is much more than just a feeling.

Our mood includes our happiness or sadness, our state of optimism or pessimism, our feelings of contentedness or dissatisfaction with our situation, and even physical feelings such as fatigue or vigor. Our mood is essentially our emotional temperature, a whole set of feelings that expresses our sense of emotional comfort or discomfort.

When individuals are in a good mood, they are confident and optimistic, relaxed and friendly, patient, interested, content. The word *happy* captures part of it, but good mood includes a lot more. People in a good mood usually feel energetic and have a sense of physical well-being; they sleep soundly and eat heartily. It's easy for them to be sociable and affectionate. The future looks bright, and the moment ripe for starting new projects. When we're in a good mood, the world seems a wonderful place to live in; it feels good to be alive.

When we're in a low mood, an opposite set of feelings takes over. We tend to turn inward and may seem preoccupied or distracted by our thoughts. The word *sad* captures some of the experience, but low mood is a bit more complicated. There may be a sense of emptiness and loss. It's difficult to think about the future very much, and when we do, it's hard not to be pessimistic or even intimidated. We may lose our temper more easily and then feel guilty about having done so. It's difficult to be affectionate or sociable, so we avoid others and prefer to be alone. Energy is low. Self-doubt takes over; we become preoccupied, worrying about how other people see us.

WHEN IS A MOOD NOT "NORMAL"?

Some of life's more common stresses and the normal human reactions to them are such common experiences that everyday terms have been coined for some mood changes—and we recognize that these mood changes are usually quite *normal*. Moving to a new community where we don't know anyone often leads to a sense of dislocation and loneliness that we know as "homesickness," an unpleasant set of feelings that may last for days or even weeks. Everyone has probably experienced these feelings at one time or another. When someone close to us dies, a profound sense of sadness and loss—the deep sorrow that we call bereavement or mourning—occurs, and it can become temporarily incapacitating. When we come to various milestones of personal achievement, we experience changes of mood in the other direction. A graduation or a wedding or the birth of a child can fill a person with joy and pride and a sense of limitless optimism that are nearly overwhelming. We wouldn't call any of these moods "abnormal," even though they may be extreme.

Like many other things we can measure in human beings—body temperature, blood pressure, and hormone levels, for example—a person's mood state normally varies within a certain range. People are not in the same mood state all the time; it is quite normal to have ups and downs.

Persons with bipolar disorder do not simply have higher ups and deeper downs. As you will see, a bipolar patient's mood swings are usually so far outside the range of normal that it doesn't take a psychiatrist to know that something is very wrong. Also, the abnormal mood states of bipolar disorder are accompanied by changes in thinking and bodily functions, changes that further indicate that they are not normal mood states. Examples of these changes include sleeplessness, alterations in appetite, impaired concentration and memory, and problems with motivation and energy level. To say that persons with bipolar disorder simply have more extreme fluctuations of mood isn't even nearly right. The symptoms of bipolar disorder, which seem to be caused by a defect in the brain's *regulation* of mood, also spill over into other areas of functioning.

Laura is a forty-year-old vice president of one of the largest banks in the country.[2] When I walked out into the waiting room to call her for our first appointment, she was sitting with a laptop balanced on her knees and a cell phone held up to her ear. "No, Steve, that's not good enough," she was saying into the phone as she nodded to me. "No, that won't work either, I need the last quarter's real numbers, not an estimate. Listen, I'm . . . ah . . . in the doctor's office. I'll call you in half an hour." I raised my eyebrows and shook my head. "Make that an hour. Bye." Click, snap, and phone and computer were both shut, and in a moment we were sitting in an interviewing room.

"I made this appointment as soon as I could after I read this." Laura handed me a pamphlet that the local chapter of the Depression and Bipolar Support Alliance had handed out at a local shopping mall during a health fair recently. "I've known for years that something was wrong, but I didn't know what. Reading this has made me think medication might help."

"What have you noticed that's 'wrong'?" I asked.

"I go into these, these things," she started. "I get this wired, can't-slow-down feeling. I've always called it 'the crazies,' and I usually crash after it's over. Sometimes I can't get out of bed for days."

"You seem to have a very high-stress job," I offered. "Maybe that's part of the problem."

"You sound like my mother. 'You don't have to take every promotion they offer you,' she says. But this isn't just stress, there's something else going on. The worst part is, I think these things are getting worse."

Laura's use of phrases like "the crazies" and "these things" seemed to indicate that she felt that these feelings were foreign, not like her normal feelings.

"Are you saying that sometimes your feelings and moods are controlling you rather than the other way around?" I asked.

Laura sat up straight in her chair. "That's the best way I could possibly describe it," she said decisively. "I can feel them coming on; it's almost physical. But I know they're . . . well, mental, I guess, is the best way to put it." Her face suddenly clouded over. "Does this mean I'm mentally ill?"

"Well," I said, "we know that there are illnesses that affect mood, and mood is certainly a mental state. But we have a lot more to talk about before I'll be able to say just what explains what you're going through."

Laura looked slightly relieved and said, "Well, that's why I'm here, for an explanation." She picked the brochure up from the edge of the desk. "This is the best explanation I've come across yet," she said thoughtfully. "And that means I can get rid of them, right? There's a treatment that will get rid of them?"

"There are many treatments for mood disorders. It may just take some time to find the one that works best."

"Then I came to the right place," she said as she sat back in her chair again. " 'You're not crazy,' my mother said. 'You don't need to see a psychiatrist.' "

"Well, I think your mother was at least half right," I said.

Laura smiled for the first time. "OK, then let's—" Suddenly a beep-beep-beep sounded from her jacket pocket. She took out her cell phone again. "If that's, um, confidential," I offered, "I can—"

Laura pushed a button, and the beeping stopped. She put the phone back in her pocket. "No, that can't possibly be as important as this. It can wait. I want to give you my undivided attention."

"Excellent!" I thought to myself. "This is a woman who understands priorities."

Imagine a person whose temperature regulation system doesn't work correctly—a person who suddenly starts shivering on a warm sunny day or breaks out into a sweat in a chilly room. This person's reactions to warm and cold are abnormal; her body "thinks" it is cold when it isn't, and she feels hot when the temperature is cool. We can think of mood disorders as problems with *emotional* temperature regulation.

In mood disorders, the mood becomes disconnected from the individual's environment, and "happy" and "sad" feelings take on rhythms and fluctuations of their own. Sometimes the fluctuations are mild, and the affected person seems to only have *more* ups and downs than other people have and to have mood fluctuations that are more difficult to understand. But because such individuals don't get profoundly depressed or irrationally "high," their problems are dismissed as being due to a difficult personality or to "immaturity." Sometimes, though, the mood states are so extremely abnormal that a person's ability to judge reality is shattered; his behavior can be bizarre and frightening. (It is in some of these cases that a diagnosis of schizophrenia can be mistakenly made, with the result that proper treatment goes wanting.) If the mood-disorder patient and his situation are examined with enough care, however, the basic underlying problem, the regulation of mood, will be found.

Because the basic problem in bipolar disorder is the normal *regulation* of mood, the disorder can present different symptoms at different times. Persons afflicted with the classic form of the illness have periods of severe *depression* as well as periods of *mania* (a mood state that is in many ways the opposite of depression). The observation that both of these mood states occur at various times during the course of the illness gave rise to the older name for the disorder: manic-depressive illness. These opposite moods occur in affected persons because the brain mechanisms that normally regulate mood don't work properly. This observation—that the mood states of affected persons move to either of the two polar opposite extremes of mood—gives the disorder its modern name, bipolar disorder. In the following sections we'll take a closer look at these opposites, or poles, of bipolar disorder, as well as an abnormal mood state in which the two opposites seem to be combined, a condition simply called a *mixed mood state*. Then, in chapter 2, we will see how the various combinations of these mood syndromes define the different forms of bipolar disorder.

A word you will frequently come across in discussions of mood disorders is *affect* (pronounced with the accent on the first syllable). To be precise, *affect* refers to the appearance of a person's mood state. *Mood* refers to the patient's inner experience, while *affect* refers to what others observe about a person's mood, the external signs of mood. (Psychiatrists talk of a patient's affect being depressed or irritable, and so forth.)

What Is "Manic Depression"?

You may have come across the terms *manic depression, manic-depressive illness* or *disorder*, or even *manic-depressive psychosis*. These are all older names for what we now call *bipolar disorder*.

In the late nineteenth century, a young German psychiatrist named Emil Kraepelin coined this term in the sixth edition of his *Textbook of Psychiatry* (Kraepelin's original German term for the illness was *Manisch-depressives Irresein*.) Kraepelin applied the term to all psychiatric illnesses characterized by recurrent episodes of abnormal mood—including cases that we would today call *major depressive disorder*.

Manic depression fell out of favor in the 1970s as it became clear that many patients with this illness never develop full-blown manic states but nevertheless have both depressed mood episodes and other abnormal mood states at the opposite "pole" of the mood scale: *hypomania*, or *mixed* mood states (explained elsewhere in this chapter). Thus, the term *bipolar disorder*.

MANIA

The manic state, or more simply *mania*, is the most extreme and dramatic of the symptom clusters of bipolar disorder.[3] Many persons who have bipolar disorder never have a full-blown manic episode. But since mania is the most unmistakable and probably the most dangerous of the abnormal mood states associated with mood disorders, it is a good place to start.

In the manic state, the mood regulator switches into "high." Mania usually starts gradually and may take weeks to develop fully. Although the symptoms may be almost imperceptible at first, they gradually become more extreme, more unpleasant, and more unmistakably pathological (table 1.1).

In the early stages of mania, the mood state of affected persons begins gradually to move "upward," and they find themselves filled with pleasant feelings of exuberance—what a physician writing over a hundred years ago called "a welling up of a sense of well-being and an overflowing of the spirits."[4] This heightened sense of well-being and confidence grows and expands and gradually evolves into euphoria. One bipolar patient described it this way:

> The world was filled with pleasure and promise; I felt great. Not just great, I felt *really* great. I felt I could do anything, that no task was too difficult. My mind seemed clear, fabulously focused, and able to make intuitive mathematical leaps that had up to that point entirely eluded me. . . . Not only did everything make perfect sense, but it all began to fit into a marvelous kind of cosmic relatedness.[5]

And here we confront one of the many ironies of this illness: at the onset of an episode of the disorder, it is not uncommon to feel *better* than usual. One manic patient said, "If I'm ill, this is the most wonderful illness I've ever had."[6]

Changes in thinking accompany the changes in mood. The feeling that one is thinking more clearly and more rationally than usual is quite common in the early stages of mania. This is an especially troublesome symptom, since such a mental state is not likely to make a person suspect

---

TABLE 1.1. Symptoms of mania

Mood symptoms	*Bodily symptoms*
Elated, euphoric mood	Increased energy level
Irritable mood	Decreased need for sleep
Grandiosity	Erratic appetite
	Increased libido
Cognitive (thinking) symptoms	
Feelings of heightened concentration	*Symptoms of psychosis*
Accelerated thinking ("racing thoughts")	Grandiose delusions
	Hallucinations

that something is wrong. Not only does thinking seem clearer than usual to the manic patient, but a feeling that mental processes are moving *faster* than usual also develops. At first there may be only a pleasant sense of nimbleness of thinking. Invariably, however, thinking processes accelerate: "quick" becomes "fast" and finally "racing." This vivid description of such an acceleration of thinking—illustrating what psychiatrists call a *flight of ideas*—comes from a collection of patient accounts written early in the twentieth century:

> My thoughts ran with lightning-like rapidity from one subject to another. All the problems of the universe came crowding into my mind, demanding instant discussion and solution—mental telepathy, hypnotism, wireless, telegraphy, Christian science, women's rights, and all the problems of medical science, religion and politics.
>
> Thoughts chased one another through my mind with lightning rapidity. I felt like a person driving a wild horse at a weak rein, who dares not use force but run[s] his course, following the line of least resistance, mad impulses rush through my brain carrying me first in one direction then in another.[7]

Racing thoughts are a symptom so typical of mania that the diagnosis becomes doubtful if this symptom is absent. This tumbling, jumbled jumping from one thought to another becomes progressively worse and more unpleasant as the episode develops.

As the manic individual's thinking speeds up, her speech does as well. Rapid, or *pressured*, speech (the term normally used by psychiatrists) is nearly always seen in mania. Manic individuals speak more and more quickly as the episode develops, attempting to express the ideas that are whirling through their consciousness at ever-faster speeds. A psychiatric text from the beginning of the twentieth century mentions one early researcher who actually counted the number of syllables per minute spoken by manic patients. He found that manic patients spoke 180 to 200 syllables per minute, compared with 122 to 150 in nonmanic persons.[8]

Sometimes racing thoughts and pressured speech lead to an outpouring of frenzied writing:

> I made notes of everything that happened, day and night. I made symbolic scrapbooks whose meaning only I could decipher. I wrote a fairy tale. . . . I noted down cryptically all that was said or done around me at the time, with special reference to relevant news bulletins and to jokes

which were broadcast in radio programs. The time, correct to the near-est minute, was written in the margin. It was all vitally important. [I was convinced that] the major work [that] would be based on this material would be accurate, original, provocative and of profound significance.[9]

The feelings of exuberance and overconfidence that characterize mania can lead to several patterns of behavior typical of the manic state: spending sprees, sexual promiscuity, and overuse of alcohol and other intoxicating substances.

Spending sprees can be extravagant and financially catastrophic, be-cause the manic person has no concern for where the money will come from to pay the bills. The increased sexual feelings of this stage of mania may lead to infatuations and even betrothals. One early psychiatric expert noted that "incomprehensible engagements, also pregnancies, are not rare in these states. I know cases in which the commencement of [mania] was repeatedly announced by a sudden engagement."[10] The loss of inhibitions typical in mania can lead to promiscuity and other uncharacteristic sexual behaviors.

We shall explore the complex relationship between bipolar disorder and substance abuse in chapter 19. Suffice it to say here that increased and un-characteristic use of intoxicating substances is frequently seen in mania.

One way to understand this hedonistic triad of mania—spending sprees, sexual overactivity, and increased substance abuse—is to group these be-haviors together as expressions of an increase in "motivated behaviors" seen in mania,[11] an exaggeration of the normal drives toward pleasurable goals.

There are almost always changes in sleeping and eating habits in mania. A decreased need for sleep is in fact one of the first symptoms to develop—often a clue for individuals who have been manic before that another episode may be starting. Food intake is usually reduced because manic individuals simply don't have time to eat. Constantly distracted by new thoughts and ideas, they feel pressed to continue to act; they just can't sit still long enough to finish a meal. The ensuing weight loss can be dramatic.

As the combination of euphoric mood and mental quickness develops, the manic individual begins to feel tremendously self-confident, even fear-less. This is the so-called *grandiosity* of the manic state. Fears of unpleasant consequences disappear altogether, and reckless enthusiasm takes over. The affected person may seek out new adventures and experiences with no regard for the possible adverse repercussions. This is one of the points at which the manic person can begin to lose touch with reality—when grandiose thinking leads the individual to start *believing* the great things he feels capable of.

In a landmark work on bipolar disorder that we'll discuss in detail in chapter 4, the German psychiatrist Emil Kraepelin recorded the symptoms and course of the illness he called *manic-depressive insanity*. (I'll be quoting Dr. Kraepelin quite a bit in this book. Not only did he write some of the most vivid and enduring descriptions of the symptoms of bipolar disorder, but his insights into the different forms and the course of the illness have proved to be correct again and again.) Kraepelin's description of the grandiose delusions of mania, written in 1896, is classic:

> The patient asserts that he is descended from a noble family. That he is a gentleman; he calls himself a genius, the Emperor William, the Emperor of Russia, Christ, he can drive out the devil. A patient suddenly cried out on the street that he was the Lord God, the devil had left him. Female patients possess eighty genuine diamonds, are leading singers, leading violinists, Queen of Bavaria, Maid of Orleans, a fairy; they are pregnant, are going to be engaged to St. Francis, are to give birth to the redeemer . . . the Messiah.[12]

Modern patients are more likely to become convinced that they are president or prime minister than king or queen, a rap star rather than a great violinist, but the feelings that lead to such beliefs are the same: a fantastic, indescribable feeling of mental power and significance. Feelings of religious inspiration are very common. Patients may believe that they are a modern prophet, the founder of a new religion, the reincarnation of Christ, even a new god. Although delusional thinking occurs in depressed states as well, it appears to be more common during manic episodes (table 1.2).

The "feeling good" stage of mania is sometimes very short lived, and the elated mood and grandiosity can be quickly replaced by an angry, irritable mood. Quoting Kraepelin again:

> The patient is dissatisfied, intolerant, faultfinding . . . even rough. Trifling external occasions may bring about extremely violent outbursts of rage. In his fury, he thrashes his wife and children, threatens to smash everything to smithereens. . . .
>
> . . . At the most trifling affront it may come to outbursts of rage of extraordinary violence . . . clamorous abuse and bellowing, to dangerous threats with shooting and stabbing, to blind destruction and actual attacks.[13]

Category of symptoms	Percentage of patients
TABLE 1.2. Delusions and hallucinations in bipolar disorder: Mania versus depression	
Delusions	
Mania	44
Depression	12
Hallucinations	
Mania	14
Depression	8

Source: Data from D. W. Black and A. Nasrallah, "Hallucinations and Delusions in 1,715 Patients with Unipolar and Bipolar Affective Disorders," *Psychopathology* 22 (1989): 28–34.

Sometimes the manic individual alternates between elation and irritability for a time, but usually the irritable, unpleasant mood becomes predominant. It is often this irritability that brings the patient to medical attention.

As the manic state continues to develop, pressured, racing thoughts; an increased energy level; and loss of inhibitions lead to more grossly disorganized and disturbed thinking and behavior. A psychiatric textbook written in the 1950s described this stage as follows:

> Driven by greater pressure of activity, terror and excitement, [the manic person] becomes violent, attacks his neighbor, begins to shout all kinds of accusations against his alleged persecutors. . . . Distortions [and] misinterpretations . . . are now elaborated into delusions of persecution accompanied by violence and panic, the patient runs down the street nude, sets fire to the house, starts an argument with the police, shoots a gun on the street or starts suddenly to preach the gospel in a frenzied manner. . . . If crossed or interfered with in any way he becomes abusive, destructive, homicidal.[14]

Thinking patterns not only spin faster and faster but also become more bizarre. Hallucinations can develop, and beliefs called *delusions* can occur. The very best modern written descriptions of the symptoms of severe mania are those of Kay Redfield Jamison. Dr. Jamison's nearly unique qualification to set them down is that she is an internationally recognized medical expert on bipolar disorder who suffers from it herself. This passage by

Dr. Jamison is what I give medical students to read so that they can learn about the symptoms of severe mania:

> Although I had been building up to this for weeks and certainly knew something was seriously wrong, there was still a definite point when I knew I was insane. My thoughts were so fast that I couldn't remember the beginning of a sentence halfway through. Fragments of ideas, images, sentences, raced around and around in my mind like the tigers in a children's story. Finally, like those tigers, they became meaningless melted pools. Nothing familiar to me was familiar. I wanted desperately to slow down but could not.[15]

These passages vividly make the point that the manic state is not pleasant—even if it may sometimes start out that way. Those unfamiliar with the illness sometimes think that persons with bipolar disorder simply experience swings of mood between "happy" and "sad." As the foregoing illustrates, this is usually not true. The full-blown manic state is not only intensely unpleasant but also dangerous. The danger arises not only from the increased risk of violence toward others (or toward the patient himself) but also from the physical stress the syndrome causes.

The combination of severe manic symptoms and the physical stress from such frenzied hyperactivity can lead to what Kraepelin called *delirious mania*, in which there is "profound clouding of consciousness and extraordinary and confused hallucinations. . . . The patients become stupefied, confused, bewildered and completely lose orientation for time and place."[16] Fortunately, it is now rare for a psychiatrist to see patients suffering from this severest form of the manic state, but in Kraepelin's time and even more recently, mania had a significant mortality rate. Persons with mania died "in a state of progressive exhaustion,"[17] suffering dehydration and cardiovascular collapse.

HYPOMANIA

In 1881 a German psychiatrist named Emanuel Mendel published a book about the manic state called *Die Manie* and in it proposed that another term be used for states of milder euphoria and hyperactivity that did not progress to full-blown mania. He called this condition *hypomania*, "similar to the state of exultation in typical mania [but] with a certain lesser grade

The "Stages" of Mania

In 1973, just as lithium, the first effective treatment for bipolar disorder, was becoming available, a study from the National Institutes of Health attempted to describe a typical manic episode from beginning to end. Patients who had been admitted to a research unit were carefully observed, and their symptoms meticulously documented and described. The authors concluded that three stages could be described in a manic episode:

[Stage I]: Increased psychomotor activity which included increased . . . rate of speech and increased physical activity. . . . Euphoria predominated, although irritability became obvious when the patients' many demands were not instantly satisfied. . . . Expansiveness, grandiosity and overconfidence [were observed]. Thoughts were coherent though sometimes [disconnected]. Also frequently observed during this stage were increased sexuality or sexual preoccupations, increased interest in religion, increased and inappropriate spending of money, increased smoking, telephone use and letter writing. Some of the patients were aware of the mood change on some level and described the feeling of "going high." At this stage the patients were not out of control.

[Stage II]: Pressure of speech and . . . activity increased still further. Mood, although euphoric at times, was now more prominently characterized by increasing [unpleasantness]. . . . The irritability observed initially had progressed to open hostility and anger, and the accompanying behavior was frequently assaultive. Racing thoughts progressed to . . . increasing disorganization. Grandiose trends [were] now apparent as frank delusions.

[Stage III]: A desperate, panic stricken, hopeless state experienced by the patient as clearly [unpleasant], accompanied by frenzied and frequently even more bizarre . . . activity. Thought processes . . . now became incoherent.*

This study on the "stages of mania" was important because investigators used modern clinical methods to document how sick patients with mania can get. Even more important, it made the researchers realize that it would be easy to misdiagnose a very disorganized patient in Stage III mania as having schizophrenia, a psychiatric illness that requires a very different treatment approach and has a different prognosis than bipolar disorder has.

*Quoted in Edward Hare, "The Two Manias: Study of the Evolution of the Modern Concept of Mania," *British Journal of Psychiatry* 138 (1981): 89–99.

of development."[18] (The prefix *hypo-* comes from the Greek word meaning "under.") Hypomania can be thought of as having only the symptoms present at the beginning of a manic episode (Stage I in the study described above): the elated mood, the increased energy level, the rapid thinking and speaking, and sometimes a bit of the irritability. Norman Endler, another psychologist who himself suffered from a mood disorder and wrote of his experiences, described hypomania this way: "Most of the time I was busy, busy, busy; taping records, playing tennis, skiing, writing manuscripts, talking . . . reading, going to movies, staying up at night, waking up early in the morning, always on the go—busy, busy, busy. Furthermore, I was boasting about all the energy I had that enabled me to keep up this fast pace. . . . Instead of occasionally 'idling' in neutral I was always in overdrive."[19]

Although persons in the hypomanic stage do not have the severe mental disorganization of mania and are by definition not agitated and frenzied to the point of violence toward themselves or others, hypomania can nevertheless have unpleasant consequences. Feelings of increased confidence can lead to foolish investments in real estate or the stock market, and patients can squander personal resources on grandiose and risky business ventures. Increased sexual feelings can lead to extramarital affairs. The irritability of hypomania can lead to arguments and disagreements with family, colleagues, or neighbors that can sour relationships, sometimes irreparably. Dr. Endler described it this way:

> As a hypomanic, I didn't stop to analyze my thoughts, feelings, or behavior. I was much too busy and didn't always stop to think about what I was doing. . . . I was critical of others and occasionally told some people off publicly. I was not so concerned about . . . the effect my behavior had on [others]. I was aggressive, talked incessantly, and interrupted others while they were speaking. Whenever I had a thought, I felt compelled to utter it, and I didn't always censor my thoughts and feelings. At times I seemed to have lost my sense of judgment. I was having a good time, I was narcissistically preoccupied with myself, but (without being aware of it) I was making my wife miserable.[20]

Persons with even mild hypomania can quit a good job in a burst of overconfidence or irritability, withdraw their life savings for a get-rich-quick scheme, or simply begin to drive their car too fast—all behaviors with potentially devastating consequences.

Words like *seductive* and *addictive* are frequently applied to hypomanic syndrome. Individuals in a hypomanic state rarely seek treatment, at least initially—remember, they are feeling *quite* well. It is only after some time of living with the illness that they can come to recognize that hypomania—as wonderful as it feels at the time—is usually a sign of trouble, presaging a crash into depression or further escalation into mania.

Because hypomanic individuals are *not* psychotic, they often cannot be involuntarily treated for their illness, because criteria for involuntary treatment insist upon "dangerous" behaviors. (We shall discuss involuntary treatment in chapter 24.) Hypomanic persons can avoid treatment for weeks, even months (table 1.3), consequently ruining their financial status, credit rating, employment history, relationships, and health.

As we shall see in a later section, some patients go through episodes of depression and hypomania only and never become completely manic. Others have both hypomanic and manic episodes. Observations about the frequency and intensity of hypomanic versus manic episodes in different individuals are beginning to suggest that the classic manic-depressive disorder with episodes of full-blown mania and depression may be only one of many forms of the illness. (We shall discuss this new way of thinking about bipolar disorder in the next chapter, in the section on "soft" bipolar disorders.)

TABLE 1.3. Length of time before hospitalization for mania in ninety-four manic patients

| | Percentage of patients | |
Time	Male	Female
14–30 days	69	62
3 months	11	11
6 months	11	10
1 year or more	6	15

Source: Data from George Winoker, *Mania and Depression: A Classification of Syndrome and Disease* (Baltimore: Johns Hopkins University Press, 1991), 13.

Note: Patients can have symptoms for many months before receiving needed treatment. During this time, hypomanic symptoms can wreak havoc on their lives.

THE SYNDROME OF DEPRESSION

The depression of bipolar disorder is both easier and more difficult to describe and discuss than mania or hypomania. It is easier to discuss because depression is a more familiar set of feelings: everyone, whether suffering from bipolar disorder or not, has gone through periods of depressed mood. But the depressive syndrome of bipolar disorder is more difficult to discuss for that very reason: it is a very different experience from "normal" depression. In modern psychiatric terminology, this abnormal depressed mood state is called *major depression* or sometimes *clinical depression* (table 1.4).

When persons who do not suffer from a mood disorder go through a period of low mood, such as after a romantic disappointment, the loss of a job, or a period of homesickness, not only is their depressed mood temporary, but they retain the normal *reactivity* of mood. If you have attended a funeral and then returned to the home of the bereaved afterward, you have probably observed this normal reactivity of mood, perhaps even in yourself. Mourners who might have been grief stricken during the service or at

---

TABLE 1.4. **Symptoms of depression**

Mood symptoms	*Bodily symptoms*
Depressed mood	Sleep disturbance:
Dysphoric mood	insomnia
Diurnal variation of mood (early-morning depression, mood improving as day goes on)	hypersomnia
Guilty feelings	Appetite disturbance:
Loss of ability to feel pleasure (anhedonia)	weight loss
Social withdrawal	weight gain
Suicidal thoughts	Loss of interest in sex
	Fatigue
Cognitive (thinking) symptoms	Constipation
Poor concentration	Headaches
Poor memory	Worsening of painful conditions
Indecision	
Slowed thinking	*Symptoms of psychosis*
	Delusional thinking
	Hallucinations
	Catatonic states

the grave site can afterward often relax, reminisce about good memories of the person they lost, and enjoy catching up with friends and relatives they haven't seen for a long time. The reactivity of mood is also retained in the lonely or homesick person who goes to the movies and loses himself in a good film. We are able to dispel feelings of bereavement, isolation, or disappointment—even if only for a few hours—if the depressed mood is a "normal" one.

"Depression" or "depression"?

A colleague of mine likes to talk about the differences between depression "with a little d" as opposed to "big D" depression. She refers to the kind of normal, expected low mood that everyone experiences from time to time as (little d) "depression" and the clinical syndrome described in this section as (big D) "Depression," or better yet "DEPRESSION." The feelings that persons with mood disorders experience when they are in a depressed state (make that DEPRESSED) are *not* simply exaggerations of the universal human experience of normal sadness.

The most significant feature of the depressed mood in the syndrome of depression is that instead of being reactive, the mood is *constricted*. Years ago, AM radio stations used to give away free radios, gifts that came with only one catch: they couldn't be tuned to any of the sponsoring station's competitors. These radios were built to receive only the signal of the station that gave them away. The mood state of the person who is suffering through a depressed episode of bipolar disorder is like one of those radios, "set" to receive only one mood signal: depression. As you will see later, the imaging studies of persons with depression have shown that this is nearly literally the case: areas of the brain where negative feelings originate are overactive in individuals with major depression, and areas that are responsible for modulating and damping down those feelings are underactive.

The mood of the syndrome of depression is a relentless, pervasive gloom that continues from one day to the next and from which the afflicted person cannot rouse herself. As Pulitzer Prize–winning novelist William Styron said of his own depression, "The weather of depression is unmodulated, its light a brownout."[21]

In these constricted mood states, depressed individuals find their thinking dominated by thoughts of sadness and loss, regret and hopelessness. Guilty ruminations are especially characteristic of the syndrome of depression, and psychiatrists often make a special point to ask about guilty feelings when they evaluate a person for depression. Ruminations on themes of guilt, shame, and regret are common in the depressed states of the mood disorders, but they are very *uncommon* in the "normal" depressed mood. Persons experiencing the normal depressed mood that comes after a personal loss attribute their bad feelings to the fact that a loss has occurred; only in unusual circumstances will they believe that they are to blame for their problem and be preoccupied by feelings of guilt or shame. The individual with a depressive syndrome, however, frequently thinks that he is to blame for his troubles, and sometimes for other people's troubles as well. The presence of guilty preoccupations is a consequential indicator for making a diagnosis of the syndrome of depression.

Feelings of inadequacy and worthlessness are similarly significant and especially common in the syndrome of major depression. Endler described how depression caused him to be tormented by feelings of incompetence even at the height of a successful academic career:

> [When I became depressed] I was positive I was a fraud and a phony and that I didn't deserve my PhD. I didn't deserve to have tenure; I didn't deserve to be a Full Professor; I didn't deserve to be a Fellow of the American Psychological Association and the Canadian Psychological Association; I didn't deserve the research grants I had been awarded; I couldn't understand how I had written the books and journal articles that I had and how they had been accepted for publication. I must have conned a lot of people.[22]

Another typical symptom of major depression is the loss of interest in usually pleasurable activities. This can be understood as another aspect of the loss of normal reactivity of mood. The depressed person is unable to derive any pleasure from listening to music, going to a movie, engaging in the sports or hobbies that usually provide enjoyment. This loss of the ability to feel pleasure has come to be called *anhedonia* (derived from the Greek word for "pleasure").

Just as the manic syndrome infuses the affected person with feelings of inexpressible joy, the syndrome of depression brings indescribable anguish. Many individuals who have suffered from depression have struggled to describe the feelings, and even great writers seem to falter in the attempt. William Styron said, "If the pain were readily describable most of the countless sufferers from this ancient affliction would have been able to confidently depict . . . their torment. Healthy people [cannot] imagine a form of torment so alien to everyday experience. For myself, the pain is most closely connected to drowning or suffocation—but even these images are off the mark."[23]

People with major depression may have a tense, irritable, miserable sort of mood called *dysphoria*. (The term *dysphoric mania* is used to describe a

---

What Is Anhedonia?

The word *anhedonia* was first coined in 1896 by the French psychologist Théodule-Armand Ribot to mean an impairment in one's ability to experience pleasure. The word comes from the Greek roots *an-* (without) and *hēdonē* (pleasure). Depressed persons are less interested in pursuing usually pleasurable activities: they complain that food has lost its taste, that colors have drained away from sunrises and landscapes, that flowers have lost their textures and perfumes—everything has become bland, dull, and lifeless.

It should come as no surprise that some of the best descriptions of anhedonia come to us from authors and artists.

Johann Wolfgang von Goethe, in his novel *The Sorrows of Young Werther*, has his main character describe his loss of responsiveness to the joys and beauty of nature: "Nature lies before me as immobile as in a little lacquered painting, and all this beauty cannot pump one drop of happiness from my heart to my brain."*

The nineteenth-century Austrian composer Hugo Wolf described a terrible sense of sorrowful isolation during his depressions, a feeling of separation from the world of ordinary pleasures—all the more painful when it occurred in springtime:

> What I suffer from . . . I am quite unable to describe. This wonderful spring with its secret life and movement troubles me unspeakably. These eternal blue skies, lasting for weeks, this continuous sprouting and budding in nature, these coaxing breezes impregnated with spring sunlight and fragrance of flowers . . . make me frantic. Everywhere this bewildering urge for life, fruitfulness, creation—and only I . . . may not take part in this festival of resurrection, at any rate not except as a spectator with grief and envy.†

*Johann Wolfgang von Goethe, *The Sorrows of Young Werther*, trans. Elizabeth Mayer and Louise Bogan (New York, Random House, 1990), 114.

†Wolf quoted in Kay Redfield Jamison, *Touched by Fire* (New York, Simon and Schuster, 1993), 21.

tense, unpleasant, irritable mood that can be seen along with the agitation and hyperactivity of the manic state.)

The changes in thinking and physical well-being caused by the syndrome of depression are perhaps easier to describe. One's energy level and thinking as well as mood are affected—in an opposite direction of polarity from that seen in mania. The depressed person experiences a slowing and inefficiency in thinking and a feebleness of memory and concentration. Information processing and reasoning falter, and simple decisions can become overwhelming dilemmas. Endler expressed it this way: "My indecisiveness was the worst of all. I couldn't decide what to eat or what to wear. I couldn't decide whether to get out of bed or to stay. I couldn't decide whether to shower or not to shower. I could never decide what to do because I didn't know myself."[24]

These *cognitive* functions (from the Latin *cognoscere*, meaning "to know") become progressively debilitated as the depression deepens, but even in milder depressions, ordinary mental tasks seem to require extraordinary effort. Kraepelin described the severe cognitive slowing he observed in his severely depressed patients: "[The patient's] thoughts are as if paralysed . . . immobile. He is no longer able to perceive or to follow the train of thought of a book or conversation. . . . He has no memory, he has no longer command of knowledge formerly familiar to him [and] must consider a long time about simple things."[25] In the elderly, these sorts of thinking problems can be so severe that depression is misdiagnosed as Alzheimer's disease.

Severe depression almost always causes a change in sleeping pattern. Depressed persons frequently suffer from insomnia—but also from its opposite, sleeping too much (*hypersomnia* is the technical term). In the depression associated with bipolar disorder, hypersomnia seems especially common, perhaps more common than in other types of clinical depression, where insomnia predominates.

Sometimes depressed persons have a peculiar rhythmic pattern of sleep disturbance and mood changes throughout the day, called *diurnal variation of mood* (*diurnal* is a word used in biology to refer to a twenty-four-hour cycle). It causes persons to fall asleep at the usual time and without much difficulty but to wake up in the wee hours of the morning after only a few hours of sleep. Lying awake hours before sunrise, they experience their lowest mood of the day, and minor problems and regrets seem magnified and overwhelming. I recall one patient who told me that during those early-morning hours, "I lie awake thinking about every stupid thing I've ever done in my life." American author F. Scott Fitzgerald, who described his struggles with depression in the 1936 autobiographical work *The Crackup*, gave a vivid account of this mood pattern. He experienced the worst of his moods during the predawn hours, recalling that "at three o'clock in the morning, a forgotten package has the same tragic importance as a death sentence." For Fitzgerald, these nocturnal agonies were the nadir of his depressions, which he called "the dark night of the soul."[26] Individuals notice a gradual lifting of their mood as sunrise approaches, and when the morning dawns, they can often rouse themselves and start their daily activities. As the day goes on, their mood continues to improve little by little, until by day's end they feel nearly back to normal. They go to bed and usually fall asleep normally, but several hours later, it's three o'clock in the morning again: they awaken depressed, and the cycle repeats itself.

Styron experienced a very striking diurnal variation in his mood during his depression, but with a reversal of the usual pattern: "While I was able to rise and function almost normally during the earlier part of the day, I began to sense the onset of the symptoms at mid-afternoon or a little later—gloom crowding in on me, a sense of dread and alienation and . . . stifling anxiety."[27]

The disruptions of various bodily rhythms that occur in depression and mania have convinced many scientists that some persons with mood disorders have a disturbance of their *chronobiology* (from *chronos*, the Greek word for "time"). Persons with mood disorders have been observed to have disturbances in the normal rhythmic pulsing of various hormone levels, in body temperature fluctuations, in the sleep-wake cycle, and in other natural rhythms. Later in this book we shall examine connections between these natural rhythms and mood and also look at other cycles: the monthly cycles of mood in women with premenstrual mood symptoms (chapter 18) and the twelve-month cycles of persons with seasonal affective disorder (chapter 15).

Appetite is also usually disturbed in depressed individuals. As with sleep problems, changes occur in both directions, and patients may eat too much or too little. They may lose or gain a significant amount of weight during periods of depression. As might be expected, the depressed person loses interest in sex; this symptom is perhaps best understood as part of the person's inability to experience pleasurable activities of any kind, the anhedonia of depression.

Of the other bodily symptoms that occur in depression, one of the most striking is a sense of fatigue with prominent low energy and listlessness. As Endler put it, "[My] fatigue [was] extreme to the point of exhaustion. I was too tired to make decisions and felt as if I had a huge weight on my back that wouldn't allow me to achieve anything. . . . No matter how long

I stayed in bed and slept I never felt rested and refreshed. . . . When I did get out of bed, I was lethargic. I was slow as molasses."[28] Headaches, constipation, and a feeling of heaviness in the chest are common, as are other more difficult-to-describe sensations of physical discomfort. Styron said, "I felt a kind of numbness, an enervation . . . an odd fragility—as if my body had actually become frail, hypersensitive and somehow disjointed and clumsy. Nothing felt quite right. . . . There were twitches and pains, sometimes intermittent, often seemingly constant, that seemed to presage all sorts of dire infirmities."[29]

It is not clear whether these symptoms are caused by depression itself or arise from the lack of restful sleep, the decrease in exercise, and the poor eating habits that depression brings on. Persons who have preexisting painful medical conditions such as arthritis or inflammatory bowel disease are usually more bothered by the physical symptoms of these illnesses when they are depressed. The connections between depression and problems with fatigue seen in chronic fatigue immunodeficiency syndrome and the painful joint and muscle disease fibromyalgia are well known but poorly understood. Depression seems to lower the pain threshold: depressed individuals are more sensitive to pain and are more distressed by it.

Some persons may be willing to seek treatment for these physical symptoms but reluctant to mention their mood problems. So sometimes patients with depression end up getting all kinds of tests and treatments for physical illnesses from their physicians, when their real problem is depression.

Just as in the syndrome of mania, persons suffering through an episode of the depression of bipolar disorder can experience the distortions of thinking that psychiatrists call *delusions*. As their view of the world and of themselves becomes increasingly colored by their pervasive mood changes, depressed individuals can come to believe that terrible things are happening all around them: "I was positive that I was going to be fired from the university because of incompetence and that [my family] would become destitute—that we would go broke," wrote Endler. "I felt guilty at the prospect of not being able to support my family."[30] In addition to such *delusions of poverty*, delusions can arise from the uncomfortable physical sensations of depression. Patients believe they have cancer, AIDS, or some other terrible illness.

Kraepelin described the increasingly bizarre *hypochondriacal delusions* he sometimes observed in his patients: "[The patient believes he is] incurably ill, half-dead, no longer a right human being, has lung disease, a tapeworm, cancer in his throat, cannot swallow, does not retain his food. . . . Face and figure have changed; there is no longer blood in his brain, he does not see any longer, must become crazy, remain his whole lifetime in an institution, die, has already died." Patients with such beliefs may refuse to eat or drink, convinced that their body cannot absorb the food. *Paranoid delusions*, beliefs that one is in danger or the victim of evil people and forces, can also occur.

> Everywhere danger threatens the patient. . . . Strange people are in the house; a suspicious motorcar drives past. People mock him, are going to thrash him, to chase him from his post in a shameful way, incarcerate him, bring him to justice, expose him publicly, deport him, throw him into the fire, drown him. The people are already standing outside; the bill of indictment is already written; the scaffold is being put up; he must wander about naked and miserable. . . . His relatives also are being tortured. . . . His family is imprisoned, his wife has drowned herself; his parents are murdered; his daughter wanders about in the snow without any clothes on.[31]

It's easy to understand why suicidal thinking and behavior are so common in the syndrome of major depression: compared with the horrors of such delusional imaginings, death may seem a welcome alternative. It's also possible to understand why delusionally depressed persons can occasionally be dangerous to others as well as to themselves: they can come to believe that those close to them are in similar danger of gruesome persecution and would be better off dead.

Hallucinations occur in severe depression but not as frequently as in mania (see table 1.1). The hallucinations are consistent with the mood and are frightening, even horrifying: "The patients see evil spirits, death, heads of animals . . . crowds of monsters . . . dead relatives. . . . The patient hears his tortured relatives screaming and lamenting. . . . His food tastes of soapy water or excrement, of corpses and mildew."[32]

Some seriously ill patients sink into a state of lethargy and despair that is called *depressive stupor*. Styron's description of this horrible condition is the best I have ever read:

> I had now reached that phase of the disorder where all sense of hope had vanished, along with the idea of a futurity; my brain . . . had become less an organ of thought than an instrument registering, minute by minute, varying degrees of its own suffering. . . . I'd feel the horror, like some poisonous fog bank, roll in upon my mind, forcing me to bed. There I would lie for as long as six hours, stuporous and virtually paralyzed, gazing at the ceiling.[33]

The Stages of Depression

A few pages back, I described the several "stages" of mania and said that many patients with bipolar disorder never progress beyond Stage I, or what you now know is called "hypomania." That is, they never experience the more severe symptoms of mania: disorganization of thinking, complete insomnia, hallucinations, or delusions.

Similarly, many patients with bipolar depression never develop the most severe symptoms of the depressive syndrome. Many persons with bipolar depression can function with symptoms for long periods because the more physical symptoms of the syndrome, such as sleep and appetite changes and impairment in energy level, are not so severe.

Only a minority of persons with bipolar depression develop the most severe symptoms of the syndrome of depression, the hallucinations and delusions that we call "psychotic" symptoms. The reason for this may be genetic: my Hopkins colleague Dr. James Potash discovered that persons with bipolar disorder who experience psychotic symptoms (hallucinations and delusions) when they are ill often have some of the same genetic markers that persons with schizophrenia have. Schizophrenia is a quite different illness characterized *mainly* by hallucinations and delusions and in which mood is relatively unaffected. It may be that the same genetic factors that put a person at risk for schizophrenia, when they occur along with whatever genetic factors predispose one to the mood symptoms, alter the symptoms seen during mood episodes to include psychotic experiences.*

*James B. Potash, Peter P. Zandi, Virginia L. Willour, Tsuo-Hung Lan, Yuqing Huo, Dimitrios Avramopoulos, Yin Y. Shugart, Dean F. MacKinnon, Sylvia G. Simpson, Francis J. McMahon, J. Raymond DePaulo Jr., and Melvin G. McInnis, "Suggestive Linkage to Chromosomal Regions 13q31 and 22q12 in Families with Psychotic Bipolar Disorder," *American Journal of Psychiatry* 160, no. 4 (2003): 680–86.

Just as few modern psychiatrists have ever seen the most extreme stage of mania, so-called *delirious mania*, it is also fortunately rare today to see a patient depressed to the point of unresponsiveness and immobility that psychiatrists call *catatonia*. Kraepelin, describing patients in an era when virtually no treatment was available for this terrible condition, starkly describes this deepest abyss of depression: "The patients lie in bed taking no interest in anything. They betray no pronounced emotion; they are mute, inaccessible; they pass their [bowel movements] under them; they stare straight in front of them with [a] vacant expression of countenance like a mask and with wide open eyes."[34]

MIXED STATES

Another type of abnormal mood can be seen in bipolar disorder. This mood, a strange combination of both the frenzied intensity of mania and the horrors of deep depression, has been called a *mixed state* (sometimes it's termed *mixed affective state*). Kay Jamison described it as the most terrible expression of the illness for her: "On occasion, these periods of total despair would be made even worse by terrible agitation. My mind would race from subject to subject, but instead of being filled with . . . exuberance and cosmic thoughts . . . it would be drenched in awful sounds and images of decay and dying; dead bodies on the beach, charred remains of animals, toe-tagged corpses in morgues."[35]

Although psychiatrists do not yet agree on the defining characteristics of this mood state, they have long recognized that symptoms of depression and mania seem to exist almost simultaneously in some patients (table 1.5). This state represents a distinct variety of abnormal moods that is separate from depression and typical mania yet combines features of both. The accelerated thinking and hyperactivity typical of the manic state remain its most striking features, but instead of a euphoric mood, these changes become combined with a depressed, despairing, desperate mood. Kraepelin described patients with "flight of ideas, excitement and anxiety" who were at the same time "anxiously despairing."[36] Other labels used for the mixed state are *mixed mania* and *dysphoric mania*.

TABLE 1.5. Symptoms in ten patients with mixed mania (dysphoric mania)

Symptoms	Percentage of patients
Depressed mood	100
Irritable mood	100
Increased activity	100
Insomnia	93
Pressured speech	93
Hostility	79
Flight of ideas	43
Anxiety attacks	43
Delusions (depressive)	36
Delusions (nondepressive)	21

Source: Data from Frederick K. Goodwin and Kay Redfield Jamison, *Manic-Depressive Illness* (New York: Oxford University Press, 1990), 49.

Just as full-blown mania is unmistakable, so is a full-blown mixed state. But in the same way that a state of mild hypomania can be difficult to distinguish from an elevated but normal mood, milder mixed states can be difficult to recognize. A mild mixed state sometimes lasts only a few hours. Whenever a patient tells me about being troubled by uncomfortable angry "rages," I suspect that he may be having mild mixed states. *Anxiety* is another word that they use to describe their experience of this mood state, although it is not the fearful fretfulness of ordinary anxiety; this state is more like a pressure cooker full of depressed emotions ready to explode.

The mixed state can be extremely dangerous because the patient has negative, depressing thought patterns together with excess energy, restlessness, and an inner sense of pressure and tension. This negative energy puts patients in mixed states at high risk for hurting themselves with suicidal behaviors. And it is often while in a mixed state that individuals are propelled into a variety of self-destructive behaviors that are not immediately life threatening. They may cut or burn themselves. Patients have told me that desperate behaviors like these help them shift a terrible inner pain and tension to "the outside" and that the physical pain is somehow easier to deal with than the painful agitation of a mixed state.

Another type of mood "mixture" occurs when, rather than a true mixture of simultaneous mania and depression, there is rapid alternation between the two states. Kraepelin described "transition periods from one state to another, which often [extended] over weeks," during which his patients seemed depressed one moment and manic nearly the next:

> Manic patients may transitorily appear not only sad and despairing, but also quiet and inhibited. A patient goes to bed moody and inhibited, suddenly wakes up with the feeling as if a veil had been drawn away from his brain, passes the day in manic delight in work, and the next morning, exhausted and with a heavy head, he again finds in himself the whole misery of his state. Or the hypomanic exultant patient quite unexpectedly makes a serious attempt at suicide.[37]

Recently, the term *ultrarapid cycling* has been proposed for such alternations in mood.

Now that you have some familiarity with the symptoms of bipolar disorder, I can talk about diagnosis. As I have already said, most people with bipolar disorder never develop all the possible symptoms of the illness. It is the presence or absence of certain symptoms as well as the pattern of mood symptoms that allows a diagnosis of a particular type of bipolar disorder.

And once a diagnosis has been made, a treatment plan can be developed. In the next chapter you'll see how the diagnostic process works.

─────────────────── KEY TAKEAWAYS ───────────────────

▶ Bipolar disorder is a *mood disorder* characterized by problems with mood regulation and sustained periods of abnormal mood.

▶ The abnormal mood states of bipolar disorder are accompanied by changes in thinking and bodily functions, such as the sleep and appetite changes, impaired concentration and memory, and problems with motivation and energy level that are seen in depression.

▶ *Mania* is characterized by euphoria, grandiosity, or irritability, along with racing thoughts, loss of inhibitions, and decreased need for sleep.

▶ *Mixed mood states* combine the physical and mental agitation of mania with the despairing mood of depression.

CHAPTER 2

The Categories of Bipolar Disorder

Diagnostic classification has two purposes in medicine: to make predictions about the course of an illness and to aid the clinician in selecting the treatment most likely to be effective. In the practice of psychiatry, since the physical basis for most psychiatric illnesses has yet to be discovered, classification systems are largely derived from studying patients with different types of symptoms and seeing whether some combinations are seen frequently and cluster together on a regular basis.

As more and more medications have become available to treat mood disorders, the classification system for bipolar mood disorders has continued to evolve. In this chapter, various subtypes of bipolar disorder are described. These are the subtypes that currently seem to make sense to clinicians because they serve one of the two purposes of diagnosis: they allow for a better prediction of the course of the illness, and they allow for a more rapid selection of effective therapy—saving the patient time that would be wasted on trying an ineffective medication.

PSYCHIATRIC DIAGNOSIS

At least once a month, it seems, I see a patient who asks to be "tested for bipolar disorder." It's certainly a very reasonable request. Unfortunately, it's not a request that can be satisfied—not just yet. There's no blood test or x-ray or biopsy that can diagnose bipolar disorder (and, for that matter, there is none that can be used to confirm the diagnosis of most of the problems psychiatrists treat).

The reason for this sorry state of affairs is that the biological and chemical basis of bipolar disorder is largely still a mystery. Despite literally hundreds of years of examining the bodily fluids and brain tissues of individuals with mood disorders—first with the naked eye, then with microscopes, later with x-rays and scanning devices, and more recently with incredibly sophisticated biochemical probes—no one has been able to definitely pin-point any abnormalities that can be accurately and reliably measured as an aid in diagnosing the disorder.

Geneticists and neuroscientists have discovered quite a few tantalizing hints—particular genetic signals in large groups of individuals with bipolar disorder, subtle brain-scan variations in persons with the illness—but none of these discoveries has translated into diagnostic tools. The clinical applications of these findings are still in the future. So modern psychiatrists are left with the same diagnostic tools that Emil Kraepelin and other nineteenth-century psychiatrists had: their eyes and ears.

We psychiatrists listen to what the patient and her family members say when they describe symptoms—their onset, course, fluctuation, and impact on the patient. Whether other members of the family suffer from a mood disorder is an important piece of information. We observe the patient for the signs of bipolar disorder described in chapter 1 by performing a *mental status examination*, the psychiatrist's equivalent of the physical examination. This examination consists of observing speech patterns and behavior, asking questions about mood and thinking processes, and evaluating other aspects of mental functioning such as concentration and memory. After this process of history taking and examination, a picture emerges of the person and of her symptoms, and the course of her illness becomes clear. A particular diagnostic category that seems to be a good fit with the clinical information is identified. Once the diagnostic category of the illness is determined, we can make predictions about the future course of the symptoms, and perhaps more important, we can select a treatment that has a good chance of relieving them. In the sections that follow, you can learn about the different forms of bipolar disorder the same way young physicians training to be psychiatrists do: by hearing from patients.

BIPOLAR I DISORDER

It had been several years since I had seen Richard in the mood-disorders clinic. He looked great. Although he was only in his late thirties, some silver tones in his hair made him look older and quite distinguished. I remembered that he had always dressed well, but today, in an obviously finely tailored suit, a crisp white shirt, and a beautiful silk tie, he looked—well, like a million. I knew that this could be a very good sign—or a very bad sign.

"That's a handsome suit you've got on, Richard. Is it new?" I asked.

"I got it about a month ago," he said proudly, "in London. A terrific shop on Savile Row, the same one Prince Harry goes to." He smiled a little mischievously. "And I know what you're thinking: no, I wasn't manic when I bought it!"

Rich certainly knew what mania was, as did several members of his family. His wealthy parents had taken control of his financial affairs in a legal guardianship proceeding for a time to prevent a financial disaster caused by manic overspending; for several years he wasn't even able to write a check at the supermarket.

Rich first developed manic symptoms during law school; he made down payments on not just one Porsche but three before a check bounced. He angrily stormed into the bank's branch office to protest, created quite a scene, and ended up in jail, where an astute nurse fortunately arranged an immediate psychiatric evaluation. Richard was admitted to a local psychiatric hospital and took his first dose of lithium before his parents even knew what had happened.

As many patients do, Rich stopped taking his lithium within a month of leaving the hospital; he started having manic symptoms almost immediately. This time his manic enthusiasm turned to travel rather than cars, and he used a credit card to buy an airline ticket to Fiji. He made it as far as Los Angeles before his mania turned dysphoric and irritable. He started yelling at and shoving a security guard who wanted to examine his luggage and wound up in jail again—this time with federal charges. After a talk with a good lawyer, another hospitalization, more lithium, a leave from law school, and a move back home, he came for treatment at the university outpatient clinic where I was training.

Richard's father also suffered from bipolar disorder and knew, from his own turbulent experiences with the illness, just how to handle the situation. A pair of scissors to the credit cards, a power of attorney, and a trip with Richard to the psychiatrist's appointments made the difference—as did the fact that Richard was an intelligent fellow who (eventually) learned from experience as well. Moreover, he learned from his father that a paternal uncle who had been killed in a car accident when Rich was a child had also actually probably died from the disease; the single-passenger accident had most likely been a suicide. Rich made the decision to take control of the illness rather than let it control him. And as with most things, once he made the decision, he stuck to it. Rich applied himself to staying well with energy and determination.

There was a time after he broke up with a girlfriend when severe depressive symptoms almost necessitated another hospitalization; Rich spent fourteen to sixteen hours in bed every day for nearly three weeks and put on almost fifty pounds. Fortunately, family support, an excellent clinical psychologist who saw him for therapy, and a higher lithium dose for several months got him through. After about a year of maintaining a stable mood, he got into a local law school to finish his studies and eventually graduated at the top of his class. He took a job in New York but now had returned home. "I couldn't pass up the opportunity to open my firm's new branch office in my hometown, could I?" he beamed.

Rich brought me up to date. Mild hypomania had occasionally emerged during the summers while he was working in New York, especially if he was working too hard and didn't watch his sleep habits. But Rich had obviously remained serious about his mental health; he monitored his moods and saw his psychiatrist regularly. Most important, he was making career decisions that reflected his knowledge of his illness. "I think the pace will be slower here than in New York. I may not become a millionaire quite as quickly," he said mischievously, "but there will also be less risk of getting sick, blowing it all, and having to start over again. So . . . I had my last lithium level done three months ago, and it was 0.8. When do you want me to get another?"

It looked as if the suit was a very good sign.

Bipolar I is the designation for the classic variety of bipolar disorder, characterized by full-blown manic attacks and deep, paralyzing depressions. In a World Health Organization survey of more than sixty-one thousand persons in eleven countries, the prevalence rate of bipolar I disorder was 0.6 percent; about six in one thousand persons suffers from bipolar I disorder.[1]

A schematic representation of the moods of bipolar I appears in figure 2.1. The pattern of abnormal mood episodes seems to vary widely, and the rhythm of the illness is almost as individual as the patient who has it. Symptoms usually begin in the late teens or early twenties (figure 2.2), although onset at later ages is not uncommon.

Bipolar I is what physicians refer to as a relapsing and remitting illness; during the course of the illness, its symptoms come and go. This feature of bipolar I—it is actually a feature of *all* mood disorders—makes it difficult to diagnose, difficult to treat, and fiendishly difficult to study.

FIGURE 2.1. Mood changes in bipolar I

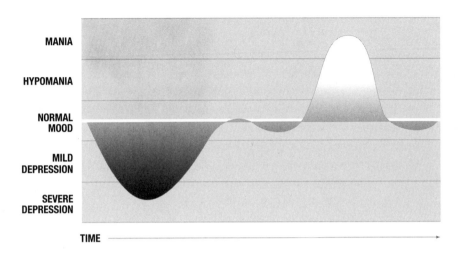

Illustration by Jenna Macfarlane

FIGURE 2.2. Age of onset of bipolar disorder in 1,304 patients

These data were compiled from ten different studies carried out between 1969 and 1984. Notice that early adulthood is the peak time for the onset of the disorder.

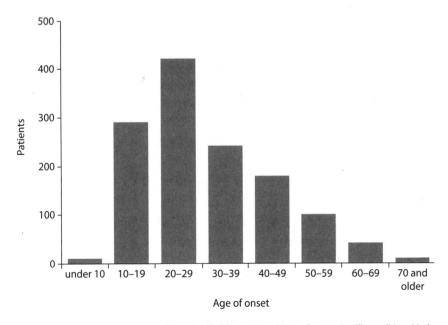

Source: Frederick K. Goodwin and Kay Redfield Jamison, *Manic-Depressive Illness* (New York: Oxford University Press, 1990), 132. Copyright © 1990 by Oxford University Press, Inc. Used by permission of Oxford University Press, Inc.

The Disease That Sleeps

When we think about illnesses of the body, we usually think of diseases that have a beginning, a middle, and an end. Take, for example, pneumonia, an infection of the lungs caused by bacteria. The disease begins when fever, cough, chest pains, and breathing problems appear. These symptoms build and worsen over a period of hours or sometimes days. Before the antibiotic era, patients reached what was called a *crisis* point, when their bodies' natural defenses had mounted their best effort against the bacterial invaders, and the patient either started getting better or died. Either the patient killed off the bacteria or vice versa, but in any case, the disease process came to an end. (Fortunately, we can now administer antibiotics that give the patient's defenses the crucial edge against the bacterial invader.)

Bipolar disorder is very different from pneumonia, because it does not simply have a beginning, a middle, and an end. Or perhaps it is more accurate to say that the illness seems to have many beginnings and endings: the symptoms of bipolar disorder can develop in an individual, and then *without any treatment at all* the symptoms may go away for years at a time—a pattern that is nearly unique among the diseases that afflict humankind.

Since most people are more familiar with diseases that end when their symptoms go away, it is often very difficult for patients and their families to understand that although the symptoms of bipolar disorder can go into *remission* after treatment (or even spontaneously), they almost inevitably will come back if treatment to prevent their return is not in place. The hallmark of bipolar illness—especially bipolar I—is the tendency to *relapse*. No matter how well the symptoms of any one episode are treated, the illness does not end but instead seems merely to hibernate—and *symptoms can come back at any time.*

Bipolar I: What to Expect

Many excellent clinical studies about the course of bipolar disorder were done in the years before effective treatments were available; these studies document and illustrate the pattern of symptoms that occurs if the bipolar disorder is not treated—what physicians call the *natural history* of the illness.[2]

Bipolar disorder usually starts in late adolescence or early adulthood with the peak onset during the third decade of life (ages twenty through twenty-nine).

How many episodes of illness did patients have in the days before treatment was available? How long did their episodes last? What was the length of time between episodes?

In a 1942 study, the records of sixty-six patients with "manic-depressive psychosis" were studied; some of these individuals were followed for up to twenty-six years. Although a few patients seemed to have had only one episode of illness in the period of study, about one-third had two to three episodes, about one-third had four to six episodes, and about one-third had more than seven (table 2.1). A few had twenty or more episodes.[3] Unfortunately, when a diagnosis of bipolar I is made, there is no way to know whether the individual will have another two or three episodes during his lifetime or more than twenty.

TABLE 2.1. **Number of episodes of illness in sixty-six patients with bipolar disorder**

Number of episodes	Percentage of patients
1	8
2-3	29
4-6	26
More than 7	37

Source: Data from Thomas A. C. Rennie, "Prognosis in Manic-Depressive Psychosis," *American Journal of Psychiatry* 98 (1942): 801-14.

Note: This study was done before any treatments were available for bipolar disorder.

How long did episodes of mania or major depression last before effective treatments were available? In the 1942 study, the average duration was about six and a half months. But we also know that depressions and manias were sometimes shorter and sometimes lasted much longer. Kraepelin, writing at a time when there were essentially no effective treatments, noted:

The duration of individual attacks is extremely varied. There are some which last only eight to fourteen days, indeed we sometimes see that states of moodiness or excitement . . . do not continue in these patients longer than one or two days or even only a few hours. For the most part, however, a simple attack usually lasts six to eight months. On the other hand, the cases are not at all rare, in which an attack continues for two, three or four years, and a double attack [can] double that time.[4]

Modern psychiatrists no longer see patients who are manic for years at a time. Effective modern treatments bring these episodes to a close, and the patient is usually better in a few days—weeks at most. Modern psychiatrists do, however, see patients who seem to become manic again and again, month after month, year after year—often every time they stop taking medication. Do these patients have many episodes, or do they have many relapses of a single episode of several years' duration? I tend to think it's the latter, but the rhythm of the illness makes research challenging.

How about the time between attacks? For many persons with bipolar disorder, modern treatments are quite effective at keeping the episodes from recurring. But how long did remissions last in the days before these treatments were available? Kraepelin noted that the time between episodes could be years, even decades—in one case forty-four years passed between one episode of illness and the next.[5]

Subsequent studies have shown that, if untreated, episodes of bipolar disorder often occur more and more frequently in individual patients (figure 2.3), and in the days before treatment was available, mood episodes seemed to be triggered more easily and tended to recur more and more frequently as patients aged.

Another finding in these studies is that many patients "switch" from a depression to a manic episode with no interval of normal mood in between. Many individuals have a period of depression lasting several weeks or months and then switch into a manic episode, again of several months' duration. Often, there is another switch and a third phase of the episode sets in: a long period of depression (see figure 2.4).

A 1969 study described the course of one hundred manic episodes and also noted the relationship of manic to depressed periods.[6] In this study, about half of the patients' manic episodes showed at least one switch—a depression either before or after a manic episode. Several studies suggest that patients who "switch" from depression to mania have a more difficult to treat form of illness than those who switch from mania to depression.[7]

Bipolar I is the classic manic-depressive illness, with fully developed manic episodes and episodes of severe depression, and it is also characterized by long periods of "hibernation" in which the symptoms temporarily disappear (table 2.2). The number of episodes varies enormously, but patients who have only one or two episodes seem to be the exception rather than the rule. Before effective treatments became available, the average length of each episode if untreated was about six months—but episodes that lasted years were not at all uncommon.

FIGURE 2.3. Acceleration of illness in one hundred patients

The cycle length of episodes of bipolar disorder (the time from the onset of one episode to the onset of the next) becomes shorter and shorter in patients whose symptoms are not well controlled and who continue to have episodes of the illness.

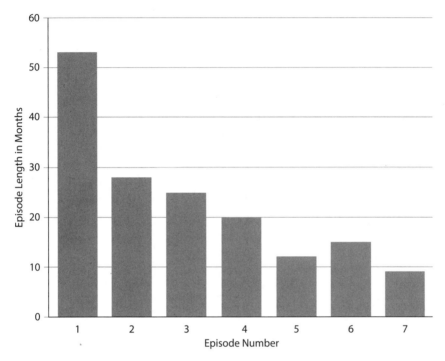

Source: Data from P. P. Roy-Burne, R. M. Post, T. W. Uhde, T. Porcu, and D. Davis, "The Longitudinal Course of Recurrent Affective Illness: Life Chart Data from Patients at the NIMH," *Acta Psychiatrica Scandinavia* 71, suppl. 317 (1985): 1–34.

About one-third of patients with bipolar I disorder have nearly complete remission of their symptoms between episodes. In fact, this illness pattern has been found to predict that an individual will have an excellent response to treatment with lithium.[8] For other patients, bipolar I is a more smoldering disorder, meaning that periods without any symptoms at all occur less frequently. The *National Institute of Mental Health (NIMH) Collaborative Study on Depression* enrolled subjects from 1979 to 1981 and followed them over time. In 2000 a report was issued that found that over the twenty years or so that they were followed, a substantial number of patients experienced fairly long periods during which they were troubled by at least some symptoms, usually mild depressive symptoms.[9]

More recently, researchers at the University of Michigan studied the illness course of 209 cases of bipolar disorder to see whether subtypes of bipolar I disorder emerged, using a sophisticated statistical method, a "Bayesian nonparametric hierarchical model with latent classes."[10] Despite the intimidating name, this technique can simply be thought of as a way of looking for patterns in a data set with no preconceptions as to what one might find

FIGURE 2.4. A triphasic mood episode, showing a period of depression followed by a period of mania and then another period of depression

It is not uncommon for psychiatrists to see patients who first sought treatment for the initial depressive phase and were put on an antidepressant, which triggered the patient's often severe first manic episode.

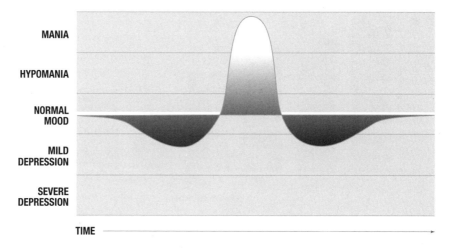

Illustration by Jenna Macfarlane

TABLE 2.2. Features of bipolar I

Mood
Fully developed manic episodes
Fully developed depressive episodes

Other features
Untreated episodes average six months
Hallucinations and delusions frequently seen
Three-phased episodes (depression, mania, depression)
Relapses more frequent as patient ages

but rather letting the data patterns "speak for themselves." The data showed that about half of the subjects had complete symptom remission between episodes and were completely free of symptoms almost 90 percent of the time; they called this the "stable" group. The remainder of the subjects fell about equally into two additional groups, both of whom spent longer periods of time symptomatic.

About one-quarter of the total group had more in the way of depressed periods and had at least some depression symptoms 23 percent of the time and therefore was called the "depressive" group. A third group was called "rapid cycling." These individuals were also found to be symptom-free 70 percent of the time, but the nearly 30 percent of symptomatic time was about evenly divided between depressive and manic symptoms. The rapid-cycling group had briefer symptomatic periods that occurred more often.

As mentioned above, the group that the Michigan researchers called "stable" has been recognized for years and is known to be more responsive to lithium. Being able to further subdivide patients who are less responsive to lithium into meaningful categories (the "depressive" and "rapid-cycling" groups) will hopefully lead to better ways to treat them as well.

FIGURE 2.5. "Data-driven" subtypes of bipolar I disorder

Using a statistical method for finding subtyping patterns in data, researchers at the University of Michigan found three categories of subjects with bipolar I disorder. This graph shows the number of patients in each of the three subtypes in a group of 209 bipolar I subjects in the Prechter Longitudinal Study of Bipolar Disorder at the University of Michigan.

Illustration by Jenna Macfarlane

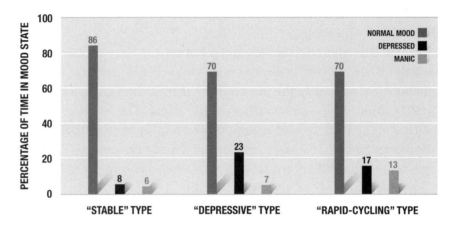

FIGURE 2.6. The proportion of time that patients in each University of Michigan subtype spent in each mood state

Note that in each subtype, patients spent more time depressed than manic.

Illustration by Jenna Macfarlane

BIPOLAR II DISORDER

Robert was a thirty-five-year-old accountant who had been seeing a psychologist for treatment of depression for about three months. Both he and his therapist were frustrated because, despite the best efforts of both, Robert's depression seemed to be getting worse.

"I can usually pull myself out of these things—or at least I can usually slog through them until they finish," he told me at our first appointment. Right away, his description of his depressions as "these things" made me feel pretty certain that this fellow had a mood disorder. Robert's moods had an alien, external quality to him; they came upon him like a fog bank rolling in, lasted for a few weeks, and then slowly dissipated. Where they came from and where they went was a complete mystery to Robert. He would sleep away the weekends, put on weight, fall behind in his work. "This has been happening to me since college," he said, "and I really want it to stop." In fact, this was not the worst his depressions had ever gotten. Shortly after graduation, Robert had such a severe depression that he spent most of the summer at home in his room. At one point he seriously contemplated suicide. The only reason he didn't get into treatment then was because he thought he was no worse off than his mother.

Robert's mother was a closet alcoholic. "There was always one of those huge bottles of wine in the refrigerator," he told me. "It always seemed either full or half full, and when I was in high school I realized that this was because she drank about a half a gallon every day." Robert's mother had never had any treatment for either her drinking problem or depression, but his description of the long "naps" she took most afternoons and the "sick headaches" that put her in bed for weeks sounded like more than alcoholism— more like a smoldering depression complicated by alcohol addiction. Another red flag for a mood-disorder diagnosis: a positive family history.

Robert had always blamed his melancholic moods on his childhood. The memories of his shame and worry about his mother seeped back into his consciousness during these times, as did guilty feelings that he had put hundreds of miles between himself and his mother now, hadn't seen her in more than two years, and could bring himself to call her only on holidays. Here was more evidence pointing to a mood disorder: guilty feelings and painful preoccupations with the past that seemed really to bother him only when his mood changed. Although I wasn't quite finished taking his history, I was already thinking about which antidepressant to recommend to him, when Robert gave me another piece of information that changed everything.

"I even feel like my thinking is slower than usual. I'll never get through tax season unless I do something to get some help—or unless one of my highs kicks in."

"One of your . . . ?"

"I call it a high. But it's not like I'm manic-depressive or anything. It's just that sometimes when things get back to normal I'm so relieved and happy that—oh, I don't know, it just feels so good not to be depressed."

"Do you find that you're especially productive during these times?" I asked.

"Oh, definitely. I can get by one two or three hours of sleep. One year I came out of a depression just in time for tax season. I didn't feel overwhelmed like I usually do. It was spring, and I wasn't depressed for a change, and I had just met the girl I was going to marry—in fact we got married that summer, and so of course things settled back down. But that was a great year."

"Do other people notice?"

"Um, yes, especially at the office. 'Slow down, Rob.' 'Take it easy, Rob.' Sometimes I get irritated by that."

I had a few more questions to ask, but I was beginning to think about how to tell this fellow that he probably had "manic depression" after all.

Bipolar II is characterized by fully developed depressive episodes and episodes of hypomania. A schematic representation of the moods of bipolar II appears in figure 2.7.

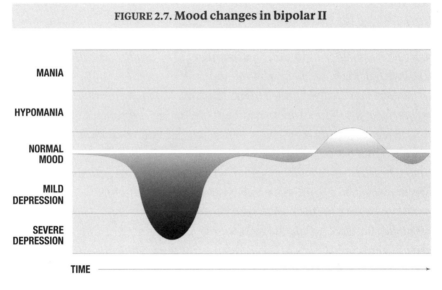

FIGURE 2.7. **Mood changes in bipolar II**

MANIA

HYPOMANIA

NORMAL MOOD

MILD DEPRESSION

SEVERE DEPRESSION

TIME

Illustration by Jenna Macfarlane

When lithium became available in the United States in the 1970s and re-searchers were trying to find better diagnostic criteria for bipolar disorder, several of them noticed that there was a large group of patients who didn't have a history of fully developed manic episodes but who seemed to be bipolar nonetheless. They had severe depressions, but their "highs" never developed into mania. Were these patients "manic depressives" who were still early in the course of their illness and simply hadn't had time to have a fully developed manic episode? Several studies attempting to answer this question concluded that these patients did *not* usually go on to fully developed mania. In one study, fewer than 5 percent of the patients with recurrent depressions and hypomania ever became manic.[11]

It is fairly clear from the research literature that bipolar II is not merely a prelude to "full-blown" manic-depressive illness—that is, bipolar II patients are not in the early stages of bipolar I. The World Health Organization estimates that the lifetime prevalence of bipolar II disorder is 0.4 percent; about four in one thousand persons develop the illness.[12]

Depression—or Bipolar Disorder?

In a study from the National Institutes of Health published in 1995, 559 patients diagnosed with a depressive disorder were followed over time, some for up to eleven years.* It was reported that almost 9 percent of them developed a hypomanic episode during the time that they were followed. That is, they turned out to have bipolar II disorder. The first hypomanic episode could usually be documented within several months of the onset of severe depression, but sometimes it took up to nine years for the correct diagnosis to become clear. A few of these 559 "depression" patients developed a manic episode—that is, they turned out to have bipolar I—but this was far less common (only 3.9 percent).

Compared with the patients with depression only, those who later developed hypomanic periods (the bipolar II patients) were about five years younger when they first developed depression. Also, their first episodes of depression were significantly longer: nearly three times as long.

The study also found that bipolar II patients had longer depressive episodes (52.2 weeks) than bipolar I patients (24.3 weeks) and that, if untreated, their symptom-free intervals were shorter.

In 2011, another report on these same patients was published, some of whom were being evaluated again more than thirty-one years since the bout of depression that brought them into the study. The researchers reevaluated 550 subjects and found that with the passage of more time nearly one in five of the patients with "depression" developed bipolar disorder (19.6 percent); 12.2 percent developed bipolar II, and 7.5 percent developed bipolar I.†

This report also noted that subjects who, at the beginning of the study, reported even a few hypomanic symptoms, symptoms that were too few or too mild to qualify for a diagnosis of bipolar disorder at the time, were at greater risk of going on to develop bipolar disorder—and the more symptoms they reported, the higher their risk.

Taken together, these studies found that persons with "depression" who go on to develop a bipolar disorder (either bipolar I or II) were

- younger when they first developed a major depression,
- more likely to have a relative with a diagnosis of bipolar disorder,
- more likely to have experienced delusional thoughts during their depressions, and
- more likely to have a few mild hypomanic symptoms.

*Hagop Akiskal, Jack Maser, Pamela Zeller, Jean Endicott, William Coryell, Martin Keller, Meredith Warshaw, Paula Clayton, and Frederick Goodwin, "Switching from 'Unipolar' to Bipolar II: An Eleven-Year Prospective Study of Clinical and Temperamental Predictors in 559 Patients," *Archives of General Psychiatry* 52 (1995): 114–23.

†J. G. Fiedorowicz, J. Endicott, A. C. Leon, D. A. Solomon, M. B. Keller, W. H. Coryell, "Subthreshold Hypomanic Symptoms in Progression from Unipolar Major Depression to Bipolar Disorder," *American Journal of Psychiatry* 168, no. 1 (2011): 40–48.

Bipolar II: What to Expect

Bipolar II is sometimes erroneously referred to as a milder form of bipolar I. But although patients with bipolar II do not develop the most severe symptoms of full-blown mania, they tend to have symptoms more of the time. Long periods of depression are typical of bipolar II disorder and can be even more debilitating than the dramatic but shorter-lived episodes of bipolar I illness.

Bipolar II disorder is often more challenging to treat than bipolar I. Why?

Several studies show that bipolar II patients often have relatives who also suffer from bipolar II disorder—but they also often have family members who have bipolar I as well as unipolar depressive disorders (that is, symptoms of depression without either mania or hypomania).[13] In one study of bipolar I and II volunteers, 26 percent of bipolar II patients had a relative with some kind of psychiatric illness (especially anxiety disorders and addiction), as compared to only 15 percent of bipolar I patients.[14] This genetic information is not of academic interest alone. As you will see in a later chapter, we can think of the brain's mood-control system as a complex and finely tuned clock with a myriad of intricate moving parts, each of which is fabricated using instructions coded in our DNA. If we can think of bipolar I as being caused by defects in a few of the bigger parts, bipolar II may be caused by many more defects in many more of the smaller parts. Because more parts need fixing, there are more complicated symptoms and a need for more complicated treatments.

And indeed, studies indicate that the symptoms and course of illness of bipolar II are different from those of bipolar I (table 2.3). Bipolar II patients

TABLE 2.3. Features of bipolar II

Mood
Fully developed depressive episodes
Hypomanic episodes

Other features
Increased sleep and appetite during depressions
Depressions sometimes more chronic
Bipolar II history in family members
Later age at first hospitalization
Fewer hospitalizations
Possible increased risk for alcoholism

have more problems with depression—in fact, the depression is sometimes so prominent that many receive a diagnosis of depressive disorder and don't get treatment for bipolar disorder at all. Persons with bipolar II are more likely to have a seasonal variation in their symptoms (they tend to get depressed in the fall and winter and feel better—or even develop hypomania—in the spring and summer), and they have more rapid cycling (see below). Whereas patients with bipolar I frequently have irritable manic symptoms, the hypomanic periods of bipolar II patients are characterized by an elated mood—irritability is less common. With regard to depressive symptoms, psychomotor agitation, guilty feelings, and thoughts of suicide were more frequently observed in bipolar II. Bipolar II patients also have a higher incidence of phobias and eating disorders.[15]

CYCLOTHYMIC DISORDER

Cyclothymic disorder (-*thymia*, from the Greek word for "mind," is used in psychiatry to refer to mood) is characterized by frequent short periods (days to weeks) of depressive symptoms and hypomania separated by only brief periods (on the order of days to weeks) of normal mood. By definition, the patient does not have either fully developed major depressive episodes or fully developed manic episodes. A schematic representation of the moods of cyclothymia appears in figure 2.8.

Emil Kraepelin described the "cyclothymic temperament" as "characterized by frequent, more or less regular fluctuations of the psychic state to the manic or to the depressive side."[16] He reported that 3 to 4 percent of his patients had the cyclothymic temperament but speculated that many more persons might have similar illnesses that "run their course outside of institutions." He believed that these "temperaments [could] be regarded as rudiments of manic-depressive insanity" that might continue "throughout the whole of life . . . without further development." This idea, that individuals with cyclothymia have a temperament or personality style characterized by nearly constant fluctuations in mood, was the predominant theory well into the twentieth century. For many years American psychiatric classification systems regarded cyclothymia more as an expression of personality than as an illness caused by an abnormality of brain chemistry. In early editions of the *Diagnostic and Statistical Manual* of the American Psychiatric Association (the *DSM*), the disorder was called *cyclothymic personality disorder*. In 1980 *cyclothymic disorder* moved over to the mood-disorder section of the manual—where it remains today.

FIGURE 2.8. Mood changes in cyclothymia

Illustration by Jenna Macfarlane

Cyclothymia is now considered a subtype of bipolar disorder, a classification supported by family-history studies. Patients with cyclothymia often have relatives with bipolar disorder but rarely have relatives suffering from depression only.[17] Treatment experiences seem to confirm this relationship: the mood swings of cyclothymic disorder often respond to many of the same treatment approaches as the bipolar disorders. This finding also confirms that cyclothymia is just as much a "chemical" problem as the other bipolar disorders.

Modern studies on community populations estimate that between 0.4 and 2.4 percent of people have cyclothymia.[18] These studies usually estimate that many with the disorder never receive treatment.

Cyclothymic Disorder: What to Expect

Kraepelin's descriptions of the symptoms of cyclothymia are lively and vivid: "These are the people who constantly oscillate . . . between the two opposite poles of mood. . . . Today lively, sparkling, beaming, full of the joy of life, the pleasure of enterprise and the pressure of activity, [but] after some time . . . depressed, enervated, ill-humored, in need of rest, and again a few months later they display the old freshness and elasticity."[19]

More recent studies, however, indicate that irritable mood is prominent in cyclothymic disorder. One expert contrasted the "sunny" hypomanic periods seen in persons with bipolar II disorder (Kraepelin's "sparkling, beaming" patients) with "dark," irritable, and risk-taking states seen more often in cyclothymic disorder.[20]

Individuals with cyclothymic disorder have frequent ups and downs of mood, with only comparatively few periods of "normal" mood (table 2.4). (This almost constant instability perhaps explains why psychiatrists thought of this as a "personality" characteristic for so long.) As might be expected, constant mood instability causes instability in many areas of the patient's life. In a 1977 study of forty-six patients with cyclothymia, the patients demonstrated a whole variety of oscillations of emotions and behavior—from sleep patterns to work habits to group affiliations (table 2.5).[21]

Cyclothymic disorder tends to begin very early in life. A study of 894 young patients (aged five to seventeen years) found that nearly three-quarters of the patients with cyclothymic disorder first experienced symptoms before age ten and, as a group, had a younger onset than patients with depression or with bipolar II disorder.[22]

Although many persons with cyclothymic disorder never develop more severe mood symptoms, a significant number eventually experience a fully developed depressive or manic episode—that is, they develop bipolar disorder. Longitudinal studies have shown that a significant number of patients diagnosed with cyclothymic disorder go on to develop a manic episode, putting them in the bipolar I category, or develop severe depression—that is, they turned out to have bipolar II. However, perhaps half of patients with the cyclothymic pattern never develop symptoms of full-blown bipolar disorder—a finding that makes cyclothymic disorder a true diagnosis in its own right.

TABLE 2.4. Features of cyclothymic disorder

Mood
Frequent alternation between mild depression and mild hypomania
Short, irregular cycles (days)
Only short periods of normal mood

Other features
Patients often wake up with mood changes
Pattern appears in late teens, early twenties
Frequently mistaken for problem with "personality"
Sometimes develops into bipolar I or II

TABLE 2.5. Mood, thinking, and behavior patterns in forty-six cyclothymic patients	
Mood	*Percentage of patients*
Irritable periods lasting a few days	50
Explosive, aggressive outbursts	50
Thinking	
Shaky self-esteem alternating between lack of self-confidence and overconfidence	75
Periods of mental confusion alternating with periods of sharpened, creative thinking	50
Activity and behavior	
Increased sleep alternating with decreased need for sleep	75
Unevenness in quantity and quality of work	75
Buying sprees, extravagance, or financial disasters	75
Repeated shifts in work, study, interest, or future plans	50
Drug or alcohol abuse	50
Extroversion alternating with introversion	50
Unexplained promiscuity or extramarital affairs	40
Joining new movement with enthusiasm, rapidly changing to disillusionment	25

Source: Data from H. Akiskal, M. K. Khani, and A. Scott-Strauss, "Cyclothymic Temperamental Disorders," *Psychiatric Clinics of North America* 2 (1979): 527–54, quoted in Frederick K. Goodwin and Kay Redfield Jamison, *Manic-Depressive Illness* (New York: Oxford University Press, 1990), 54.

"SOFT" BIPOLAR DISORDERS

If you look at the end of the section on bipolar disorders in the fifth edition of the *DSM*, you will see the category "bipolar disorder not elsewhere classified" (also, simply, "bipolar NEC"). This odd category exists because the developers of the *DSM* recognized that there are patients who seem to have some kind of bipolar disorder but who don't meet the diagnostic criteria for bipolar I or II or cyclothymia.

Maria is a violinist in the local symphony orchestra. She is close to seventy but looks much younger. Born in what is now the Czech Republic, she defected to the United States during a tour of a chamber music group in the 1980s. Maria found herself in New York with only a small suitcase of clothes, her violin, and a charming European accent. She credits the latter two with her success in finding good work with several American orchestras over the years.

"I must tell you, Doctor, that my son has started taking Lamictal, just like me. His psychiatrist asked him about my medications and put my son on the same one. It's so good to know he's being treated by a psychiatrist as brilliant as you."

"Now, now, it was hardly brilliant of me to—"

"Oh, yes, so humble, so modest you are, just like all great men."

This was a little game we had played for years, ever since I had put her on a mood stabilizer instead of an antidepressant.

Because she moved to a new city every five years or so, Maria had seen a number of different professionals for her mood problems—mostly depression. For many of those years she received no treatment at all but simply slogged through her periods of depression on her own. She took several antidepressants, but they never seemed to be very helpful, and after a time, Maria would stop taking them. One physician gave her a prescription for the tranquilizer Valium, and although it didn't treat her depression very well, it numbed Maria's feelings enough to keep her going. When she moved to a new community, she was able to get more prescriptions for Valium by reporting to her new doctor that it helped her—which, after a fashion, it did. During the really bad times, Maria used alcohol to augment the Valium's effect. By the time she was in her midforties, she was well on her way to chemical dependency. One terrible year, she lost a job because of missing several rehearsals and an important concert while in a week-long alcohol- and Valium-induced fog during a period of depression. Her husband left her, and a month later she got word that her son, also a talented musician, had dropped out of the prestigious conservatory he was attending and disappeared.

Maria's depression worsened to the point that she took a nearly fatal overdose of Valium and alcohol. It was only because the manager of the apartment building where she was living happened to go into her apartment that particular day that she ended up in a hospital rather than in the state medical examiners' facility.

In the psychiatric hospital, a newly available antidepressant was started. Effexor seemed to be helpful after a few days, and she was sent home. But a week later, it seemed that it was perhaps making things worse rather than better. Maria started to feel "wired" and agitated and couldn't sleep.

It was at this point that we first saw Maria in the clinic. The psychiatric resident took an excellent history from Maria, and by asking about her family history found out that Maria's father had twice been in a psychiatric hospital in Europe. "The doctors said he had manic depression, but he went for years without any treatment and was fine," *Maria said,* "so we didn't believe them."

After the resident had finished presenting Maria's case to me, I asked the young doctor whether she thought Maria's illness had any indications of a bipolar disorder. "Well," *she said,* "it sounds like the father probably had bipolar disorder."

"Right," *I said.* "Anything else?"

"She became overstimulated after starting on the Effexor, but . . ."

"But?"

"But she took antidepressants before and didn't have that reaction; they just didn't help with her depression."

"That can happen," *I responded, then asked,* "Did she mention any periods of hyperactivity?"

"I asked her about that," *the resident continued.* "She said that she when she was younger, she sometimes had a few hours or maybe a day of more energy than usual and being more productive but they never lasted four days or longer."

"Four days?"

"According to the DSM, a period of hyperactivity has to last at least four days to be considered hypomania."

"Don't believe everything you read in the DSM," *I said with a smile.* "Let's go see the patient and decide what to do."

We stopped Maria's new antidepressant and started her on lamotrigine. In a few days the agitation stopped. It took much longer for her depression to lift completely, but it eventually did.

What was Maria's diagnosis? She suffered from long-standing depression. She sometimes had brief periods of mild hypomanic symptoms but had never had any manic or hypomanic episodes (strictly defined, at least) that would make her fit the bipolar I or II diagnosis. She didn't have the "constant oscillations" of mood that are typical of cyclothymic disorder. But her illness nevertheless had some bipolar features: a family history of bipolar disorder and the period of agitation and insomnia that occurred after she started on the most recent antidepressant. She didn't fit any DSM bipolar categories— but she clearly had some type *of bipolar disorder.*

Psychiatrists have long recognized that there are many forms of bipolar disorder. Kraepelin noted that "it is fundamentally and practically impossible to keep apart in any way" the various forms of bipolar disorder; "everywhere there are transitions."[23]

For many years clinicians have described various types of "soft" bipolar disorder, mostly in patients who came to them to be treated for depression but whose illness seemed related to bipolar disorder.[24] Terms like *pseudo-unipolar depression* and *bipolar III* have been coined to describe various types of severe depressions that have some features of bipolar disorder but do not fall into traditional categories for bipolar diagnoses.

As more treatments for bipolar disorder become available and as more research on mood disorders is done, it is becoming clear that many patients who suffer from mostly depressive symptoms can benefit from treatment with medications for bipolar disorders and may in fact have a type of bipolar disorder.

For about a half century, psychiatry divided mood disorders into cases of unipolar depression, an illness characterized by only depressive symptoms, and bipolar disorders, in which patients suffer depressive episodes but also manic, hypomanic, or mixed states as well.

"Soft" bipolar disorders seem to challenge this way of thinking; many of these patients have an illness that is dominated by depressive symptoms and shows only the slightest colorings of mania. Sometimes, a family history of bipolar disorder is the only hint. More frequently, they have brief periods of elevated mood that they don't consider particularly abnormal but that, when examined more closely, bear the hallmarks of hypomania: decreased need for sleep, increased energy, uncharacteristic overconfidence, and loss of inhibitions. They can have periods of agitation and irritability that last only a few hours and may represent mild mixed states.

I have seen many patients who have been unsuccessfully treated with one antidepressant after another for what they have been told is "unipolar

---

TABLE 2.6. Indicators of "soft" bipolar disorders

Family history of bipolar disorder

History of mania or hypomania caused by treatment with antidepressants

History of "mixed" mood states

Depressive, "hyper," or cycling temperament

Recurrent depressions

depression." For many of these patients, there are bipolar features in their illness that haven't been recognized as such. When one of the medications more typically used to treat bipolar disorder is prescribed, these patients frequently have a significant improvement in their depressive symptoms.

Some patients with this kind of problem become upset when I try to explain that a better approach to their depression might be to treat it as a form of bipolar disorder; they worry that a diagnosis of bipolar disorder means that they have a more serious problem than "just depression" or that they are "really crazy." This reaction overlooks a couple of facts: first, depression is always a serious illness, and second, many, perhaps most, people with bipolar disorder never develop full-blown mania or psychotic symptoms (which is what most people are thinking of when they use the pejorative term *crazy*). I sometimes use the term *complicated depression* to talk about these illnesses.

Dr. Kraepelin Makes a Comeback: The Mood Disorder Spectrum

Emil Kraepelin argued for collecting all mood disorders into one big category that he called "manic-depressive disorder," an idea that fell out of favor in the first half of the twentieth century. Many mood disorder researchers now maintain that Kraepelin's idea is more accurate and that mood disorders vary along a *spectrum*, with pure depressive disorders at one end and bipolar I disorder at the other.

A review paper published in 2007 found more than eleven hundred articles that argue for and against this idea.* I would argue that most psychiatrists who treat patients with mood disorders agree with Dr. Kraepelin—they see patients everyday who don't fit neatly into a *DSM* category.

FIGURE 2.9. The "spectrum" of mood disorders from bipolar I to pure "unipolar" depression

BIPOLAR I · BIPOLAR II · "SOFT" BIPOLAR DISORDERS · UNIPOLAR DEPRESSION

BIPOLAR DISORDERS   **PURE DEPRESSIVE DISORDERS**

Illustration by Jenna Macfarlane

*F. Benazzi, "Is There a Continuity between Bipolar and Depressive Disorders?" *Psychotherapy and Psychosomatics* 76, no. 2 (2007): 70–76.

The important point to remember is that, despite what you might gather from reading short newspaper or magazine articles about depression and bipolar disorder, we haven't yet figured out how to classify these illnesses. It is becoming clear that many cases that seem to be "just depression" are related in some way to bipolar disorder. Many depressed patients who don't seem to have classic manic-depressive illness will nevertheless benefit from medications used to treat bipolar disorder.

SCHIZOAFFECTIVE DISORDER

Some patients have an illness with features both of mood disorders and of a very different psychiatric illness: schizophrenia. In addition to mood-disorder symptoms such as depression, hypomania, or mania, these patients have the hallucinations, delusions, and other mental experiences typical of schizophrenia; they often receive the diagnosis of schizoaffective disorder.

As we saw in chapter 1, some patients with bipolar disorder develop delusional beliefs or hallucinations. But in the mood disorders, these symptoms can usually be understood as arising out of the mood state. For example, in a severe depression a patient might have the delusional belief that she has a terrible illness or has lost all of her money or that family members are being tortured by kidnappers, beliefs that are, well, depressing. Manic patients may hear the singing of angels or the voice of God—again, hallucinations that can be understood as coming out of the expansive, grandiose mood of mania. Delusions (false beliefs and ideas) and hallucinations (false sensory perceptions such as hearing voices) are said to be *mood congruent* when they can be understood as being part of the abnormal mood.

Persons with schizophrenia have bizarre delusions and hallucinations too, but they don't usually seem to bear any relation to a change in mood. Examples of schizophrenic delusions include the belief that one's next-door neighbors are pumping poisonous gas into one's house, or that one's real spouse and children have been replaced by exact replicas, or that the FBI has implanted a transmitter in one's brain. Patients with schizophrenia sometimes believe that other people are reading their minds or putting into their heads thoughts that are not theirs. They might hear their own thoughts repeated to them aloud or hear the voices of unseen commentators describing their actions to other unseen persons. None of these symptoms has much relationship to mood changes. More importantly, persons with schizophrenia do not experience episodes of sustained abnormal changes in mood. When a person has bizarre delusions or hallucinations like these or has these kinds of symptoms during times when they do not seem to be in an episode of abnormal mood, the diagnosis of schizoaffective disorder is often made.

What is this disorder, and where does it belong in the classification of psychiatric disease? These are questions that have plagued psychiatry for many years; we still don't have very good answers.

Is schizoaffective disorder truly a separate disorder, an illness that shares symptoms with mood disorders and schizophrenia but is neither? If it is, it has been quite difficult for researchers to agree on its defining symptoms. In an earlier version of the *DSM*, the diagnostic category of schizoaffective disorder was included without *any* listing of the symptoms that defined it.

If one does a search on "schizoaffective disorder" on PubMed, the online database of medical research articles hosted by the National Library of Medicine, many of the articles that come up are arguments about whether the disorder even exists. Many others are studies showing that psychiatrists often do not agree on the diagnosis in individual patients.

I have seen patients who have been diagnosed with schizoaffective disorder by other clinicians who seemed to me instead to have a severe case of a mood disorder that has been difficult to treat. I have seen patients diagnosed with schizoaffective disorder because they have prominent paranoid symptoms—that is, they believe they are being watched or followed or talked about. Although paranoid symptoms are very common in some types of schizophrenia and not as common in the mood disorders, close questioning often reveals the mood component in these patients. In a book written during the twentieth century called *A Mind That Found Itself*, Clifford Beers described his battle with a mental illness that was almost certainly bipolar disorder. In one scene he describes a train ride to the psychiatric hospital. As the train passed through the stations along the way, Beers noticed people standing on the station platforms reading the newspaper. He became convinced that they were reading about him. At first glance, this symptom doesn't seem to have any mood component, and in fact it is a rather typical symptom of schizophrenia called an *idea of reference*. Fortunately, however, Beers described this symptom in great detail in his book and wrote that he thought the people on the train platforms were reading about his long history of mental illness and about what a failure he had been. With this added detail—the themes of shame and failure in the symptom—the mood component becomes obvious, and the real diagnosis clear: a mood disorder.

Another possible explanation for the mingling of symptoms of a mood disorder and schizophrenia in one patient is that the patient may suffer from *both* illnesses. If one considers that bipolar I affects about 1 percent of the population and that about 1 percent of the population suffers from schizophrenia, then obviously, if there are no other factors operating to prevent the illnesses from occurring together, as many as 0.01 percent of the population will suffer from both disorders—that is, one in ten thousand. If one adds other mood disorders such as bipolar II, cyclothymia, and the "soft" bipolar disorders, the numbers of persons with schizophrenia who also have a mood disorder is even greater. Treatment experience would seem to support this idea: patients with a diagnosis of schizoaffective disorder seem to be most effectively treated with medications for mood disorders used in combination with medications for schizophrenia.

Indeed, some patients' illness definitely seems to combine two disorders: they have the kind of bizarre delusions common in schizophrenia, which seem to have nothing to do with an abnormal mood, but also have clear-cut episodes of depression and mania. This seems to be a rare occurrence, but it is important not to miss it. I have occasionally seen patients whose psychiatrist seemed reluctant to make the diagnosis of schizoaffective disorder, perhaps not wanting to frighten patients and families with the diagnosis of an illness that is usually more impairing and difficult to treat than a bipolar disorder. This reluctance to diagnose, however, can result in not treating the illness aggressively enough.

I once saw a patient whose psychiatrist had referred him for consultation because what had been diagnosed as severe bipolar depression with psychotic symptoms had responded poorly to many different treatments for mood disorders. This patient was certainly depressed, but his illness—which had required multiple hospitalizations and had become so disabling that he could no longer work or even live in his own apartment—had other features consistent with schizophrenia. For this patient, treatment for depression was helpful just up to a point. Only when he was also prescribed clozapine (Clozaril), a medication usually reserved for patients with severe schizophrenia who have failed to benefit from other medications, did he have a substantial recovery. Making a change in diagnosis and recommending a radically different treatment approach was upsetting for this patient and his family at first—for just the reasons mentioned above. But the patient's parents also admitted that they had long suspected that their son had "more than just bipolar disorder," and after more careful explanation of my reasoning and further discussions with the patient and his family, we shifted the course of the treatment plan, ultimately with positive results.

This is a lesson in the importance of making the correct diagnosis in mood disorders.

A diagnosis of schizoaffective disorder is in many ways more serious than that of bipolar disorder, since this illness shares some of the features of schizophrenia and some of the treatment challenges of that illness. Delusions and hallucinations may respond incompletely to medication treatment, and more severe (and sometimes progressive) social and occupational impairment is not uncommon. For this very reason, however, it is even more important, if a diagnosis of schizoaffective disorder is being considered, to be extra careful in reviewing the symptoms and course of illness and to use information from as many sources as possible.

KEY TAKEAWAYS

▶ There are many forms of bipolar disorder, and almost no two cases are exactly alike.

▶ For many persons who turn out to benefit from medications for bipolar disorder, symptoms of depression dominate the clinical picture, making diagnosis difficult.

CHAPTER 3

Bipolar Disorder and the *DSM-5*

Individuals who are being treated by a mental-health professional and who read their diagnosis in their medical records or insurance statements often have questions about the diagnostic categories and terms that are used. Psychiatry is one of the few medical specialties that has a more or less official list of disorders and diagnoses, and in this chapter we'll take a closer look at the latest version of this list, the fifth edition of the *Diagnostic and Statistical Manual of Mental Disorders* (the *DSM-5*), developed and published by the American Psychiatric Association. I'll present a brief overview of the *DSM* and explain some of the diagnostic terminology for bipolar disorder.

WHAT IS THE *DSM*?

Perhaps the most valuable use of the *DSM* is in research into the causes and treatment of mental illnesses. Use of the *DSM* in research means that when you find a study of some particular psychiatric disorder in a professional journal and read that "the patients met the *DSM* diagnostic criteria" for that disorder, you can be sure that the patients all had a certain well-defined collection of symptoms and other characteristics in common, that the researchers were not mixing, as it were, psychiatric apples and oranges in their study.

There are problems with the *DSM*, however, and many experts have been extremely critical of it. In recent years, even its use in research has begun to wane.

The *DSM* is essentially a collection of checklists of *symptoms* for each diagnostic category and is not based on an understanding of the *causes* of emotional problems. This might seem like a quibbling academic question at first, but it's not. As an example, a *DSM*-type classification system for physical illnesses might classify diseases based on the severity and location of symptoms such as pain or fever. A moment's thought reveals how useless such a system would be. Patients coming to an emergency department with symptoms of abdominal pain and a fever might be diagnosed with "Hot Painful Belly Disorder." But since these same symptoms can be caused by a myriad of different problems, ranging from appendicitis to gall stones to porphyria, a diagnosis of "Hot Painful Belly Disorder" is completely useless for deciding how to treat the patient. Switching back to psychiatric diagnosis, good clinicians know that two patients might have nearly identical symptoms of depression from many different causes that range from normal bereavement, to reactions to long-term depressing life circumstances such as poverty or ongoing physical abuse, to biologically and genetically caused mood disorders—or even hormonal problems. Cataloging the *symptoms* is only a first step in deciding what to do for the patient. A list of symptoms doesn't help decide whether the patient needs grief counseling, social work, domestic violence intervention, or a prescription for an antidepressant.

Because the *DSM* contains a list of psychiatric diagnoses followed by succinct and clearly written "criteria" for making those diagnoses, it also has the unfortunate effect of making psychiatric diagnosis look deceptively easy. It is tempting for individuals who have no psychiatric training to use this series of symptom checklists to diagnose mental illness. Well, why not?

First of all, it is only with an enormous amount of training and experience that one can gain an appreciation of the expansive range of *normal* emotions and behaviors and have a sense of what falls outside this normal range. Significant clinical experience and judgment are needed to decide what constitutes an "expansive mood" or an "increase in energy" that is clinically significant. I have been called to see "manic" patients referred by their counselors or their family members and found that the patients, though a bit more intense in manner than most people, have a mood state perfectly within the normal range. The *DSM* is full of diagnostic criteria that use qualifiers like "clinically significant," "marked impairment," and "excessive involvement in . . . ," all of which require judgment based on experience to make a determination. Even many counseling and therapy professionals, if they have not trained in a setting where they have had the opportunity to see severely depressed or manic patients, may not have an appreciation for what constitutes *severe*. Nonprofessionals will, of course, usually have even less experience with the range of normal and abnormal moods. Without the experience of seeing many patients with severe mental illnesses and treating them, it is impossible to accurately separate normal from abnormal mental experiences or "clinically significant" mood changes

The *DSM*: A Short History

The roots of the *DSM-5* go back at least as far as the US Census of 1840, which included the category of "idiocy/insanity" in its system for classifying American citizens. By 1880 there were seven categories into which persons with mental illness could be placed: mania, melancholia, monomania, paresis, dementia, dipsomania, and epilepsy (which at the time was considered a mental illness). In 1917 the American Medico-Psychological Association—the forerunner of the American Psychiatric Association—developed a statistical manual for use in mental hospitals that included various categories of diagnoses to help the hospitals record the number of patients they were caring for with different conditions. As time went on, other organizations interested in the statistics of mental illness, such as the Veterans Administration and the US Army, developed their own statistical manuals. After World War II, the World Health Organization included a long section on mental disorders in the sixth edition of its *International Classification of Diseases* (the *ICD-6*).

In 1952 the American Psychiatric Association published the *Diagnostic and Statistical Manual: Mental Disorders* (the *DSM-1*), which differed from previous statistical manuals in that it contained a glossary describing the symptoms of the different disorders. Thus, in addition to an official list of categories of mental illness, the *DSM-1* provided guidance to the clinician in making psychiatric diagnoses. By the time the third edition of the manual appeared in 1980, each category of psychiatric disorders had a list of *diagnostic criteria*—the symptoms and other characteristics of each disorder that were thought to define it and set it apart from other psychiatric disorders.

The current edition, the *DSM-5*, was published in 2013, almost twenty years after the previous edition, the *DSM-4*. The twelve-year revision process included "an intensive 6-year process [that] involved conducting literature reviews and secondary analyses, publishing research reports in scientific journals, developing draft diagnostic criteria, posting preliminary drafts on the *DSM-5* web site for public comment, presenting preliminary findings at professional meetings, performing field trials, and revising criteria and text."*

*American Psychiatric Association, *Diagnostic and Statistical Manual of Mental Disorders: DSM-5* (Arlington, VA: American Psychiatric Association), introduction.

from those that are within the range of the normal. In psychiatry as perhaps in no other field, the dictum "A little learning is a dangerous thing" holds quite true. To their credit, the authors of the *DSM* acknowledge this problem, stating in the introduction to the *DSM-5*, "The diagnostic criteria identify symptoms, behaviors, cognitive functions, personality traits, physical signs, syndrome combinations, and durations that require clinical expertise to differentiate from normal life variation and transient responses to stress."

Another issue is that many *medical* conditions can mimic abnormal mood states, dozens of pharmaceuticals can cause depression or euphoric states in some persons, and drugs of abuse can cause all kinds of abnormal mood states and psychoses in almost anyone. Almost all the *DSM* diagnoses contain "exclusion criteria" for medical conditions, such as "the symptoms are not due to a general medical condition." A physician will probably notice the abnormalities in the facial appearance of a patient with Graves's disease or Cushing's syndrome as soon as the patient walks into the room; the nonphysician probably has never heard of these illnesses and doesn't know that they can cause psychiatric symptoms practically identical to those of a major depression episode. The physician knows well the typical walk of a patient with Parkinson's disease and the subtle language problems of the patient who has had a silent stroke—both neurological conditions that can cause mood symptoms. Obviously, only a clinician trained in the diagnosis and treatment of physical illness will be able to pick up on these signs.

Finally, just as the range of normal experiences and behaviors is enormous, so is the range (and complexity) of abnormal mental experiences and behaviors; they cannot be contained in any one book and certainly cannot all be described in a few dozen diagnostic categories. Alfred Kinsey, a great student of human behavior and a pioneering researcher on sexuality, once said, "The world is not divided into sheep and goats. . . . Nature rarely deals with discrete categories. Only the human mind invents categories and tries to force facts into separated pigeonholes."[1] To paraphrase Kinsey, bipolar disorder is probably not divided simply into bipolar I and bipolar II, either—and patients often don't fit into *DSM* pigeonholes. Again, to the credit of its authors, the *DSM-5* acknowledges this, stating in the introduction, "It is well recognized that this set of categorical diagnoses does not fully describe the full range of mental disorders that individuals experience and present to clinicians on a daily basis throughout the world."

There is also the fact that many patients with one psychiatric disorder also suffer from another—patients with mood disorders often have addiction problems, patients with developmental disorders such as autism frequently get depressed or anxious—not to mention that symptoms of one disorder are often seen in another: the "criteria" for attention-deficit hyperactivity disorder (ADHD) are nearly identical to those of hypomania, for example. Many patients with bipolar disorder also have panic attacks, but to say that these patients suffer from a mood disorder *and* an anxiety disorder simply isn't accurate. In fact, treating anxious and depressed patients with antianxiety medications such as clonazepam (Klonopin) and other sedatives can make things worse rather than better.

For all these reasons, just as in the prior three editions of this book, I am not going to list the *DSM* diagnostic criteria for the bipolar disorders. I don't want to tempt nonclinicians to engage in self-diagnosis or diagnosis of family members. The *DSM* is easily available in libraries, but it should be considered a reference book for researchers and clinicians, not a textbook of psychiatry.

BIPOLAR CATEGORIES IN THE *DSM-5*

Only two subtypes of bipolar disorder have been characterized well enough to have been assigned their own *DSM* categories: bipolar I and bipolar II. Cyclothymic disorder is included in the *DSM-5* as a diagnosis as well. As we saw in chapter 2, in the section on "soft" bipolar disorders, there are probably other forms of the illness that will eventually be described and understood well enough to be demarcated with their own labels as well, but for now a patient having one of the "soft" bipolar disorders would be diagnosed with "bipolar disorder not elsewhere classified (bipolar disorder NEC)," according to the *DSM*.

——————————— KEY TAKEAWAYS ———————————

▶ The *DSM* is *not* the "bible" for psychiatrists. It should be thought of as research tool that helps to categorize psychiatric problems but is of little use for diagnosing a particular patient.

CHAPTER 4

The Mood Disease
Some History

Having reviewed the many symptoms of bipolar disorder and the many forms the illness can take, I want to pause for a moment to review just how far we've come in our understanding of this illness—and where we've come *from*. I think the understanding of any subject is incomplete unless you know a little about its history, and the history of thinking about bipolar disorder not only is a fascinating story in its own right but also will provide valuable insights into how psychiatrists view the diagnostic process and approach the treatment of psychiatric disorders. (This is a chapter that may be of more interest to students and mental-health professionals than to patients and their families. You can skip it without any loss of continuity.)

BEFORE "BIPOLAR"

The ancient Greeks believed that all maladies of mind and body were caused by imbalances among four vital bodily fluids, or "humors." One of the terms we still use to describe depression, *melancholia*, is derived from the Greek word for one of these humors: black bile. According to humoral theory, depression was thought to be caused by an excess of black bile and mania by an excess of yellow bile.

Although they were incorrect about the causes of the two opposite mood states, several ancient physicians had remarkable insight into the connection between them. Aretaius of Cappadocia (ca. 150) described the syndrome of depression in which patients became "peevish, dispirited, sleepless" and "complain[ed] of life and desire[d] to die." In other patients he described manic symptoms: "At the height of [their] disease [they] have impure dreams, and irresistible desire[s]. . . . If roused to anger by admonition or restraint, they become wholly mad." But, most remarkably, he stated, "In my opinion, melancholia is without any doubt the beginning and even part of the disorder called mania."[1] Paul of Aegina (625–690) made a similar connection between the two syndromes, basing his thinking on humoral theory. Like other Greeks, Paul assumed that melancholia was caused by too much ordinary black bile, but he postulated that mania was caused by an excess of "yellow bile which, by too much heat," had become burned black bile.[2]

Considerations of possible physical causes for the symptoms of bipolar disorder more or less ceased after the fall of the Roman Empire, and the symptoms and behaviors that we now recognize as arising from psychiatric conditions were usually attributed to witchcraft or demonic possession rather than to disruptions of a person's physiology. When medieval times gave way to the Renaissance and the Enlightenment, mental illness again became the purview of physicians rather than priests, and modern attempts to understand and classify diseases began. Melancholia and mania were often considered to be two separate disorders by these early physicians. However, a few insightful clinicians, such as the English physician Robert James (1705–1776), connected the two syndromes: "There is an absolute Necessity for reducing Melancholy and Madness [mania] to one Species of Disorder, and consequently considering them in one joint View. . . . We find, that they both arise from the same common Cause and Origin, that is, an excessive Congestion of the Blood in the Brain. . . . We find that melancholic Patients . . . easily fall into Madness, which, when removed, the Melancholy again discovers itself."[3] This idea put James in the minority among his peer physicians writing about mental disease, who thought that melancholics were predisposed to "madness" and vice versa but the two conditions were nevertheless entirely different.

Not until the middle of the nineteenth century did the idea that depression and mania might be expressions of a single mental illness gain wide attention. It was suggested by two French *alienists* (a term—from *aliéné*, the French word for "insane"—that was used in France and in English-speaking countries at one time to denote physicians specializing in mental disorders). Jules Baillarger (1809–1890) published a paper in 1854 describing an illness he called *la folie à double forme*, and two weeks later Jean-Pierre Falret (1794–1870) rushed a paper into print in the same journal in which he insisted that he had been teaching his students about *la folie circulaire* at the Salpetrière hospital for ten years. (This was, incidentally, the same hospital where several years later the young Sigmund Freud began to formulate his own theories about mental phenomena.) Both men described a mental illness characterized by alternating periods of melancholia and mania that were often separated by periods of normal mood. After the appearance of their original papers, Baillarger and Falret wrote several "me first!" "no, *me* first!" letters to the *Bulletin* of the Imperial Academy of Medicine, each claiming to be the originator of this idea. Which deserves credit as the first to describe bipolar disorder is a matter upon which scholars still disagree.[4] But medical historians do *not* disagree about the identity of the psychiatrist who published the first comprehensive description of the mood disorders and established the basis of the classification system for mental illnesses that we still use today.

DR. KRAEPELIN AND "MANIC-DEPRESSIVE INSANITY"

FIGURE 4.1. **Emil Kraepelin**

Source: Wellcome Collection. CC BY 4.0

It was the German psychiatrist Emil Kraepelin (1856–1926) who, in 1899, solidified the modern concept of bipolar disorder in the sixth edition of his enormously influential textbook on mental illnesses, *Psychiatrie: Ein Lehrbuch für Studirende und Ärzte*. Kraepelin had been working for several years to develop a logical and comprehensive classification system for major mental illnesses, and successive editions of his *Textbook of Psychiatry* document the development of his thinking (table 4.1).

In the fifth edition, he divided severe forms of mental illness into two broad categories: those that had a deteriorating course of illness and those that were "periodic." These two groups are still recognizable in modern classifications of psychiatric disorders, the "deteriorating" group containing the various forms of schizophrenia and related disorders, and the "periodic" group containing the mood disorders. Although he was not the first to suggest that mania and depression were both expressions of one disorder, Kraepelin was the first to articulate, clearly and convincingly, the idea that *all* disorders of mood were related to one another: "Manic-depressive insanity . . . includes on the one hand the whole domain of so-called periodic and circular insanity, on the other hand simple mania, [and] the greater part of the morbid states termed melancholia. . . . In the course of the years I have become more and more convinced that all the above-mentioned states only represent manifestations of a single morbid process."[5] Although others had already arrived at this

| TABLE 4.1. The Evolution of a Concept: "Manic-Depressive Illness" |

The evolution of Kraepelin's thinking about mood disorders is reflected in the different editions of his textbook of psychiatry. In early editions, he considered the "circular form" of periodic mood illnesses, what is now called bipolar disorder, only one of six subtypes. In succeeding editions of his textbook, he moved away from classifying the different patterns of mood episodes as separate illnesses, until in the seventh edition, Kraepelin collapsed all disorders characterized by recurrent mood episodes into one category, for which he coined the term "manic-depressive insanity."

Early editions, 1893–1899	5th edition, 1893	6th edition, 1896	7th edition, 1899
Melancholia	Melancholia	Periodic insanity:	*Manic-depressive illness*
Mania	Mania	Manic form	
Periodic illnesses:	Periodic illnesses:	Depressive form	
Delirious form	Manic form	*Circular form*	
Manic form	Depressive form		
Depressive form	*Circular form*		
Circular form			

same conclusion, it was Kraepelin's "manic-depressive synthesis" that has come to be considered the beginning of the modern classification system for major mental illnesses. Some have argued that it was the simplicity of Kraepelin's diagnostic system, rather than any new insights into psychiatric illness, that resulted in the influence of his diagnostic schema.[6] But, whatever the reason, "Kraepelinian" thinking has come to dominate the field of psychiatric diagnostic classification.

In contrast to many of the other prominent psychiatrists of his time who focused on studying the brain in their laboratories, Kraepelin spent much of his time taking care of patients. A clinician who saw enormous numbers of patients and treated them over many years, he came to consider course of illness as an important factor for classification purposes, and so he recorded his observations of his patients' illnesses in superb detail. As you know from reading them in previous chapters, his descriptions of the symptoms of bipolar disorder are vivid and insightful, and they have never been surpassed. A former professor once told me that "anyone who thinks they've discovered something new in psychiatry simply hasn't read the German psychiatric literature." I think it's fair to say that anyone who thinks he has discovered something new about bipolar disorder—at least, about its symptoms and diagnosis—simply hasn't read Kraepelin.

Kraepelin's contributions, although tremendously significant for those interested in the classification of mental disorders, offered little practical benefit in his time to those afflicted with them. I would imagine that Dr. Kraepelin's patients were more accurately informed about their illness than most patients of that time and had more reliable prognostic information, but there was really nothing he could do to help them with their symptoms. There was still no treatment for *any* psychiatric condition that offered much hope of alleviating the symptoms or altering the course of the disease. Although the English translation of the chapter on "manic-depressive insanity" in the eighth edition of Kraepelin's textbook is more than two hundred pages long, the "Treatment" section is less than five pages long—and most of that consists of warnings about the suicidal behaviors of depressed patients and cautions against discharging them too soon from the hospital. In the absence of treatments for manic-depressive illness, patients spent months, even years, in hospitals and asylums.

As more and more powerful microscopes were invented and special tissue stains were developed for brain tissues, various microscopic structures of the brain—the many different types of neurons and the microscopic architecture of the different parts of the brain—became visible for the first time. Anatomical and chemical abnormalities were found to characterize several other diseases with prominent mental symptoms. In 1906 the Swiss neuropathologist Alois Alzheimer, who was a student of Kraepelin, discovered abnormal microscopic plaques and tangles of cellular debris in the brains of persons who had died from the progressive brain disease that was eventually named for him. Individuals with *cretinism*, a particularly severe form of intellectual disability, were found to have abnormally low levels of thyroid hormones. In 1915 *pellagra*, another mysterious disease characterized by skin lesions and gradual mental deterioration, was discovered to be caused by a deficiency of vitamin B.

But blood tests and brain studies revealed nothing about manic-depressive illness. Try as they might, pathologists and anatomists, using the tools that were available to them at the time, could find nothing abnormal in the brain structures of individuals with bipolar disorder.

New ways of thinking seemed necessary to understand the mental illnesses for which no physical cause could be found, and shortly after the beginning of the twentieth century, new theories were advanced, most

A New Test for Psychiatric Disease (ca. 1906)

As the study of mental disorders entered the twentieth century, hopes for more effective treatment of psychiatric disorders rose when scientific discoveries shed light on the causes of several mental illnesses. In 1906 the German microbiologist August Wassermann discovered a method to detect in human spinal fluid antibodies to the microorganism that causes syphilis. This may not sound like a discovery that had anything to do with psychiatry, unless you know that syphilitic infection of the central nervous system was at this time one of the most common causes of severe psychiatric symptoms, and that nearly half of the patients in mental institutions suffered from "general paresis of the insane," as syphilis with psychiatric manifestations was known. With the development of the Wassermann test, it became possible to diagnose the illness with a very high degree of reliability. For the first time, a cause of a form of "madness" had been discovered. That same year another German microbiologist, Paul Ehrlich, developed the first effective treatment for syphilis, using arsenic compounds. Although the treatment was crude and dangerous, it was effective enough in the early stages of the disease to reduce the incidence of the illness by 50 percent in several European countries.

We hardly think of syphilis as a mental illness today, but patients with syphilitic infection of the brain can suffer hallucinations, delusions, and mood changes not very different from those seen in bipolar disorder and schizophrenia. An early twentieth-century psychiatric text describes the mania-like excitement that was sometimes seen in persons with central nervous system syphilis: "The intensity of the excitement is extreme; there is absolute sleeplessness [and] incessant restlessness. The grandiose delusions are the controlling feature of the paretic's thought. The patient . . . comes before us tremulous with emotion, his eye bright, as the overpowering visions of wealth and grandeur float before his mind."[*] The discovery of reliable and effective diagnostic techniques for general paresis of the insane—unfortunately, arsenicals had little effect on the advanced central nervous system disease—was seen by many as an enormous advance in the understanding of psychiatric disorders. Clinicians charged with the care of psychiatric patients had great hopes that the causes of other psychiatric disorders would soon be found.

[*]Henry J. Berkley, *A Treatise on Mental Disorders* (1900; reprint, New York: Arno Press, 1980), 179.

notably by Sigmund Freud, that seemed to have considerable power to explain the basis of these still-mysterious illnesses. These theories, boiled down to their essence, held that mental symptoms were reactions to life events in vulnerable individuals—not disease states caused by disruptions in biological functioning. The new theories of mental illness instructed psychiatrists to use "talking cures" to treat their patients.

By carefully exploring patients' biographies in minute detail, physicians attempted to understand what conflicts and life events their patients were reacting to with symptoms of depression or mania. It was the expectation that the proper combination of understanding, reinterpretation, and encouragement could alleviate patients' symptoms. Freud, more than any other early psychiatrist, developed elaborate theories about normal and abnormal childhood psychological development that he believed could explain why some people developed extreme psychological symptoms in response to difficult life situations and events while others did not. Manic-depressive illness and schizophrenia came to be called *functional illnesses* because it was believed that patients with depression or mania or symptoms of schizophrenia had *normal* brain and nervous system functioning. Although Freud and his disciples did not totally discount biological agents as having some role in the causation of these problems, they did not see their patients as suffering from *diseases*. A "functional illness" was believed to be an illness of the mind, not of the brain. These concepts dominated American psychiatry until well into the 1960s.

During these decades most psychiatrists believed that abnormal mental phenomena were caused by traumatic childhood events, poor parenting, repressed sexual feelings, and interpersonal conflicts. They lost interest in the classification and categorization of psychiatric illnesses; the very idea of trying to make a diagnosis in a psychiatric patient seemed a waste of time because the form as well as the cause of a psychiatric problem seemed to be as individual as the biography of the patient in whom it occurred. Then in 1949 an unknown Australian psychiatrist published an article in the *Medical Journal of Australia* called "Lithium Salts in the Treatment of Psychotic Excitement."

DR. CADE AND LITHIUM

By the 1930s and 1940s, most physicians interested in the treatment of mental disorders had joined psychoanalytic institutes to learn the theory and practice of psychiatry according to the teachings of Freud and his followers. They trained and practiced mostly in the big cities, mostly treating patients with mild depression or anxiety, patients who had the time, motivation, and money to attend therapy sessions four or five days a week to explore their past and reinterpret their present to become healthier, happier, and better "adjusted." Freud's theories revolutionized the understanding of many aspects of human behavior, and they continue to form the basis for the practice of psychotherapy. But there were many patients who benefited little from these new ideas. They were the patients Dr. Kraepelin had cared for: the victims of schizophrenia and manic-depressive illness.

For these patients, housed for months or years in (mostly public) hospitals and asylums, the therapeutic armamentarium had not changed much in two hundred years: bed rest for the depressed; physical restraint for the agitated; baths, tranquilization with morphine and bromides, and the use of other substances thought to have beneficial effects, among them quinine and even cod-liver oil. None of these interventions had any but the most insignificant effects on serious mental illness.

John F. J. Cade, MD, senior medical officer in the Mental Hygiene Department of Victoria, Australia, was convinced that manic-depressive illness was a biological disorder, not a psychological one (figure 4.2). Working in his laboratory to determine whether some toxin might be present in the urine of patients with manic-depressive illness, Cade became especially interested in urea and uric acid, by-products of protein metabolism found in urine. He was testing the toxicity of these compounds by injecting small amounts of them into guinea pigs.

FIGURE 4.2. **John Cade**

Source: State Library of Victoria

One of the technical problems with this work was that uric acid is rather insoluble in water, making it difficult to prepare injectable solutions at high concentrations. Looking for a soluble urate salt to use instead of uric acid, Cade consulted prior research and discovered that uric acid was easiest to dissolve in water when it was combined with a lithium ion as lithium urate. He injected small amounts of lithium urate into the guinea pigs and noticed that uric acid seemed to be less toxic in this form. This suggested to Cade that the lithium component of the compound might have some sort of protective effect against urate toxicity. To determine what the effect of the lithium ion might be, he injected them with lithium carbonate—the carbonate ion is harmless and is found in substances such as baking soda—and discovered that "after a latent period of about two hours the animals, although fully conscious, became extremely lethargic and unresponsive to stimuli for one to two hours before once again becoming normally active."[7]

Cade admitted in his original paper that "it may seem a long distance from lethargy in guinea pigs to excitement in psychotics," but asylum doctors of the time were desperate for new treatment possibilities, so Cade decided to administer lithium preparations to several patients who were chronically agitated. The effect on patients with mania was dramatic.

Of the ten patients that Cade treated with lithium, all experienced dramatic improvement in their symptoms. He had also given lithium to six patients with "dementia praecox" (schizophrenia) and three patients with "chronic depressive psychoses" but with less effect. The agitated patients with schizophrenia became less agitated but had "no fundamental improvement"; the depressed patients had "no improvement."

One would think that the news of Cade's discovery would have spread like wildfire. It did not. In fact, several decades elapsed before lithium was approved for the treatment of bipolar disorder by the US Food and Drug Administration. Why this incredible delay?

The Discovery of Lithium: No Accident

It is often emphasized in textbooks and articles on the history of lithium treatment that Cade's discovery of lithium's efficacy in bipolar disorder was pure accident—an observation that misses an important point. Cade, like many hospital psychiatrists, but unlike perhaps many other psychiatrists of his time, was pursuing a biological intervention for what he believed was a biological disorder. His case descriptions reveal that even though he had little specific therapy to offer them, he had taken a complete history of his patients' course of illness, carefully examined them, and, following in the footsteps of Emil Kraepelin, made a *diagnosis* based on his examination and history taking. Cade's approach to these severely ill patients—his assumption that they suffered from diseases rather than from emotional reactions—provided the theoretical underpinning that made his discovery possible. A psychiatrist who believed in "reactions" and "functional illness" would have been unlikely to divide patients into the diagnostic categories of mania, schizophrenia, and depressive psychosis and report on the differential efficacy of a pharmaceutical in each group. Such a psychiatrist would have been even less likely to look for toxins in the urine of patients with mania.

The First Lithium Patients

Unlike the often dry-as-dust research papers that appear in today's medical journals, full of data and statistics, research reports in the 1940s, especially in psychiatric journals, often contained detailed case histories and vivid descriptions of symptoms. In his landmark paper describing his treatment of patients with bipolar disorder with lithium, Cade's descriptions rival those of Kraepelin:

Case I—W.B., a male aged fifty-one years, who had been in a state of chronic manic excitement for five years, restless, dirty, destructive, mischievous and interfering, had long been regarded as the most troublesome patient in the ward. His response was highly gratifying. From the start of treatment on March 29, 1948, with lithium citrate he steadily settled down and in three weeks was enjoying the unaccustomed surroundings of the convalescent ward. As he had been ill so long and confined to a "chronic ward," he found normal surroundings and liberty of movement strange at first. He remained perfectly well and left the hospital on indefinite leave with instructions to take a dose of lithium carbonate, five grains, twice a day. He was soon back working at his old job. However, he became more lackadaisical about his medicine and finally ceased taking it. His relatives reported that he had not taken any for at least six weeks prior to his readmission on January 30, 1949, and was becoming steadily more irritable and erratic. On readmission to the hospital he was at once started on lithium carbonate, ten grains three times a day, and in a fortnight had again settled down to normal. He is now (February 28, 1949) ready to return to home and work.

Case VIII—W.M., a man of fifty years, was suffering from an attack of recurrent mania, the first of which he had had at the age of twenty. The present attack had lasted two months and showed no signs of abating. He was garrulous, euphoric, restless and unkempt when he started taking lithium. Two days later he was reported to be quieter. By the ninth day he was definitely settling down and the following day commenced work in the garden. By the end of two weeks he was practically normal— quiet, tidy, rational, with insight into his previous condition. This was in marked contrast to his condition a fortnight before when he had to be locked in a single room at night . . . and was too restless to eat in the dining room owing to his unsettling effect on the other patients.*

*John F. J. Cade, "Lithium Salts in the Treatment of Psychotic Excitement," *Medical Journal of Australia* 36 (1949): 349–52.

Part of the reason was the state of world psychiatry following the end of World War II. German psychiatry, which had produced superb clinicians like Kraepelin and Freud and many other pioneers in the science of mental disorders, was in ruins, literally and figuratively. The German psychiatric establishment had been mesmerized by the Nazi movement, and prominent German psychiatrists had enthusiastically participated in the expulsion of Jewish colleagues from the profession and even in the murder of the patients they had been charged to care for. Thousands of intellectually disabled and mentally ill individuals were gassed in the years leading up to and during the war. When Cade wrote of his work with lithium, Germany was no longer providing leaders in psychiatric medicine; rather, German psychiatry was in dire need of rehabilitation.[8]

In the United States and England, psychoanalytic theories had replaced the traditional medical practices of evaluation, diagnosis, and treatment with the prescription of the "talking cure" for all emotional problems. Accurate psychiatric diagnosis simply didn't exist; any patient with severe symptoms was usually called "schizophrenic" and admitted to a state psychiatric hospital for little more than custodial care. Ronald Fieve, the American psychiatrist who championed the use of lithium in the United States in the 1970s and who was instrumental in getting American psychiatrists to prescribe it for their patients, observed that during the late 1940s and the 1950s in New York, he "rarely met with the diagnosis of manic-depression. . . . It had virtually disappeared. Most cases of excitable, talkative, and elated behavior were being diagnosed as schizophrenia."[9]

But a Danish psychiatrist, Morgans Schou, realized that Cade's discovery represented a real breakthrough. He noted in a 1954 paper, "It is rather astonishing that [Cade's] observation has failed to arouse greater general interest among psychiatrists."[10] Schou and his colleagues did the careful clinical trials that eventually resulted in the development of recommended dosages and preparations of lithium for the treatment of symptoms of bipolar disorder. Perhaps more than any other clinical researcher, Schou established the efficacy of lithium treatment for mania. Even more important was his discovery that lithium could prevent the recurrence of symptoms in patients with bipolar disorder.

In 1957 another breakthrough occurred in the treatment of mood disorders when Roland Kuhn, a Swiss psychiatrist, described how a compound originally developed as an antihistamine had remarkable effects on depressed patients. He reported his results in a Swiss medical journal, and his paper was reprinted the next year in English as "The Treatment of Depressive States with G 22355 (Imipramine Hydrochloride)." But Kuhn also

Lithium before Cade: The Forgotten Lange Brothers

It turns out that John Cade was not the first psychiatrist to give lithium to patients with mood disorders. More than fifty years earlier, the Danish psychiatrist brothers Carl and Friedrich Lange had used lithium salts to treat patients with depression and had seen some success.* Carl, the older brother, had described "periodic depressive states" in 1886 and attributed the condition to an excess of uric acid in the body. His younger brother, Frederik, reported his success in treating thirty-five patients with depression several years later.

Unfortunately, because the Lange brothers wrote about their discoveries in a German psychiatric research journal that was never translated into other languages, their reports did not garner much attention. The Lange brothers' work was essentially forgotten by the time Cade started his investigation into lithium and mood disorders seventy years later.

*Edward Shorter, "The History of Lithium Therapy," *Bipolar Disorders* 11, suppl. 2 (2009): 4-9.

noticed that in some patients imipramine simply replaced one mood problem with another: "In marked manic-depressive psychosis, i.e., if the depressions are easily and frequently replaced by manic-like phases or actual manic states, the reaction is less favorable. . . . The tendency arises for the depression to switch over into a manic phase."[11]

In one of their first papers on the use of lithium in manic patients, Schou and his colleagues pointed out that "the beneficial effect of lithium in cases of mania appears to offer new possibilities for a study of the *pathophysiology* [i.e., the disease mechanism] of the manic-depressive psychoses."[12] The discovery of the therapeutic effects of imipramine on depressed patients and the observation that it could precipitate mania in patients with "manic-depressive psychosis" were two more clues that bipolar disorder might be more than a psychological "reaction."

The fact that a chemical (lithium) made the symptoms of mania go away indicated that mania had at least some biochemical basis. The discovery of the different effects of imipramine on depressed persons with and without a history of mania reinforced the disease model for bipolar disorder. Persons with a history of mania became manic if they took imipramine; persons who did not have a history of mania (usually) did not. Imipramine was not simply a "manio-genic" drug, a drug that produced euphoria in everyone who took it. The fact that only bipolar individuals became manic from it suggested that their illness had a different biochemical basis from that of other cases of depression. The modern age of psychiatry had begun, as had the search for more and better pharmaceutical treatments and for the physical basis of these disorders.

KEY TAKEAWAYS

▶ Although physicians who wrote about mental illness had suspected for centuries that there was a connection between depressive and manic mood states, the German psychiatrist Emil Kraepelin firmly established this concept in his textbook of psychiatry in the 1890s and coined the term *manic-depressive illness*.

▶ The Australian psychiatrist Dr. John Cade discovered and reported on the specific therapeutic effect of lithium on the symptoms of mania in 1949, helping to usher in modern psychopharmacology.

PART II

The Treatment of Bipolar Disorder

Although there have been effective medications for the treatment of bipolar disorder for decades, the underlying biology of this illness remains so mysterious that deciding which available medication will work best for a particular patient is more art than science. I would argue that no other group of medical specialists has so little definitive science to guide their treatment decisions than do psychiatrists.

You may know that penicillin was discovered quite accidentally when Sir Alexander Fleming returned from a summer vacation to discover that a fungus had contaminated the petri dishes in which he was growing the deadly bacterium *Staphylococcus aureus*. He observed a bacteria-free halo around the contaminating fungus and realized that the mold (*Penicillium notatum*) was exuding something that prevented the bacteria from growing. The age of antibiotics had begun.

As you will discover in the next chapters, nearly *every* medication that psychiatrists prescribe was similarly discovered by some happy accident, as in the case of lithium and valproate (Depakote), or by trial and error (the antidepressant imipramine and several anticonvulsant mood stabilizers). However, despite this lack definitive knowledge of how these medications work in the brain to bring about their beneficial effects, clinical research has shown that medications *do* help a substantial proportion of bipolar patients. We've learned how to prescribe these medications safely, and we have some indications of which bipolar symptom patterns predict that a particular medication will help.

In the following chapters, I will discuss treatment approaches for bipolar disorder. As you have already seen from the previous section, the symptoms and course of illness of bipolar disorder vary tremendously from one patient to another. Almost no two persons with the illness seem to have exactly the same disease. And as you will read in part III, "What Causes Bipolar Disorder?," it's also likely that there are subtly different causal factors in different patients. Both of these facts explain why there is, presently at least, no "best" treatment for bipolar disorder and why the treatment of bipolar disorder also varies greatly from one patient to another.

All of the treatment approaches in this section have been shown to help *some* subgroup of persons with bipolar disorder, and we are getting better at matching treatments to patients based on their symptoms and the pattern of their illness.

CHAPTER 5

Mood-Stabilizing Medications

M ood stabilizers are medications that have both antimanic and antidepressant effects. Perhaps an even more important effect of this class of medications is their ability to decrease the frequency and severity of episodes of the illness. Thus, the majority of patients with bipolar disorder are treated with one or another of these medications, and sometimes with several.

LITHIUM

In the second century AD, the Greek physician Seranus Ephisios recommended that physicians who treated patients suffering from mania should prescribe "natural waters, such as [from] alkaline springs."[1] We now know that the water from many alkaline springs is rich in lithium. Roman physicians recommended that their patients "take the waters" at various springs for various physical and mental ailments. Down through the centuries, centers for healing grew up around natural springs all over Europe, from the little town in eastern Belgium called Spa to Bath in England, Wiesbaden in Germany, and dozens of other towns in Italy and Greece.

In the 1950s, the Danish psychiatrist Morgans Schou began what turned out to be his life's work: building on Cade's discovery of the therapeutic effect of lithium for bipolar disorder and refining the therapeutic use of lithium and establishing its effectiveness in these patients. Schou became convinced of the effectiveness of lithium in treating acute mania soon after he started to prescribe it to patients, and he was one of the first clinical researchers to become convinced of another therapeutic effect of the drug: its ability to prevent further episodes of illness (lithium's preventive, or *prophylactic*, effect). Schou had a harder time convincing his colleagues around the world that lithium could prevent recurrences of bipolar disorder, that patients should take it even after their acute symptoms subside. In

1967 Schou and his colleague Paul Christian Baalstrup reported on eighty-eight patients who had taken lithium for several years and who had a dramatic reduction in the frequency and duration of their mood episodes (figure 5.1 shows a sample of their results). Several patients who had been sick for several weeks out of every year experienced a complete remission of their illness that lasted more than five years; their bipolar disorder had essentially ceased.[2]

As they treated more and more patients with the medication, it became so apparent to Schou and his colleagues that lithium favorably altered the course of bipolar illness that they had ethical qualms about doing a more rigorous placebo-controlled study—one in which bipolar patients would be divided into two groups, some to receive lithium and the others a placebo ("sugar pill"). In a rather cranky 1968 article titled "Prophylactic Lithium: Another Therapeutic Myth?," several British psychiatrists scolded the Danes for reporting their results without a placebo group.[3] So Baalstrup and Schou did a lithium discontinuation study in which they took patients who had been stable on lithium for at least a year, divided them into two roughly equal groups, and in one group substituted a placebo for the lithium.

FIGURE 5.1. Data from six patients in Baalstrup and Schou's early study on the prophylactic effects of lithium on bipolar symptoms

Each line represents the symptom course of one patient. In all these patients, when lithium was started, episodes of mania and depression stopped completely.

Depression

Mania

Lithium administration

Source: Data from Paul Baalstrup and Morgans Schou, "Lithium as a Prophylactic Agent: Its Effect against Recurrent Depressions and Manic-Depressive Psychosis," *Archives of General Psychiatry* 16, no. 2 (1967): 162–72.

This was a *double-blind study*, the most powerful type of clinical trial possible—and now a required test for new medications. In this type of study, patients who are similar in age, diagnosis, severity of illness, and so forth and who agree to be in the study are divided into two groups. One group gets the medication that is being tested, and the other group (the *control* group) gets a placebo (or in some studies the control group receives a standard medication for the disorder in question). The patients do not know whether they are taking the new medication or the placebo, and neither do the clinicians who examine them for improvement; hence the term *double*-blind. It is only after the trial is over that the group membership of the patients is revealed and the results of the two groups compared. Improvement is measured objectively by using checklists of symptoms and various rating severity scales that have been verified as reliable and valid.

The results of the Baalstrup and Schou study were dramatic: of the thirty-nine patients whose lithium was replaced with the placebo, twenty-one relapsed within five months; of the forty-five other patients, those whose lithium was not replaced, *none* had a relapse. In 1970 Baalstrup and Schou published their results in the same British journal in which their critics' paper had appeared, establishing once and for all that lithium's prophylactic effect on bipolar disorder was no myth.[4]

Lithium's Robust "Anti-suicide" Effect

Persons with bipolar disorder are at high risk of suicide; their suicide rate is twenty to thirty times higher than that of the general population. Half of those with an early age of onset have a history of suicide attempts. Fortunately, in addition to its ability to prevent illness episodes, lithium has a specific "anti-suicide" effect.

Many research studies have shown that lithium has a significant effect on the reduction of suicide attempts and deaths by suicide in comparison to antidepressants or other mood stabilizers in persons with bipolar disorder. Long-term treatment with lithium reduces suicide attempts by about 10 percent and deaths by suicide by about 20 percent.

A 2016 review of these studies in the French psychiatry journal *L'Encéphale* concluded that it is "crucial for . . . suicide prevention" to maintain lithium blood levels in the therapeutic range over the long term.* Lithium has a modulating effect on serotonin circuits in the brain that are involved with impulsiveness and aggressiveness, and these are vulnerability factors that put persons with bipolar disorder at higher risk of suicide.

*V. Benard, G. Vaiva, M. Masson, and P. A. Geoffroy, "Lithium and Suicide Prevention in Bipolar Disorder," *L'Encéphale* 42, no. 3 (2016): 234–41.

Therapeutic Profile

It has now been shown in many more studies that lithium is not only effective in the treatment of mania and depression; it also reduces the severity, duration, and frequency of manic and depressive episodes of bipolar patients.

Lithium is a naturally occurring element found in mineral springs, seawater, and certain ores. Like its close cousin sodium, it is never found in its pure form in nature but only combined with other ions as a salt of one type or another. It is mined on an industrial scale for use in the manufacture of ceramics and batteries. Therapeutic lithium preparations usually contain lithium carbonate (the carbonate ion combined with lithium; when the carbonate ion is combined with the closely related sodium, it forms sodium carbonate, which is common baking soda).

Because it is an element, lithium is not chemically transformed (metabolized) within the body, and because lithium atoms are so similar to sodium atoms, the body handles lithium in much the same way it handles sodium. Lithium is rapidly absorbed through the gastrointestinal tract, enters the bloodstream, and is filtered through the kidneys and eliminated from the body.

Descriptions of the effects of a pharmaceutical in the body always include one vital statistic: the medication's *half-life*. This is a measure of how quickly the body gets rid of the medication. Specifically, it is the time required for half the amount of the drug to be eliminated or metabolized by the body. Put another way, it is the time it takes for the body to reduce the level of the medication by half. The half-life of lithium in adults is between fourteen and thirty hours.[5] Another useful number that can be derived from the half-life statistic for any medication is the time it takes for the level of medication to build up to a constant level in the body, or in other words the time it takes for the amount being taken in to equal the amount being

---

TABLE 5.1. Therapeutic profile of lithium

Medication class:	Mood stabilizer
Brand names:	Eskalith, Eskalith CR, Lithobid, Lithonate, Lithotabs
Half-life:	14–30 hours
Metabolism:	None
Elimination:	Kidneys
Other considerations:	Blood levels extremely important

eliminated: the *equilibrium point*. By a series of mathematical steps that we don't need to detail here, it can be shown that the equilibrium point is always the same for all medications: five half-lives. This means that since the half-life of lithium is roughly one day, it will take roughly five days for a patient who starts on lithium to reach a steady level of lithium in the bloodstream. It also means that if the lithium dose is changed, it will take about five days for the blood level to stabilize at the new level.

Because of the toxicity and even deaths that were reported when heart patients sprinkled it freely on their food as a salt substitute, there was a significant delay in the acceptance of lithium as a therapeutic agent. Lithium is a powerful pharmaceutical, one that must be treated with respect. It has a very low *therapeutic index*, meaning that the difference between the therapeutic dose and a toxic dose is small.[6] Fortunately, lithium can be measured in the bloodstream accurately and cheaply, and the dosage can be adjusted according to the results.

It is important to pay attention to lithium blood levels not only to prevent toxicity but also because it has been clearly demonstrated in clinical studies that lithium needs to be present in the bloodstream at a certain level to be effective in most patients. (We speak of a "therapeutic level" in discussing the effective range of lithium in the bloodstream for treatment, not a "normal level." Lithium is a trace element in the body, normally present in undetectable concentrations. Bipolar disorder is not a lithium deficiency!) Just what that level should be has been a matter of debate, and the definition has shifted over the years. But an important study from Massachusetts General Hospital found that a level of between 0.8 and 1.0 meq/L (this stands for milliequivalents per liter and is a chemical measure

TABLE 5.2. Comparison of higher and lower lithium levels in relapse rates of bipolar disorder

Treatment group	Any relapse	Depressed	Manic/ mixed	Hypomanic	Withdrew from study
Standard range (0.8–1.0 meq/L)	6 (12%)	3 (6%)	3 (6%)	0	24 (51%)
Low range (0.4–0.6 meq/L)	21 (44%)	1 (2%)	17 (36%)	3 (6%)	11 (23%)

Source: Data from Alan Gelenberg, John Kane, Martin Keller, Phillip Lavori, Jerrold Rosenbaum, Karyl Cole, and Janet Lavelle, "Comparison of Standard and Low Levels of Lithium for Maintenance Treatment of Bipolar Disorder," *New England Journal of Medicine* 321, no. 22 (1989): 1489-93.

of concentration) was most effective.[7] In this double-blind study, bipolar patients were divided into two groups, a "standard-dose" group, whose lithium levels were kept between 0.8 and 1.0 meq/L, and a "low-dose" group, whose levels were maintained between 0.4 and 0.6 meq/L. The researchers found that the relapse rate in the "low-dose" group was more than double that in the "standard-dose" group (table 5.2).

There's more to these data than may initially meet the eye, however. Many more patients from the "standard-dose" group than from the "low-dose" group dropped out of the study because of side effects. The take-home message seems to be that levels closer to 1.0 meq/L are more protective—but that many people have trouble taking that high a dose because of side effects. Many psychiatrists compromise and try to maintain their patients at levels between the "standard" and the "low" range. Dr. Schou, whom many consider to be the father of lithium therapy, recommended levels of 0.5 to 0.8 meq/L.[8] However, it's clear that some people have good control of their symptoms on even lower levels—elderly patients, for example. Lithium levels thus need to be individualized to the patient, and Dr. Schou also

What Is the Optimum Lithium Blood Level for Controlling Bipolar Disorder?

After analyzing the research literature and taking a survey of fifty international experts in the treatment of bipolar disorder, a joint task force of the International Society for Bipolar Disorders (ISBD) and the International Study Group on Lithium (IGSLI) published the following recommendations in 2019:

- For adults, children, and adolescents: standard levels of 0.6–0.8 meq/L with option to reduce to 0.4–0.6 in the case of good response but poor tolerance to this level.

- Increasing to 0.8–1.0 meq/L in case of poor response.

- Adults aged sixty-five to seventy-nine: standard levels of 0.4–0.6 meq/L with option of going up to 0.7–0.8 meq/L.

- Adults aged eighty and up: standard levels of 0.4–0.6 meq/L with option of going up to a maximum of 0.7 meq/L.*

*W. A. Nolen, R. W. Licht, A. H. Young, G. S. Malhi, M. Tohen, E. Vieta, R. W. Kupka, C. Zarate, R. E. Nielsen, R. J. Baldessarini, and E. Severus (ISBD/IGSLI Task Force on the treatment with lithium), "What Is the Optimal Serum Level for Lithium in the Maintenance Treatment of Bipolar Disorder? A Systematic Review and Recommendations from the ISBD/IGSLI Task Force on Treatment with Lithium," *Bipolar Disorders* 21 no. 5 (2019): 394–409.

pointed out that "changes in lithium levels as small as 0.1 to 0.2 [meq/L], upward or downward, may substantially improve patients' quality of life during maintenance treatment."[9]

The lithium level in the bloodstream rises after every dose, peaks in about two hours, then begins to fall again. If a patient takes his lithium two or three times a day, there will be several peaks and valleys. Because the level is rising and falling throughout the day, it is important that the blood for a lithium-level test be drawn at a time when it can be correctly

Symptoms of Lithium Toxicity

Because the difference between therapeutic blood levels and toxic levels of lithium is significantly smaller than with most other drugs, it is important that persons taking lithium be familiar with the symptoms of too much lithium in the bloodstream, or *lithium toxicity*. Older patients are especially vulnerable to lithium toxicity. It's useful to divide the kinds of lithium toxicity into two types:

Acute toxicity occurs when a person's lithium level is *suddenly* too high, such as when a person mistakenly takes an extra dose, is significantly dehydrated, or intentionally overdoses. The symptoms are mainly in the digestive tract:

- Diarrhea

- Nausea and vomiting

- Stomach pains

- Dizziness

- Muscle weakness

Chronic toxicity occurs when the lithium level has slowly risen over time to toxic levels, as when a person's dose has changed or kidney problems are developing. Digestive symptoms are less common and nervous system issues predominate:

- Slowed thinking or confusion

- Severe tremor (shaking, usually most noticeably in the hands)

- Slurred speech

- Unsteady walk or problems with balance

In either type of toxicity, excessively high lithium levels can lead to coma or even be fatal, so significant signs of lithium toxicity may represent a medical emergency worth a trip to the emergency room for treatment.

interpreted. The convention that has been adopted is to use a twelve-hour level, making it convenient to draw blood in the mornings. For most patients this means getting to the lab twelve hours after their bedtime dose—for example, by 11:00 a.m. if the bedtime dose was taken at 11:00 p.m. the night before—with their usual morning dose in their pocket or purse.

Lithium is uniquely effective for some patients with bipolar disorder, for whom it is truly a miracle drug. In many of these patients, other medications simply don't control their symptoms as well. At the consultation clinic at Johns Hopkins, we regularly see patients who have been told they can no longer take lithium because of medical issues (usually because they have developed kidney disease, a complication of high blood pressure and diabetes as well as other medical disorders). Many of these patients have taken it for decades with complete control of their illness. Some have been so stable that they haven't seen a psychiatrist in years, getting their lithium treatment and monitoring from their family doctor instead. These patients come to us desperate to start taking it again because other medications they've tried since stopping lithium simply haven't kept them well. Fortunately, most can resume lithium treatment despite their kidney disease (there have even been case reports of patients with such severe kidney failure that they require dialysis being safely treated with the drug).[10] Their desperation and the great lengths these patients go to in order to get back on lithium are explained by its unique effectiveness for them. Usually they are patients with classic bipolar I disorder, characterized by severe manias requiring hospitalization, often with psychotic features. Another illness characteristic is that their between-episode recovery is usually quite complete, that is, they do not have smoldering residual mood symptoms for long periods when they are not acutely ill. This group of patients, for whom lithium is fantastically effective and for whom nothing else works quite so well, has prompted a number of research projects searching for genetic markers for its therapeutic effect. The hope is that this research will eventually lead to a test that will help physicians select medications for individual patients with mood disorders. In this case, physicians want a test that will predict whether a particular patient is likely to benefit from taking lithium.

Side Effects

Individuals vary widely in their sensitivity to the side effects of lithium (and all other medications, for that matter). Some patients will have no side effects; others will have several. Fortunately, almost all the side effects of lithium can be eliminated or managed (table 5.3).

Lithium Maintenance: Not as Effective the Second Time Around?

For years, there were reports that if patients stopped taking lithium to prevent their bipolar symptoms from returning and later decided to restart it after a relapse, lithium didn't work quite as well. There was a bit of research evidence to support this view, but there was conflicting evidence, so it was more "clinical lore" than proven fact.

But a 2017 paper coauthored by distinguished mood disorders expert Dr. Robert Post presented strong evidence that this is indeed the case.* From a large group of patients with bipolar disorder, Dr. Post and colleagues reviewed the records of sixty-five lithium-responsive patients who stopped taking lithium for at least four weeks; they were then followed for an average of four years after restarting lithium. The researchers reported that over a quarter of the patients had "attenuated" (decreased) responsiveness to the medication on restarting it. In about half of these patients, lithium completely lost its effectiveness.

They found that the patients whose lithium responsiveness was attenuated after discontinuation shared several characteristics:

- The longer patients were off lithium, the more likely they were to have an attenuated response when they restarted it.

- Patients who had only a partial response during the time they took lithium were more likely to become even less responsive after a period off it.

- Patients who had an episode during the period they were off lithium were more likely to show decreased responsiveness.

The authors concluded that "the results of this study should provide a cautionary warning for physicians and patients that discontinuation of lithium can result in loss of its effectiveness and that careful evaluation of the risk/benefit ratio for stopping lithium is required."

*S. Cakir, O. Yazici, and R. M. Post, "Decreased Responsiveness following Lithium Discontinuation in Bipolar Disorder: A Naturalistic Observation Study," *Psychiatry Research* 247 (2017): 305–9.

Many of lithium's side effects are *dose related*, meaning that the higher the dose, the more severe the side effect. One side-effect management strategy, then, is to lower the lithium dose. The advantages of higher levels are clear, as noted above, but most physicians will try to maintain patients at the lowest dose that controls their symptoms.

TABLE 5.3. Treatable side effects of lithium	
Side effect	*Remedy*
Nausea, diarrhea	Take immediately after meals
	Switch preparations
Weight gain	Diet and exercise
Thirst, frequent urination	Diuretics helpful but must be prescribed by an MD (see text)
Tremor	Beta blockers
Flareup of preexisting dermatologic conditions	Dermatologic preparations
Hypothyroidism	Thyroid medications

Because of its similarity to sodium, lithium has some of the same effects that an increased sodium (salt) intake would have: increased thirst, increased urination, and water retention. These side effects are often temporary and subside as the body adjusts to the medication. Many patients notice this slight and temporary increase in urination and thirst when they start taking lithium. For some patients, however, it's after taking lithium for many years that they notice they need to urinate much more often and find that they are frequently thirsty. This occurs because lithium can affect the functioning of the kidneys over time. Remember that the kidneys' job is to remove waste products from the bloodstream; they filter nearly twenty gallons of blood every hour to do this, and they recycle nearly all of this fluid back into the bloodstream. When taken for many years, lithium can impair this recycling function, so that large amounts of urine are produced. The term for this problem is *diabetes insipidus* (which has nothing to do with diabetes mellitus, the common "sugar diabetes"). This problem develops slowly, is easy to diagnose with a few laboratory tests, and is treatable with amiloride, a drug that changes how the kidneys reabsorb water and other agents. When caught early on, this problem is usually completely reversible, so it's critical that patients taking lithium let their doctor know if they find themselves awakening more often to urinate during the night.

When lithium was first prescribed, concern arose based on case reports that lithium disrupted the kidneys' filtering system, causing the kind of damage that can result in the need for dialysis. This has now been shown to be extremely rare, occurring almost entirely in persons who are already at risk for kidney damage from other causes, such as poorly controlled high blood pressure or diabetes. Fortunately, this problem usually takes decades to slowly develop.[11]

Because of these potential problems, blood tests that measure kidney function are routinely ordered for patients taking lithium, in addition to blood tests to monitor their lithium blood levels.

Lithium is irritating to the gastrointestinal tract and can cause nausea or diarrhea. Taking it on a full stomach can ease these problems considerably. A fine shaking in the hands (tremor) can occur at higher dosage levels. These problems can sometimes be alleviated with slow-release preparations, which reduce the peak blood level that occurs after each dose. Medications used to treat tremors, called *beta blockers*, are frequently prescribed and can be very helpful. Weight gain can be an annoying side effect and unfortunately has an equally annoying remedy: diet and exercise.

Between 5 and 35 percent of patients treated with lithium develop depressed thyroid gland functioning (hypothyroidism).[12] When hypothyroidism develops, it may cause an increase in mood cycling in addition to the symptoms of too little thyroid hormone (low energy, dry skin, sensitivity to heat, and puffiness around the eyes are some of the early signs). If a person's lithium seems to "stop working"—that is, if the person suddenly seems to have an acceleration in her illness—hypothyroidism should be suspected. When it does occur, hypothyroidism can be treated by thyroid-replacement medications. A test of thyroid functioning is the third in the battery of blood tests routinely ordered for lithium patients.

Lithium can cause flare-ups of preexisting skin conditions but only rarely causes new dermatological problems. Patients with psoriasis, acne, and other such problems may need closer follow-up from their dermatologist.

Another side effect that troubles a significant number of patients taking lithium is a noticeable dulling of mental functioning and coordination. Patients complain that their ability to memorize and learn is affected and that they have a difficult-to-explain sense of mental sluggishness. For years these complaints were downplayed by clinicians, many of whom tossed them off as coming from patients who simply weren't used to feeling "normal," who missed the mental alacrity of hypomania. This view seemed to be supported by research using psychological tests on bipolar patients taking lithium, research that has been inconclusive. But when nonpatient volunteers were given lithium and similarly tested, there was a small but definite drop-off in their performance, proving that lithium-induced mental sluggishness is a significant problem for some patients.[13] This is a dose-related side effect and is another reason to strive for the lowest possible maintenance dose of lithium that still controls mood symptoms adequately.

Lithium has been associated with birth defects, especially certain heart defects. At one time, it was recommended that women never get pregnant while taking lithium, but more recent research has shown that while lithium increases the risk of serious heart problems in the fetus, the risk is still quite low. What to do about taking lithium during pregnancy is a complicated decision that should be discussed well beforehand with your psychiatrist and your obstetrician. (See chapter 18 for a more complete discussion of medications and pregnancy.) Lithium is secreted in breast milk, so patients taking lithium should not breastfeed.

─────────── KEY LITHIUM TAKEAWAYS ───────────

▶ Lithium continues to be the gold standard treatment for bipolar disorder, especially for persons with bipolar I.

▶ Lithium's "anti-suicide" effect makes it an especially valuable intervention.

▶ Lithium is the "magic bullet" for many bipolar I patients: both necessary and sufficient to keep them well.

▶ Lithium blood tests are important, but interpreting the results is best left to an expert. The optimal level for an individual patient depends on factors such as illness phase, severity of symptoms, and age.

▶ Women in the childbearing years taking lithium should have a pregnancy-planning discussion with their prescriber. Many women decide that the effects of an illness episode on the baby outweighs the very low risk of birth defects.

LAMOTRIGINE (LAMICTAL)

Several years ago, I was in a cab with a colleague of mine returning to our hotels after a day at an international conference on bipolar disorder in Pittsburgh. We were talking about the seminars we had attended, discussing how we might better classify bipolar disorders, whether lithium is safe during pregnancy, and other bipolar topics of the day's sessions. During a pause in our conversation, the cab driver looked back at us in his rearview mirror and asked, "Do either of you guys prescribe Lamictal?" We were both a bit surprised by the question, since lamotrigine had not yet been approved by the Food and Drug Administration (FDA) to treat bipolar disorder, but we replied that yes, we had prescribed the new drug for several of our patients at Johns Hopkins. The cabbie paused for a short moment and then said, "That's good. . . . Ya know, Lamictal saved my life."

Lamotrigine (brand name Lamictal) is something of a child prodigy among medications used to treat bipolar disorder. Unlike other medications, which became common treatments for bipolar disorder only after many years of investigation and testing, lamotrigine proved its value in treating bipolar disorder in short order. As a result, it went from an uncommonly used drug prescribed mostly at research medical centers to a mainstay of the treatment of bipolar disorder in only a few years. Like several other medications I will discuss, lamotrigine was introduced as a medication to treat seizure disorders. The first studies on lamotrigine appeared in the 1980s, describing it as a useful "add-on" therapy for epilepsy patients who were already taking other antiseizure medications. During the early investigations of this use, researchers noted that patients who took lamotrigine for seizure control reported an improvement in their mood and sense of well-being—even if it hadn't helped much with their seizures. These observations led to clinical trials in patients with mood disorders, which quickly revealed that lamotrigine is an effective medication for many such patients.

Lamotrigine has several effects on the brain that might explain its efficacy in bipolar disorder. It inhibits the release of the neurotransmitter glutamate, an amino acid that causes stimulation of various neural circuits. Glutamate is also the signal that the nervous system uses to trigger a kind of cellular suicide called *apoptosis* that inactivates and removes malfunctioning neurons. There is evidence that abnormally high levels of glutamate are present in several brain areas of persons with bipolar disorder, suggesting that lamotrigine's effectiveness is due to a dialing back of glutamate activity in the brain to more normal levels.[14]

Therapeutic Profile

The most exciting aspect of lamotrigine's profile is its effectiveness in bipolar depression. One of the first reports on its use in the treatment of bipolar disorder told of a patient who had suffered from rapid-cycling bipolar I disorder since he was fourteen years old.[15] In the year before starting lamotrigine, he had been either depressed or manic continuously, with no period of normal mood. When the research team first saw him, he was severely depressed and had not responded to lithium, to other mood stabilizers, or even to antidepressants. After beginning to take lamotrigine, his depressive symptoms gradually improved, and eleven months later he'd had no recurrence of either depressive or manic symptoms. Case reports and studies of lamotrigine as a medication added to other agents started to accumulate and continued to look promising.

In 2003 two large studies were published that compared the efficacy of lamotrigine with lithium (and also with a placebo) in keeping patients with bipolar disorder from having another mood episode; each study lasted eighteen months. In one study, the patients were recovering from a manic or mixed episode as they entered the study; in the other, patients were recovering from a depression.[16] In the section on lithium, I mentioned that the best way to tell whether a medication is truly effective is to do a double-blind, placebo-controlled study. Both of these studies comparing lamotrigine with lithium and a placebo were carried out in just this way; they also were large studies that included hundreds of patients, and they lasted for a year and a half—much longer than most medication trials. So when both studies reported that lamotrigine was just as effective as lithium in keeping patients well, this new medication suddenly came into the spotlight and became one of the foundations of the treatment of bipolar disorder.

The exciting finding from these studies was that lamotrigine is especially effective against depression in bipolar disorder—extremely good news. This was such an important finding because, as you will see later, the depression in bipolar disorder is much more difficult to treat than manic or mixed states (see "Treating Bipolar Depression" in chapter 7). You may remember from chapter 2 that individuals with bipolar II disorder have more problems with depression than with mania and that these depressions can be especially long, debilitating, and difficult to treat. Lamotrigine can often fill an important therapeutic need for these patients, because for them lithium is often less effective. Conversely, lamotrigine appears to be less effective than lithium for patients with bipolar I disorder.[17]

Lamotrigine has a half-life of about twenty-four hours, and its metabolism is affected by taking carbamazepine and valproate (table 5.4). Blood-level tests are not routinely ordered for lamotrigine because of its low toxicity and because therapeutic effects have not been correlated with particular amounts in the blood.

Side Effects

In contrast to the other mood stabilizers, lamotrigine causes only minimal side effects. Patients taking it may have some initial nausea or gastrointestinal upset and the sort of side effects that many medications affecting the brain can cause: sleepiness, light-headedness or dizziness, and headaches. At higher doses, some patients complain of concentration problems similar to those often reported by patients taking lithium. In my experience, lowering the dose usually takes care of this problem.

TABLE 5.4. Therapeutic profile of lamotrigine	
Medication class:	Mood stabilizer (anticonvulsant)
Brand name:	Lamictal
Half-life:	15–24 hours
Metabolism:	Affected by carbamazepine, valproate
Elimination:	Liver
Other considerations:	Rarely causes severe skin rashes but otherwise has a good side-effect profile

A rare but serious problem that has been associated with lamotrigine is a dangerous type of allergic skin rash called *toxic epidermal necrosis* (TED). TED is the most extreme form of a group of allergic skin reactions that are lumped together under the term *erythema multiforme*. These problems were reported right after lamotrigine was introduced as a treatment for epilepsy in the early 1990s. When research was done to see which patients were at highest risk for these serious reactions, it was discovered that children and patients who started the drug at high doses were more likely than others to develop a serious rash. Subsequently, the drug's manufacturer recommended against prescribing lamotrigine to children except under special circumstances and also changed the dosing recommendations for starting the drug in adults. Now patients start lamotrigine at a low dose (about one-tenth of the ultimate therapeutic dose) and gradually increase it over a period of weeks, a process often referred to as lamotrigine *induction*. Although this means that it may take five weeks or more to get to the usual therapeutic dose of 200 to 400 mg/day, the risk of serious skin reactions to lamotrigine has virtually been eliminated. Since these dosing recommendations were put into effect, the rate at which patients developed serious rashes has dropped to that seen in the general population. In the pivotal clinical trials where lamotrigine was prescribed to several thousand patients for the treatment of bipolar disorder, none of the patients developed a serious rash.[18]

Nevertheless, many individuals develop minor skin reactions to medications and lots of other things as well, so it's important when a person starts taking lamotrigine to take precautions against developing a rash from another source. If a rash develops in a patient taking lamotrigine, it presents something of a therapeutic dilemma: Is the patient's rash erythema multiforme or a minor skin reaction? If the rash is a serious one, is lamotrigine the culprit? The patient might be told to stop the drug unnecessarily, perhaps missing out on a medication that might be highly effective. For this reason, patients starting on lamotrigine should consider the protocol developed at Stanford University to prevent skin rashes from other sources (table 5.5). I had one patient who had been told by her previous psychiatrist to stop lamotrigine, which up to that point had seemed very helpful for her bipolar depression, because she had developed what in retrospect was probably a reaction to poison ivy. She was able to restart lamotrigine and move up to a therapeutic dose with no problems. I tell my patients as I hand them the prescription, "No gardening, no hiking, no new restaurants or shampoos or clothes detergents; stay out of the sun and take care of your skin!"

Occasionally, I have seen patients with bipolar disorder who have appeared to greatly benefit from taking lamotrigine but who developed mild erythema multiforme while on it. Several studies have shown—and I have seen—that these patients can sometimes, by starting at a tiny dose and increasing more slowly than usual, safely get to a therapeutic dose and stay on it. Obviously, a careful risk versus benefit discussion needs to occur before embarking on such a plan, and very close monitoring is needed.

A corollary to the start-low protocol for lamotrigine is that a person who stops taking it for a period of time should not resume taking it at the same dose. Experts recommend that patients who are off lamotrigine for one week or more should restart the drug at the low beginning dose.

TABLE 5.5. The Stanford Protocol for patients starting lamotrigine

Do not start lamotrigine within 2 weeks of any rash, viral infection, or vaccination.

Take precautions outdoors to prevent sunburn and contact with poison ivy, oak, and sumac.

During the first 3 months of treatment avoid exposure as much as possible to any new

medicines;

foods;

soaps, cosmetics, conditioners, deodorants; and

detergents, fabric softeners.

────────── KEY LAMOTRIGINE TAKEAWAYS ──────────

▶ Lamotrigine appears to be especially effective for bipolar depression in bipolar II patients.

▶ The side-effect profile is excellent.

▶ The risk of serious dermatological reactions is real but quite low; following the Stanford Protocol for avoiding rashes is well worth the effort.

▶ Even patients who develop a rash can often have a "re-challenge" and take lamotrigine.

▶ Patients taking lamotrigine who go without it for more than a week should restart the induction process at a low dose.

CARBAMAZEPINE (TEGRETOL, EQUETRO, EPITOL)

After the introduction of carbamazepine for the control of epilepsy in the 1960s, several reports appeared indicating that epilepsy patients taking carbamazepine who also had mood problems not only had good control of their seizures but had improvement in their psychiatric symptoms as well. It was a small step to test carbamazepine in patients with mood problems who did not have epilepsy. Much of the early work on the use of carbamazepine in bipolar disorder was done by Japanese clinicians looking for an alternative to lithium, which was not approved for use in Japan until years after it was available in the United States. In 1980 a study appeared in the *American Journal of Psychiatry* titled "Carbamazepine in Manic-Depressive Illness: A New Treatment," and the race was on to refine the use of this medication in bipolar disorder and to define the group or groups of patients whom it helped the most.[19]

Therapeutic Profile

Although carbamazepine has been used to treat bipolar disorder for several decades, less research has been done on its efficacy in this illness than for other medications. This gap is slowly being filled, however, and newer studies have appeared, prompted by the development of a sustained-release preparation of carbamazepine.

Every once in a while, a patient of mine requests that I prescribe the "best" mood stabilizer or antidepressant medication there is. I usually respond by saying that if there were a "best" medication in a particular class of medications, it would be the only pharmaceutical manufactured and prescribed. What would be the point of using anything else? The reason there are so many drugs of a particular type is that some work better or have fewer side effects in particular patients. Many newer medications don't seem to be more effective than available ones when studied in large groups of patients, but they are clearly better for certain patients who can't take or don't respond to an older agent.

Carbamazepine is one such medication: it doesn't seem to have any big advantage in most studies of groups of patients, but it works *very* well—in fact, it works when other medications do not—for some patients. In one well-designed double-blind study, manic patients who took carbamazepine actually seemed to do worse than patients taking lithium.[20] But most psychiatrists have had a patient like "Ms. B.," whose case history was reported in a paper from the National Institute of Mental Health (NIMH) in 1983:

> Ms. B., a 53-year-old woman, had a history of treatment resistant, rapid cycling manic-depressive illness that required continuous state hospitalization from 1956 to her admission to NIMH in 1978. She had been non-responsive to [antipsychotic medications, tricyclic antidepressants] and lithium. . . . After institution of carbamazepine, both mood phases improved dramatically and she was able to be discharged. . . . During a subsequent hospitalization her severe mania again did not respond to [antipsychotic medications] and she was not able to leave the hospital until she was treated with carbamazepine.[21]

In this study the authors noted that "additional improvement appeared to occur when [antipsychotic medications] were used in conjunction with carbamazepine or when lithium and carbamazepine were used in combination." This had become carbamazepine's niche: a second-line mood-stabilizing agent for patients who do not respond to other agents; it was often used in combination with other agents. However, at least one placebo-controlled study using carbamazepine alone to treat patients hospitalized with mania supported the idea that this medication may be underused and can be helpful for many patients.[22]

Like the other mood-stabilizing medications, carbamazepine can be measured in the bloodstream, and blood-level tests can be used to adjust the dose. Unfortunately, not much work has been done on carbamazepine blood levels in bipolar patients, so the therapeutic range used for the treatment of epilepsy is usually the target that psychiatrists aim for in their patients.

TABLE 5.6. **Therapeutic profile of carbamazepine**	
Medication class:	Mood stabilizer (anticonvulsant)
Brand names:	Tegretol, Equetro, Epitol
Half-life:	18–15 hours (shortens over time)
Metabolism:	Complex; affects and is affected by other drugs
Elimination:	Liver
Other considerations:	Blood-level tests helpful; blood tests for liver inflammation and blood abnormalities needed

Carbamazepine is metabolized in the liver (table 5.6), and like some other drugs, it causes the liver to increase the level of the enzymes that metabolize it. This means that the longer a person takes carbamazepine, the more quickly the liver gets rid of it. So after a few weeks, the blood levels may go down, and the dose may need to be increased. This increase in liver enzymes can also affect other medications that the patient might be taking, including certain tranquilizers, certain antidepressants, other epilepsy medications, and some hormones. The change in hormonal levels is very important for women using birth control, since some oral contraceptives that use low hormone levels lose their effectiveness if taken with carbamazepine. It is critical that all physicians involved in a person's care know when the person has started taking carbamazepine so that dosage adjustments for other medications can be made.

Side Effects

Carbamazepine can cause the same sort of general side effects as many other medications that affect the brain do: sleepiness, light-headedness, and some initial nausea. These problems tend to be short lived and dose related.

There have been rare cases of liver problems associated with carbamazepine, so blood tests for liver inflammation are routinely done. There have been even rarer reports of dangerous changes in blood counts, so blood cell counts are also done, especially in the first several weeks of therapy. Cases of a dangerous skin reaction called Stevens-Johnson syndrome have been attributed to carbamazepine; this is another of the severe variants of erythema multiforme that I mentioned in the discussion of lamotrigine. All these problems are quite rare, but patients should be on the watch for the development of a rash, jaundice, water retention, bleeding or bruising, or signs of infection.

OXCARBAZEPINE (TRILEPTAL)

As its name suggests, oxcarbazepine (brand name Trileptal) is closely related to carbamazepine. It is another medication used to treat epilepsy, and it seems to work similarly to carbamazepine but has several impressive advantages. Oxcarbazepine is not associated with the blood-count problems that can be caused by carbamazepine or with the changes in liver enzymes that affect the metabolism of other drugs. This makes it significantly easier to take, with less need for monitoring blood tests and changes in dosage. It also appears less likely to cause Stevens-Johnson syndrome. Much of the early work on oxcarbazepine in bipolar disorder was done in Europe, and studies by German investigators in the mid-1980s suggested it was as beneficial as carbamazepine in treating mania. More recently, many other research papers have been published that support its safety and efficacy, especially as an "add-on" to other mood stabilizers. The effectiveness of oxcarbazepine for breakthrough manic symptoms has been especially well established,[23] and reports of it being effective when taken alone have also been published.

Many clinicians have been reluctant to prescribe oxcarbazepine's parent compound, carbamazepine, because of the possibility of severe adverse reactions. Given the fewer significant problems associated with oxcarbazepine, we will probably see it prescribed more often and studied more closely.

——— KEY CARBAMAZEPINE/OXCARBAZEPINE ——— TAKEAWAYS

▶ Both drugs have been shown to be effective in some patients with bipolar disorder, but neither has been studied as well as lithium or lamotrigine.

▶ Both drugs have been shown to help with breakthrough symptoms when added to other medications.

▶ Published case reports support the efficacy of both these drugs taken alone as a patient's only mood stabilizer.

▶ Oxcarbazepine (Trileptal) may be as effective as carbamazepine (Tegretol) in bipolar disorder but with a lower risk of serious side effects.

VALPROATE (DEPAKOTE, DEPAKENE, EPIVAL)

Valproic acid is a carbon compound similar to others that are found in animal fats and vegetable oils: it is a fatty acid. It was first synthesized in 1882 and was used for many years as an organic solvent for a variety of purposes. Valproate was approved by the Food and Drug Administration for use in treating epilepsy in 1978.[24] After the discovery that carbamazepine, also an antiepileptic medication, was effective in treating mania, interest in using valproate in bipolar disorder grew. In the mid-1980s, American psychiatrists conducted several studies on the use of valproate in treating bipolar disorder, and ten years later valproate became a frequently used medication for bipolar disorder.

As you will see, however, not only does valproate appear to be less effective than the drugs already discussed in this chapter (one can argue that it shouldn't even be called a "mood stabilizer") but also it has a number of very serious side-effect problems.

Therapeutic Profile

The half-life of valproate is between six and sixteen hours in adults (table 5.7). Thus, it reaches equilibrium in the body more quickly than lithium does, in two to three days. Valproate seems to have some advantages over lithium in the treatment of acute manic episodes. First, it appears to work more quickly. Whereas lithium may take up to three weeks to have its full effect, valproate has been shown to start working within five days. Second, valproate also seems to be more effective for certain subgroups of manic patients: patients with rapid cycling (four or more mood episodes per year) and patients with mixed mania (a mixture of manic hyperactivity and pressured thinking with depressed or unpleasant mood).[25] Third, valproate is much less toxic.

TABLE 5.7. **Therapeutic profile of valproate**

Medication class:	Mood stabilizer (anticonvulsant)
Brand names:	Depakene, Depakote, Epival
Half-life:	6–16 hours
Metabolism:	Affected by other antiepilepsy drugs
Elimination:	Liver
Other considerations:	Blood-level tests helpful; blood tests for liver inflammation are needed

Controlled studies of the use of valproate to treat acute depression and to prevent recurrences of bipolar disorder have been less impressive.[26] In fact, if one sticks to the more rigorous controlled studies, it can be argued that valproate should be used only to treat acute mania and that the lack of strong evidence for its benefit in depression or for maintenance treatment argues against any other use in bipolar disorder.[27] Nevertheless, any psychiatrist with experience in treating mood-disorder patients will tell you that some patients need and benefit from valproate and that for them it is extremely and sometimes uniquely effective. It may be that these patients have an unusual variant of bipolar disorder and that the benefit of valproate for these patients gets lost in large studies, where they are vastly outnumbered by patients who do not respond to valproate.

Like lithium, valproate can be measured in the bloodstream; blood levels above 45 mcg/ml (micrograms per milliliter) have been shown to be necessary for the therapeutic effect to occur, and side effects become more problematic at levels greater than 125 mcg/ml.[28] Several studies have shown that valproate is helpful in cyclothymia, bipolar II, and "soft" bipolar disorders and that lower doses and lower blood levels are required for these illnesses than in the treatment of bipolar I.[29] As with lithium, blood for a test of valproate levels should be drawn twelve hours after the last dose.

Side Effects

Side effects that are common as a patient starts taking valproate include stomach upset and some sleepiness. These problems usually go away quickly. Increased appetite and weight gain are perhaps the most serious side effects. Mild tremor occurs as well and can be treated with beta blockers. A few patients report hair loss, usually temporary, which resolves even more quickly with the use of shampoos and vitamin preparations containing the minerals zinc and selenium.[30]

Cases of severe liver problems have been reported in patients taking valproate, but they have occurred almost exclusively in children taking the drug for control of epilepsy, most of whom had other medical problems and were taking several different medications. A 1989 review article stated that no fatalities from liver problems caused by valproate were ever reported in patients over the age of ten who were taking only valproate. Just to be on the safe side, however, patients taking valproate for the first time are given a blood test to detect liver inflammation, and the test is repeated at appropriate intervals while they are taking it. Since valproate can also, in rare cases, cause a drop in blood counts, a complete blood count is usually done as well. These are rare problems, and when they do occur, they develop slowly and usually during the first six months of therapy. Thus, they can be detected with routine blood tests. Nevertheless, patients on valproate should be on the lookout for signs of liver or blood-count problems, which include unusual bleeding and bruising, jaundice (yellowing of the eyes and skin), fever, and water retention.

Valproate has been associated with the development of polycystic ovarian syndrome in women. The components of this syndrome are irregular menstrual periods, the development of facial hair and male-pattern hair loss, obesity, and ovarian cysts.

Valproate has been associated with birth defects, and women of child-bearing age should practice birth control while taking valproate if there is any possibility of becoming pregnant.

─────────── **KEY VALPROATE TAKEAWAYS** ───────────

▶ It's questionable whether valproate should be considered a "mood stabilizer," as it has only been clearly proven to be effective in treating acute mania. Evidence for prescribing it to treat bipolar depression and to prevent future episodes (prophylaxis) is weak.

▶ There is a substantial risk of weight gain, especially in women, in whom it can also cause significant gynecological and hormonal problems (polycystic ovarian syndrome).

OTHER MOOD STABILIZERS

Several other agents show promise for the treatment of bipolar disorder. For the most part, the potential of these medications is based on clinical trials in which the medication is added to the regimen of patients already taking an established mood stabilizer such as lithium, but sometimes a few case reports of a therapeutic effect are enough to attract the attention of psychiatrists.

Pramipexole (Mirapex) is a medication that is usually used to treat Parkinson's disease and restless leg syndrome; it activates dopamine circuits in the brain. Several studies have shown pramipexole to be an effective add-on treatment for bipolar depression not responding to mood stabilizers alone.[31] As with other treatments that are especially helpful for bipolar depression, there is a risk of developing hypomanic or manic symptoms.

The FDA and "Off-Label Prescribing"

Pharmaceutical companies must demonstrate to the Food and Drug Administration that a medication that they wish to market in the United States is safe and effective for the treatment of a medical condition before it can be prescribed. They do this by studying the drug in hundreds or thousands of persons with a condition, comparing its efficacy with a placebo or against another medication already approved for that condition. If the new medication works better than a placebo for the condition or as well as (and hopefully better than) an already approved medication, an application with these data is submitted to the FDA, which decides about approval. It is then referred to as "indicated" for that condition. The FDA also makes a judgment about whether the benefits of the medications outweigh the risks from side effects. The drug manufacturer and the FDA also negotiate the content of the drug's "label," actually a pamphlet-sized document called the "package insert" that essentially contains instructions for prescribers.*

The costs of studies required to generate enough data for the FDA to approve a drug are exorbitant, tens or even hundreds of millions of dollars to carry out. Most often the studies of a new medication focus on one condition, that is, for one indication, even though it may be effective for several. This means that the term *FDA approved* must be interpreted with caution. The fact that a medication is not FDA approved for a condition may not mean that it is ineffective for that condition. Just as likely, the pharmaceutical company has made a business decision that the cost of doing efficacy studies to get labeling for another indication simply isn't worth the increased profit that FDA labeling might mean for that condition.

A good example of this issue is the medication gabapentin. The FDA labeling of Pfizer's brand of gabapentin, Neurontin, includes "post-herpetic neuralgia," a painful condition that some people develop following a bout of "shingles" (herpes zoster). In these individuals, the infection damages the affected nerves, which continue to send pain signals to the brain for months or even years after the shingles rash has cleared. This type of pain is called "neuropathic" pain because it appears to be caused by damaged nerves. There are many other types of neuropathic pain, probably the most common being that caused by uncontrolled diabetes (diabetic peripheral neuropathy). It turns out that gabapentin is extremely effective for diabetic neuropathy, is widely prescribed in the United States for this condition, and is even approved for that indication in Great Britain by the British equivalent of the FDA. So why isn't Neurontin "FDA approved" for diabetic neuropathy? Most likely because Pfizer decided that Neurontin is already an established treatment for diabetic neuropathy and that the investment of multiple millions of dollars on additional studies and preparing an FDA application for approval for this indication won't increase sales.

Another factor in these decisions is whether the company's patent on the drug has expired (or is about to expire). Once a company's patent expires, any drug manufacturer may begin producing the drug. Obviously, a pharmaceutical company isn't going to invest millions of dollars for a new indication if it will have to share the profits with other companies.

Once a medication has been approved to treat one disorder, physicians are allowed to prescribe it to any patients for whom they judge it to be medically appropriate, including patients with another disorder. The FDA does not regulate the practice of medicine; physicians may prescribe any available drug for other conditions if, based on their review of available research and their judgment and experience, the drug is appropriate to treat the patient. When used to treat a condition not listed in the FDA "label," this practice is called *off-label prescribing*.

All this means that just because a medication isn't "FDA approved" for a condition doesn't mean that it hasn't been extensively evaluated by researchers or won't be safe and effective. If taking a medication for an off-label disorder seems risky, it may reassure you to learn that most new mood stabilizers, including lamotrigine, were widely prescribed "off label" for years before they received FDA labeling for bipolar disorder.

*Food and Drug Administration, "How Drugs Are Developed and Approved," www .fda.gov/drugs/development-approval-process-drugs/how-drugs-are-developed -and-approved.

There is evidence that N-acetyl cysteine (NAC), an amino acid available as a nutritional supplement, may be useful as a mood stabilizer.[32] A number of studies examining NAC as an add-on medication to other mood stabilizers have shown promising results, especially in bipolar depression. This discovery is especially exciting because the mechanism of action of NAC is completely different from that of any other mood stabilizer. NAC is a metabolic precursor to glutathione, a powerful antioxidant that occurs in brain tissue, suggesting that NAC, like other mood stabilizers, may work through neuroprotective mechanisms. (More on NAC in chapter 9.)

Tiagabine (Gabitril) and zonisamide (Zonegran) are other antiepilepsy drugs that have attracted the interest of clinical researchers on bipolar disorder. Ongoing work may result in these drugs also being introduced as mood-stabilizing medications.

——————————————— KEY TAKEAWAYS ———————————————

▶ A medication is considered "mood stabilizer" if it is effective in treating manic episodes and depressive episodes and prevents future episodes from occurring.

▶ Lithium is arguably the gold standard for treatment for bipolar I disorder.

▶ Several medications originally developed to treat epilepsy have been re-purposed to treat bipolar disorder and can be more effective than lithium for some patients.

CHAPTER 6

Antipsychotic Medications

A difficulty that immediately arises in discussing this group of medications is their unfortunate name, as they are used to treat problems other than psychosis.

A psychosis can be thought of as a mental state or disorder in which the affected person's ability to comprehend his or her environment and react to it appropriately is severely impaired. The layperson's definition of *psychotic* might be "out of touch with reality." Someone who is hearing voices (having hallucinations) or who has bizarre idiosyncratic beliefs (delusions) is psychotic. The word also connotes a severe disorganization of thinking and behavior, usually with restlessness and agitation. The full-blown manic syndrome is a good example of a state of psychosis, and we have already talked about "psychotic features" in depression.

These medications are the mainstays of treatment for schizophrenia, a psychiatric illness in which hallucinations and delusions are the principle symptoms and mood is relatively unaffected.

Although these medications are certainly effective for psychotic symptoms in those persons with bipolar disorder who develop them, they have additional antimanic and antidepressant effects that make them extremely helpful for the many patients who never do.

BEYOND "ANTIPSYCHOTIC"

As we saw in part I of this book, episodes of bipolar disorder—both depression and mania—can sometimes include extremely frightening mental symptoms and dangerously disturbed behaviors. And, as we saw in the previous chapter, mood stabilizers sometimes take weeks to begin working. What can be done to slow down the racing, pressured thoughts, the bursting overactivity of the manic patient before lithium starts working? This is where antipsychotic medications have been useful. Because their calming effects begin almost immediately, these medications are especially useful in acute mania and are frequently part of the treatment for the severely ill manic patient. In cases of depression where the patient is highly restless and agitated, they can have similar beneficial effects.

Thorazine and Beyond

In the 1930s a group of pharmaceutical compounds called *phenothiazines* were synthesized in Europe and were found to have antihistamine and sedative properties that were attributed to their blockade of the receptors for the neurotransmitter *dopamine*. One in particular, chlorpromazine (Thorazine), was found to be useful in surgical anesthesia because it deepened anesthetic sedation more safely than other available agents did. In the early 1950s, two French psychiatrists carried out several clinical trials using chlorpromazine to treat highly agitated patients suffering from schizophrenia and mania. They hoped the drug would provide sedation for these profoundly ill patients, which it did—but these astute clinicians noticed that the medication did much more.

In addition to its quieting and sleep-promoting effects, chlorpromazine made the hallucinations and bizarre delusional beliefs of many patients with schizophrenia practically disappear. It also decreased the severity of disorganized thinking and agitation seen in patients with acute mania. Chlorpromazine, in other words, had a *specific* effect on the cluster of symptoms often referred to as "psychotic" symptoms, and thus the name for this group came about: *antipsychotic medications*. Occasionally they are still referred to as *neuroleptic medications* (or *neuroleptics*), from *neuroleptique*, the French word (coined from Greek roots) that means roughly "affecting the nervous system." The term *major tranquilizers* was frequently used for these medications at one time (with the term *minor tranquilizers* used for sleep and anxiety medications), but these agents are much more than just "tranquilizers," and this term has, fortunately, fallen out of favor.

In the 1980s, new antipsychotic medications were developed that had much more effect on the brain's serotonin circuits than the older antipsychotics did, and clinical trials with these new drugs demonstrated that they are effective not only for psychotic mania but also for hypomania and depression. Some clinicians (including this one) think of these medications as mood stabilizers in their own right.

Antipsychotic medications are usually divided into two groups, the original group of medications (like chlorpromazine), the *typical antipsychotics*; and the newer group, the *atypical antipsychotics*, which have more effect on the serotonin system than their predecessors do.

The main chemical effect of antipsychotic medications is to block dopamine receptors in the brain. Neural circuits that use dopamine as their neurotransmitter may be dysfunctional in some way in people with schizophrenia, and this situation may cause the bizarre hallucinations and disorders of thinking typical of that illness. Antipsychotic medications may work by affecting these systems in some as yet unknown way.

How Is the Brain Like a House?

You have probably read comparisons between the human brain and the computer, but in a rather interesting way, the brain is also like a house.

If your house is like mine, behind its walls are a number of circuits. The network of wiring that brings electricity into every room is the most obvious, but there are others as well. There's a network of piping that supplies water to the bathrooms and the kitchen—a network that has two subdivisions: hot water and cold water. The HVAC system has a network of ducts to circulate warm air in the winter and cool air in the summer. All these networks work together to make your house a comfortable environment to live in.

Like your house, the brain has different circuits that work together to control bodily functions and mental experiences. The brain's circuitry is, of course, tremendously more complex than anything in your house, with many, many more circuits and with complicated connections between circuits. Just like your house, however, each circuit has a different purpose and function. But unlike your house, in which different circuits are made of different materials (e.g., copper wires, plastic pipes, aluminum ductwork), different brain circuits differ not in what they are made of but in the chemical messengers that each circuit uses to send messages.

These chemical messengers are called *neurotransmitters*. You may have heard of one of them, *serotonin*, that is especially important in mood circuitry, called *serotonergic* systems or circuits. There are other neurotransmitters that are probably just as important: *norepinephrine* and *dopamine* are two, and there are many more.

As you read through the next several chapters, you will learn that the medications that we use in psychiatry mainly work through their effects on neurotransmitters—sometimes by increasing neurotransmitter levels, sometimes by blocking their effects—and that these effects appear to modulate one or another circuit. For those interested in understanding more of the details of all this, I'll be discussing them in part III of this book.

Newer antipsychotic medications are called *atypical antipsychotic medications* (you may also see them referred to as *second-generation antipsychotics*) to differentiate them from the older antipsychotic medications that had more potent effects on dopamine and less effect on the serotonin system in the brain. The original antipsychotic medications are now often referred to as *typical antipsychotics*. They are used only rarely now in the treatment of mood disorders, mainly in cases of severe mania with agitation and even in those cases, for only short periods of time. The main reasons for this are the side effects that they cause.

TABLE 6.1. Atypical antipsychotic medications	
Pharmaceutical name	*Brand name(s)*
Aripiprazole	Abilify
Asenapine	Saphris
Brexpiprazole	Rexulti
Clozapine	Clozaril
Iloperidone	Fanapt
Lurasidone	Latuda
Olanzapine	Zyprexa, Zyprexa Zydis
Melperone*	Bunil, Buronil, Eunerpan
Paliperidone	Invega
Quetiapine	Seroquel
Risperidone	Risperdal
Sulpiride*	Dogmatil
Ziprasidone	Geodon

*Not approved for use or not available in the United States.

Therapeutic Profile

The first atypical antipsychotic, *clozapine*, was synthesized in the laboratory in the 1960s but was not marketed in the United States until 1990. One of the reasons it took so long to get onto the market is that, in about 1 percent of patients who take it, it causes a dangerous drop in the number of white blood cells (called *agranulocytosis*).[1] This problem might have meant the end for clozapine as a new medication, except that it was found to be highly effective in treating patients with schizophrenia who had derived little benefit from traditional antipsychotic medications. Dramatic case studies of patients with chronic treatment-resistant schizophrenia who basically "awakened" from years of unrelenting psychotic symptoms after they started clozapine sustained the interest of clinicians and pharmaceutical researchers. When it was discovered that the risk of agranulocytosis could be substantially reduced if the patient had her white blood cell count monitored closely, clozapine treatment became available to larger groups of patients, and before long, treatment-resistant mood-disorder patients were treated with it as well.

A 1996 research article reported on the use of clozapine in twenty-five acutely manic patients "for whom lithium, anticonvulsants and [traditional] neuroleptics had been ineffective, had produced intolerable side effects, or both."[2] Almost three-quarters of the patients had "marked improvement" in their manic symptoms. The answer to the question posed in a 1995 article title, "Is Clozapine a Mood Stabilizer?" seems to be an emphatic yes.[3]

After the introduction of clozapine and the appearance of research papers describing its effectiveness for the treatment of mood disorders, drug developers got to work developing medications with the same benefits that did not cause the blood count problems associated with clozapine. Many more atypicals have now come along, and their introduction substantially expanded the number of treatment options for bipolar disorder.

It is now very clear that the atypical antipsychotic medications are helpful in all phases of bipolar disorder—mania *and* depression—as well as for ongoing treatment to prevent relapse (sometimes known as maintenance treatment). The really good news is that these medications have significant antidepressant effects in many patients (another reason why calling them "antipsychotic" medications is inaccurate). In 2002, just after the first atypicals introduced after clozapine appeared, the *Journal of Clinical Psychopharmacology* published a letter to the editor titled "Are the Atypical Antipsychotic Drugs Antidepressants?"[4] Once again the answer is a definite yes, and in subsequent years, this fact has been borne out in study after study.

Practicing psychiatrists (including this one) will tell you that some of the atypicals seem to be more antimanic and others more antidepressant in their effect. Unfortunately, research that might bear this out by comparing the effects of different atypicals for mania and for bipolar depression has not been done.

Side Effects

The most significant side-effect problem with atypical antipsychotic medications is their tendency to make some individuals gain weight and develop such obesity-related problems as high cholesterol and even diabetes.

These problems are more common in individuals who develop *metabolic syndrome* while taking these medications. Not all individuals develop these problems, but attention to diet and weight issues is very important for persons taking these medications, especially for patients who take them long term. One cause of the weight gain associated with the atypical antipsychotics is stimulation of the appetite center of the brain, although recent research indicates that these medications probably affect several hormones that control how the body handles calories and stores fat.[5]

Atypicals and Metabolic Syndrome

The term *metabolic syndrome* refers to a collection of factors that put a person at higher risk of developing cardiovascular disease, such as heart attacks and stroke:

- Obesity

- Increased blood sugar levels (prediabetes or diabetes)

- Increased levels of cholesterol and triglycerides ("lipid," or fat, molecules in the blood)

- Hypertension (high blood pressure)

There is evidence that the first of these factors, obesity, causes the development of the other three in many persons. While several atypicals cause significant increases in appetite that often lead to weight gain, studies have shown that they cause disturbances in glucose metabolism independent of that caused by weight gain.

It's important that persons taking an atypical antipsychotic and their prescribers stay on the lookout for the development of metabolic syndrome by tracking weight, testing for high blood sugar and lipid levels, and monitoring blood pressure. The American Diabetes Association also recommends measuring waist circumference annually and making a note of any family history of diabetes.

Although several medications have been reported to reduce the risk of developing metabolic syndrome, the diabetes drug *metformin* (Glucophage) has the most consistently positive results. Although helpful all by itself, it's been shown that patients taking metformin lose the most weight when they also make healthy lifestyle changes like adopting a healthier diet and exercising regularly.*

P. Pramyothin and L. Khaodhiar, "Metabolic Syndrome with the Atypical Antipsychotics," *Current Opinion in Endocrinology, Diabetes and Obesity* 17, no. 5 (2010): 460–66.

Some of the atypical antipsychotics are less likely to cause weight gain than others; in fact, several are weight neutral—that is, they seem to have little or no effect on weight.

TABLE 6.2. **Weight gain risks of some atypical antipsychotics**	
Higher risk	Clozapine
	Olanzapine
	Quetiapine
↑	Risperidone
	Ziprasidone*
Lower risk	Aripiprazole*

Source: Data from T. Baptista, N. M. Kin, S. Beaulieu, and E. A. de Baptista, "Obesity and Related Metabolic Abnormalities during Drug Administration: Mechanisms, Management, and Research Perspectives," *Pharmacopsychiatry* 35, no. 6 (2002): 205–19.

*Negligible effect on weight.

The weight-neutral agents are preferable for already obese patients and for patients with diabetes or a family history of diabetes. Blood tests for diabetes and high cholesterol are often done at the beginning of treatment and regularly thereafter in patients taking antipsychotics for maintenance treatment, and they are also weighed regularly. All patients taking atypical antipsychotics should take steps to control possible weight gain by paying attention to their diet and getting regular exercise.

A rare but serious side effect of the atypical antipsychotic medications is the development of problems with heart rhythm. Normally, a burst of electrical activity originating in the heart's natural pacemaker flows smoothly through the heart muscle, causing it to contract in an organized way to pump blood through the body's blood vessels. These medications can cause the electrical activity of the heart to change in such a way that it takes longer for the heart muscle to "reset" electrically between heart beats, a phenomenon called *QT prolongation*. The letters *Q* and *T* refer to points on an electrocardiogram (ECG or EKG). QT prolongation is dangerous because it can lead to much more serious changes in the heart's electrical activities such that the heartbeat becomes disorganized. This can cause a fainting spell, a stroke, or even sudden death. This happens because the abnormally long time to "reset" can trigger a switch from a normal rhythm to a disorganized, rapid, and inefficient heartbeat that shows up on an EKG as a series of spiky waves called *torsades de pointes* (TdP). Fortunately, only a minority of persons who develop QT prolongation go one to develop TdP. Most of those who do have other underlying risk factors that can be identified and sometimes corrected.[6]

Another issue with this group of drugs is their potential side effects on muscle function. This was a serious issue with their predecessors, the drugs now referred to as *typical antipsychotics*. In fact, it was the search for antipsychotic drugs that didn't have this effect that led to the development of the atypicals. Muscle stiffness, restlessness, and abnormal movements are some of the problems the drugs in this category can cause.

The development of the atypicals was one of two dramatic advancements in the treatment of mood disorders that occurred in the 1990s. The other was the development of the selective serotonin reuptake inhibitor (SSRI) antidepressants, starting with fluoxetine (Prozac). I would argue that the introduction of the atypicals was the more important of the two, as it arguably resulted in a new group of mood-stabilizing drugs. If a mood stabilizer doesn't completely control bipolar symptoms or an antidepressant doesn't completely control unipolar depression symptoms, one of the first interventions is usually to add an atypical, probably making them some of the most frequently prescribed medications in psychiatric practice.

QT Prolongation and Risk Factors for Torsades de Pointes

- Older than sixty-five years of age
- Abnormally slow heart rate
- Congenital (inherited) prolonged QT syndrome
- Treatment with diuretics ("fluid pills")
- Abnormally low blood levels of potassium, calcium, and/or magnesium
- Female gender
- Genetic predisposition
- Preexisting heart disease: history of myocardial infarction (heart attack) or congestive heart failure.
- Advanced liver disease
- Treatment with multiple drugs that also cause prolonged QT interval*

*Modified from M. Li and L. G. Ramos, "Drug-Induced QT Prolongation and Torsades de Pointes," *Pharmacy and Therapeutics* 42, no. 7 (2017): 473-77.

Movement and Muscle Tone Side Effects

The antipsychotic medications discussed in this chapter have the potential for negative effects on muscle tone and movement as a consequence of the dopamine blockade that they cause. In textbook discussions of these medications, you will see these problems referred to as *extrapyramidal symptoms*, or *EPS*. Dopamine is the main neurotransmitter used in a complex circuit of brain areas called the *extrapyramidal system*, which coordinates movement. (The term *extrapyramidal* contrasts this system with another, called the *pyramidal system* because its main fibers are carried in triangular bundles into the spinal cord [the "spinal pyramids" or "pyramidal tract"].) The pyramidal system controls the quick, accurate execution of fine muscle movement, and the extrapyramidal system makes sure that the rest of the body moves as needed for the smooth and graceful execution of these movements. Antipsychotic medications, by blocking the dopamine receptors in these centers, can cause a variety of side effects that affect movement.

One of these is *pseudo-Parkinsonism*. You may know that persons suffering from Parkinson's disease have a slowed and shuffling walk, seem to lose facial expression because of stiffness of their facial muscles, and have trembling of their hands. Pseudo-parkinsonism consists of these same symptoms.

Another extrapyramidal side effect is the *acute dystonic reaction*. This is a sudden muscular spasm, more common in young males, that usually involves the tongue and facial and neck muscles. People taking antipsychotic medications can also develop a very distressing restlessness called *akathisia*. This is felt mostly in the legs, so that the individual feels the need to walk or pace.

Fortunately, all these side effects are treatable, either by lowering the dose of medication or by adding one of several medications that are used to treat Parkinson's disease. Although uncomfortable, these side effects are not dangerous and usually respond quickly to treatment once they are encountered and identified.

Most of the typical antipsychotic medications can, over a period of years, cause a side effect called *tardive dyskinesia*, or *TD* for short. This consists of repetitive involuntary movements, usually of the facial muscles—most often chewing, blinking, or lip-pursing movements. TD movements sometimes resolve simply by reducing the dose of medication, and there are now several prescription medications available to treat TD. We used to worry a lot about TD because some patients who developed it seemed to continue to have these movements even after the medication was stopped.

(continued)

But two factors are calming these worries: the discovery that most TD symptoms *do* eventually go away with time and, more importantly, the development of the atypical antipsychotic medications, which do not seem to cause TD very often.

I want to emphasize that extrapyramidal symptoms are usually easily treated and are not dangerous. But the symptoms of bipolar disorder that the antipsychotic medications are usually used to treat *are* extremely dangerous. These medications are powerful agents, and they need to be used carefully and for the shortest period of time possible, but for the present, at least, they are nearly irreplaceable in treating the most dangerous and most terrible symptoms of severe mania and psychotic depression.

KEY TAKEAWAYS

▶ Atypical antipsychotic medications offer both antimanic and antidepressant effects and are usually "add-on" medications in treatment mood disorders.

▶ Some, though not all, atypicals cause increased appetite, which can lead to weight gain and even obesity, putting the patient at higher risk of developing obesity-related problems such as high blood pressure and type II diabetes.

▶ A rare but potentially life-threatening heart rhythm problem can affect some individuals who take these medications, and persons with a history of heart disease should be screened for risk factors and closely monitored while taking them.

CHAPTER 7

Antidepressant Medications

T he role of antidepressant medications in treating the depression of bipolar disorder has been debated for decades. This is because these medications can push a bipolar patient from depression into a manic state, and in some patients, antidepressants seem to increase the cycling of their illness.

However, despite the risks associated with antidepressants for persons with bipolar illness, some patients with bipolar disorder appear to benefit from them and can take them safely. Unfortunately, we don't yet have any way of identifying those patients, so caution is the byword when it comes to prescribing these drugs.

The antidepressants can be divided into groups according to what chemical effects they have in the brain, making for some tongue-twisting labels. By and large their effects are on *neurotransmitters*, the chemical messengers that that brain cells (*neurons*) use to communicate with each other. In a later chapter, I will discuss these important molecules in more detail and explain why changing the amounts of these chemicals in the brain makes the symptoms of depression better.

TRICYCLIC ANTIDEPRESSANTS

Although tricyclics are now less frequently used as antidepressants, our discussion starts with this group because they were among the first antidepressant medications developed and because they still provide the standard by which all promising new pharmaceuticals for the treatment of depression are judged.

These drugs are called *tricyclics* because of the three rings in their chemical structure. The effect of tricyclics on *norepinephrine*, one of the chemical messengers in brain cells, was one of the first chemical effects of a medication active in the brain to be measured in the laboratory. The observation that tricyclics *increased* norepinephrine levels in the brain, along with the discovery that certain other medications used to treat high blood pressure that *lowered* norepinephrine levels were observed to cause depression in some patients led to the early "amine hypothesis" of the mood disorders: that depression is caused by too little norepinephrine, and mania, presumably, by too much. However, further research indicated that tricyclics increased amines in the synapse within *hours* of taking them but took *weeks* to begin to help with depressive symptoms, which led to a search for an alternative explanation. Table 7.1 lists the common tricyclics.

The principal reason that tricyclic antidepressants are now less frequently prescribed is their many side effects. As with all medications, some patients can take tricyclics easily and without unpleasant side effects, but many patients have to put up with a few days or even weeks of troublesome side effects to get the benefits. Fortunately, all the side effects are dose related, and most are temporary.

Tricyclics block another of the body's chemical messengers, called *acetylcholine*, which is used in the part of the nervous system that regulates many "automatic" functions of the body such as digestion. These *anticholinergic* side effects include a slowing down of the gastrointestinal tract, causing constipation and dry mouth. The focusing of the lens of the eye and emptying of the urinary bladder are also controlled by this system, and tricyclics can cause blurry vision and urination difficulties also, although usually only at high doses. Patients with a history of glaucoma or urinary tract problems should be monitored closely by their physician while taking these medications. Tricyclics also cause weight gain in many patients.

TABLE 7.1. Tricyclic antidepressants

Pharmaceutical name	Brand name
Amitriptyline	Elavil
Amoxapine	Asendin
Clomipramine	Anafranil
Desipramine	Norpramin
Doxepin	Sinequan
Imipramine	Tofranil
Maprotiline	Ludiomil
Nortriptyline	Pamelor
Protriptyline	Vivactil

Tricyclics are toxic in larger amounts, and overdoses can be deadly. Although the lethal overdose is up to twenty times the normal dose for an adult, children are more sensitive to the toxic effects of these medications; just a handful of tablets can be fatal in a small child. For this reason, tricyclic medications must be scrupulously safeguarded in households with children.

SELECTIVE SEROTONIN REUPTAKE INHIBITORS (SSRIs)

It will come as no surprise that a new pharmaceutical that had none of the tricyclic side effects listed above and was not toxic in overdose caused something of a sensation when it was introduced in 1988. That pharmaceutical was fluoxetine (Prozac). For a time it seemed that everyone you talked to was either taking Prozac or reading about it. A Prozac capsule showed up on the covers of *Newsweek* and *New York* magazines, and the drug was featured in innumerable other magazine and newspaper articles.

Unlike the tricyclics, this class of antidepressants has little direct effect on norepinephrine in the brain but instead blocks the reuptake of another neurotransmitter, *serotonin*, into neurons. The potent and specific serotonin-reuptake-blocking effects of these agents give this class its name: *selective serotonin reuptake inhibitors*, or *SSRIs* (table 7.2).

The side-effect profile of the SSRIs is very benign, and because of this they are usually considered first-line treatment. This means that if a prescriber decides that a patient may benefit from taking an antidepressant, she will often prescribe an SSRI.

TABLE 7.2. Selective serotonin reuptake inhibitors

Pharmaceutical name	Brand name(s)
Citalopram	Celexa (Cipramil)
Escitalopram	Lexapro (Cipralex)
Fluoxetine	Prozac, Sarafem (Erocap, Fluohexal, Lovan, Zactin, and others)
Fluvoxamine	Luvox
Paroxetine	Paxil, Paxil CR* (Aropax, Seroxat, and others)
Sertraline	Zoloft (Altruline, Aremis, Gladem, Besitran, Lustral, Sealdin, and others)

Note: Names in parentheses are brands marketed outside the United States.

*Slow-release preparation.

Some patients experience nausea for the first couple of days after starting one of the SSRIs, and a very few have diarrhea or vomiting. Headaches are not uncommon at first, but they usually last only a day or two. These problems can often be alleviated by restarting the medication at a lower dose and increasing slowly. SSRIs can have a caffeine-like effect in some people, and while this energy boost is just what is needed by some depressed patients, others feel unpleasantly nervous or "wired" when taking these medications. The converse can also be seen, and sleepiness is sometimes a side effect. Many patients report that SSRIs seem to curb their appetite a bit and notice some weight loss, especially soon after they begin taking them. Weight gain can also be a problem, however. If they are going to occur, these side effects are usually noticed by patients pretty much immediately; none sneak up after a person has been on an SSRI for weeks or months.

One problem that might not be noticeable to patients until they've been taking an SSRI for weeks or months is a change in sexual functioning, specifically a noticeable decrease in sexual interest (loss of libido) or a difficulty in reaching or inability to reach orgasm. This is a significant problem affecting about one-third of patients. A variety of strategies are available for dealing with these problems when they occur, so they should be reported to the physician. Weekend "vacations" from the medication have been reported to be helpful, as well as the addition of other medications that seem to block these effects, but sometimes a switch to an antidepressant in another class is the only solution.

When I asked one of my male patients whether he was having any sexual dysfunction from his new antidepressant, he replied that he thought fluoxetine had *improved* his sex life, increasing his sexual stamina and causing him to have more intense orgasms—a reminder that a list of potential medication side effects should never be a reason not to try a particular medication. Pleasant surprises sometimes do occur. Also, a medication effect that causes problems for some patients can actually be helpful for others; for example, SSRIs have been reported to be helpful in treating premature ejaculation.[1]

SELECTIVE SEROTONIN NOREPINEPHRINE REUPTAKE INHIBITORS (SNRIs)

As you might guess from the name of this group of antidepressants, their activity in the brain involves effects on two neurotransmitter systems: serotonin circuits and norepinephrine circuits.

TABLE 7.3. Selective serotonin norepinephrine reuptake inhibitors (SNRIs)	
Pharmaceutical name	*Brand name(s)*
Desvenlafaxine	Pristiq
Duloxetine	Cymbalta (Davedax, Xeristar, Yentreve, and others)
Levomilnacipran	Fetzima
Milnacipran*	Savella*
Venlafaxine	Effexor, Effexor XR† (Efexor, Efexor XR,† and others)

Note: Names in parentheses are brands marketed outside the United States.

*FDA labeled only for treatment of fibromyalgia

†Slow-release preparation.

A feature that these medications all share is their ability to treat certain pain problems. These include *neuropathic* pain, a chronic pain problem resulting from damage to the nerves, most commonly caused by poorly controlled diabetes. Another is *fibromyalgia*, a little-understood disorder characterized by pain in the muscles and joints that also appears to be caused by a malfunction in the nervous system's pain circuitry. Several SNRIs have FDA labeling for the treatment of these conditions as well as for depression, and one, milnacipran (Savella), is labeled for the treatment of fibromyalgia but not depression. Remember that getting FDA approval (or, really, FDA labeling) for a medication to treat a particular condition is an expensive process and that a medication may have research showing its effectiveness for one condition but not be FDA labeled for treatment of another.

The side-effect profile of the SNRIs is similar to that of the SSRIs. There are indications that the *discontinuation syndrome* for SNRIs can be more severe than for SSRIs.

MORE ANTIDEPRESSANTS

Since the early 1990s, many other new antidepressants have come onto the market that do not fall into any of the foregoing categories. Since most of these pharmaceuticals don't share many common features, there is no good class name for them, although you'll sometimes see many of them listed as *atypical* or *second-generation* antidepressants (table 7.4). They have a variety of effects on norepinephrine, serotonin, and other neurotransmitters. Some have more than one effect on these systems, and so they are thought to provide different ways of manipulating the chemical systems in the brain that are concerned with mood. Bupropion is most active on a different neurotransmitter altogether, dopamine. The side-effect profiles of these medications vary widely. Some have a profile more like that of tricyclics, others more like that of SSRIs.

TABLE 7.4. Second-generation antidepressants

Pharmaceutical name	Brand name(s)
Agomelatine*	(Melitor, Thymanax, Valdoxan)
Bupropion	Wellbutrin, Wellbutrin SR,† Wellbutrin XR†
Mirtazapine	Remeron
Vilazodone	Viibryd
Vortioxetine	Trintellix

Note: Names in parentheses are brands marketed outside the United States.
*Not available in the United States.
†Slow-release preparations.

Antidepressant Discontinuation Syndrome

You should never stop taking an antidepressant suddenly, especially if you have been taking a higher dose. Doing so runs the risk of developing a collection of uncomfortable symptoms that have been called *discontinuation syndrome*. Fortunately, preventing the problem is easy and simply done: by tapering the medication slowly. The antidote to the problem if it develops is also simple one: restart the medication and then taper.

Some medications cause more symptoms than others. The SNRIs can be especially troublesome in this regard, while some of the newer agents, like vortioxetine, rarely cause any discontinuation symptoms.

Symptoms of antidepressant discontinuation syndrome include the following:

- Flu-like symptoms (lethargy, fatigue, headache, achiness, sweating)
- Insomnia (with vivid dreams or nightmares)
- Nausea (sometimes vomiting)
- Imbalance (dizziness, vertigo, light-headedness)
- Sensory disturbances ("brain zaps," "tingling," "electric-like" or "shock-like" sensations)
- Feeling overstimulated (anxiety, irritability, agitation, jerkiness)

MONOAMINE OXIDASE INHIBITORS (MAOIs)

In the early 1950s, a new drug that developed for the treatment of tuberculosis was observed to cause mood elevation in some patients who took it for their lung disease. Several years later, numerous research papers confirmed the therapeutic effects of this medication, iproniazid, in patients suffering from depression. Shortly afterward it was discovered that iproniazid deactivates an enzyme in the body that metabolizes amine compounds in the nervous system. This enzyme, called *monoamine oxidase*, is responsible for gobbling up molecules of norepinephrine, serotonin, and several other neurotransmitters. Inactivating monoamine oxidase has the effect of increasing the amounts of these neurotransmitters in the nervous system, and this effect—in some as yet poorly understood way—may be how these medications alleviate the symptoms of depression. This class of pharmaceuticals is called *monoamine oxidase inhibitors, or MAOIs* (table 7.5).

There are two forms of monoamine oxidase in the body, MAO-A and MAO-B. Until recently, all of the pharmaceuticals used to treat depression were active in blocking MAO-A. In addition to its activity in the nervous system, MAO-A is also present in the lining of the intestine. Some naturally occurring substances in foods are close enough chemically to norepinephrine to need deactivation before they are absorbed into the bloodstream, and intestinal MAO-A serves this purpose. The importance of this becomes clear when I tell you that another name for norepinephrine is *adrenaline*—a name that is probably more familiar to you. Tyramine, an amino acid that has adrenaline-like effects on blood pressure and heart rate, is present in high enough concentrations in some foods to cause dangerous cardiovascular problems in individuals taking MAOIs. Numerous pharmaceuticals, including the ingredients of many over-the-counter remedies, also have adrenaline-like effects. People taking MAOIs therefore need to observe certain dietary restrictions and, even more importantly, must *scrupulously* read the labels of any over-the-counter medication they are considering—or better yet, consult their pharmacist before taking any pharmaceutical they buy over the counter.

MAOIs also interact with other medications that are prescribed or commonly used in emergency rooms for various problems. People taking MAOIs must be sure to inform all physicians who treat them that they are on this type of medication. And they should consider wearing an alert bracelet in case they are brought into an emergency room unconscious or otherwise unable to communicate.

TABLE 7.5. Monoamine oxidase inhibitors (MAOIs)	
Pharmaceutical name	*Brand name(s)*
Phenelzine	Nardil
Tranylcypromine	Parnate
Selegiline	Eldepryl, Emsam transdermal system*

*The selegiline patch.

Years after the MAOIs first became available, a pharmaceutical was developed that blocks primarily MAO-B. MAO-B is present almost entirely in the brain and is not involved in blocking tyramine absorption in the intestine. The big advantage of an MAO-B inhibitor over an MAO-A inhibitor, then, is that persons taking it don't have to be on a special diet. This drug, called *selegiline*, had already been used for the treatment of Parkinson's disease for several years. There were attempts at the time to use it as an antidepressant, but it was discovered that the required doses were so high when taken in pill form that selegiline affected *both* forms of MAO (A and B)—no advantage there! Then someone came up with the idea of making a selegiline *patch*, so that the drug is absorbed through the skin rather than taken orally. The patch turns out to have two important advantages. First, because the selegiline is more directly absorbed into the bloodstream, it can be given at a lower dose and maintain its specificity for MAO-B. Second, since it doesn't travel through the intestine, it doesn't affect the MAO-A located there nearly as much as the older MAOIs did. Thus, the selegiline patch is an easier way of taking an MAOI, with fewer side effects and less worry about tyramine-rich foods.

MAOIs can have other side effects, too. They can be stimulating and cause insomnia. For this reason, taking the oral preparations at bedtime should be avoided. Dizzy spells, especially when one suddenly gets up from lying down, can occur. MAOIs block a reflex that maintains blood pressure when we stand up, preventing the sudden drop in blood pressure on standing (called *orthostatic hypotension*) that causes light-headedness. Weight gain and sexual dysfunction are other side effects.

Because of these issues, MAOIs are most often prescribed to patients who have failed to benefit from other antidepressants. This said, they are sometimes uniquely effective, indeed, are "miracle drugs" for some patients. I think every psychiatrist I've ever spoken with has had the experience of effectively treating a particular patient with an MAOI after no other antidepressant had helped.

TREATING BIPOLAR DEPRESSION

The observation that antidepressants can cause manic symptoms in persons with bipolar disorder has been confirmed again and again. Perhaps more worrisome is the observation that antidepressants may cause an acceleration of the illness in some patients. Some persons with bipolar disorder experience increased cycling of their mood episodes and even switch to a period of rapid cycling.

In the late 1990s, the National Institute of Mental Health sponsored a large, multicenter study of the treatment of bipolar disorder called the Systematic Treatment Enhancement Program for Bipolar Disorder (STEP-BD).

Antidepressants and the Risk of Mania

In one of the first research papers on an antidepressant, "The Treatment of Depressive States with G 22355 (Imipramine Hydrochloride)," the author noted that "in individuals who are predisposed" the drug could "give rise to manic-like states or even a manic state." This observation has been thoroughly confirmed since this paper was published in 1958, and the "predisposed individuals" are now recognized to be persons with bipolar disorder.[*]

It is also clear that antidepressant do not have this effect on all patients with bipolar disorder. A rule of thumb seems to be that the more severe the manic or hypomanic symptoms that a patient has had previously, the higher the risk of developing manic symptoms from taking an antidepressant. Thus, bipolar I patients are at higher risk than are bipolar II patients.

Some antidepressants are more likely than others to trigger manic symptoms in a person with bipolar disorder. This is one proposed ranking of this risk:[†]

Higher risk of mania ↑ Tricyclic antidepressants

SNRIs

SSRIs

Lower risk Bupropion

[*]Roland Kuhn, "The Treatment of Depressive States with G 22355 (Imipramine Hydrochloride)," *American Journal of Psychiatry* 115 (1958): 461.

[†]R. M. Post, L. L. Altshuler, M. A. Frye, T. Suppes, A. J. Rush, P. E. Keck Jr., S. L. McElroy, K. D. Denicoff, G. S. Leverich, R. Kupka, and W. A. Nolen, "Rate of Switch in Bipolar Patients Prospectively Treated with Second-Generation Antidepressants as Augmentation to Mood Stabilizers," *Bipolar Disorders* 3, no. 5 (2001): 259–65.

This study enrolled more than four thousand people with bipolar disorder, followed them over several years while they were receiving treatment, and evaluated the success or failure of various interventions. One surprising finding was in a subgroup of 350 patients who developed depression during the course of the study. About half of these patients were then prescribed an antidepressant in addition to their mood stabilizer, while the others stayed on the mood stabilizer alone. At the end of about six months, antidepressant medications appeared to have offered no benefit whatsoever—nor did the patients who took an antidepressant have any more problems with manic symptoms than the patients who took only a mood stabilizer.[2] Now, this seems to fly in the face of decades of research and clinical experience demonstrating what I said at the beginning of this chapter—that some bipolar patients need, benefit from, and can safely take antidepressants. But it makes the point strongly that those patients are the exception, not the rule, and that most bipolar patients should probably avoid taking antidepressant medications.

Studies on the issue of increasing mania and rapid cycling indicate that some patients are at more risk than others of aggravating their condition

Beware of ACID

Another instructive finding from the STEP-BD study was that after patients with bipolar disorder take antidepressants and appear to recover from depression, some of them start having more problems getting to sleep and notice the feelings of tense uneasiness that psychiatrists call "dysphoria," along with a smoldering irritability. The STEP-BD researchers referred to this set of symptoms as "ACID," short for *antidepressant-associated chronic irritable dysphoria*, and they found that these patients were quite impaired by these symptoms. The researchers already suspected that antidepressants were the cause of this problem, so they looked through the records of STEP-BD patients with the triad of chronic irritability, dysphoria, and sleep disturbances, noting who had or had not taken an antidepressant along with a mood stabilizer. The results were unequivocal. They found that the patients with these symptoms who had taken an antidepressant outnumbered patients taking only a mood stabilizer by ten to one.*

*Post et al., "Rate of Switch"; and R. S. El-Mallakh, S. N. Ghaemi, K. Sagduyu, M. E. Thase, S. R. Wisniewski, A. A. Nierenberg, H. W. Zhang, T. A. Pardo, and G. Sachs (STEP-BD Investigators), "Antidepressant-Associated Chronic Irritable Dysphoria (ACID) in STEP-BD Patients," *Journal of Affective Disorders* 111, nos. 2-3 (2008): 372-77.

with antidepressant treatment. Unfortunately, it is not possible to say with certainty who is and who is not at risk. Bipolar I patients seem to be at greater risk than are bipolar II patients; women are at greater risk than men; and patients who already have a history of more rapid cycling—either more full-blown episodes or a tendency toward cyclothymia (continuous low-amplitude cycling) between full-blown episodes—are at greater risk. Moreover, a few studies indicate that some antidepressant medications seem to be safer than others—that is, less likely to precipitate mania (and, by implication, perhaps less likely to increase cycling).

So what do we conclude from all this? I think a reasonable approach is to recommend a cautious and closely observed trial of one of the safer antidepressants for patients who still have serious depression despite optimization of mood-stabilizer treatment, but only if they have never had a previous problem with an antidepressant. At the first sign of irritability, dysphoria, or sleep disturbance, strong consideration should be given to stopping the antidepressant. I think it's also fair to conclude that trying one antidepressant after another in bipolar patients should be avoided; the research literature really does support the idea that most bipolar patients will *not* benefit from an antidepressant.

Perhaps more than any other treatment issues, the questions surrounding the use of antidepressants in bipolar disorder emphasize the need for individualization of treatment for every patient. There are no hard-and-fast rules for when, why, or how to use an antidepressant for bipolar patients. Patient and physician need to communicate clearly and honestly about every aspect of symptoms and treatment to achieve the best treatment outcome.

―――――――――――― KEY TAKEAWAYS ――――――――――――

▶ The prescription of antidepressants to persons with bipolar is controversial and not without risk.

▶ There is significant research evidence that antidepressants can trigger mania, induce mixed states, and increase mood cycling in some patients with bipolar disorder.

▶ One of the results of the STEP-BD study was that *as a group*, patients with bipolar disorder do not benefit from antidepressants in the long term. However, there is likely a subgroup of bipolar patients who benefit from and can safely take antidepressants.

CHAPTER 8

New (and Old) Medications and Pipeline Drugs

I n the past decade, science has made almost unbelievable progress in understanding the intricate workings of the human brain. This means that, for the first time, pharmaceuticals are being developed based on how they interact with specific biological systems in the brain. Thanks to work in the fields of genetics and neuroscience, molecular pathways have been identified that seem to be involved in the development of the symptoms of mood disorders. New pharmaceutical agents are now often selected for testing because they are known to have certain molecular effects. In some cases, clinical trials are being carried out on older medications that have been used for decades to treat other medical problems. No one suspected that these pharmaceuticals might help persons with bipolar disorder, but they are substances that are known to work through some particular biochemical process that we now know can go awry in mood-disorder patients.

THE DOPE ON DOPAMINE

A number of recent studies support the idea that the neurotransmitter dopamine is important for mood regulation. One of the brain's main dopamine systems is concerned with coordination and movement, and so this molecule was pretty much ignored when it came to mood-disorders research. However, it has been known since the 1960s that problems in the dopamine system are the cause of Parkinson's disease, a progressive neurological disorder characterized by problems with movement and balance, so quite a few pharmaceuticals that work through this system have been developed over the years.[1]

Starting in the 1980s, several different lines of research demonstrated that dopamine circuitry is important for the brain's pleasure/reward response, suggesting that the dopamine system might be important as a cause for depression. So it is not surprising that drugs affecting dopamine circuitry (called *dopaminergic* drugs) appear to be beneficial for some patients with bipolar disorder, especially bipolar depression.

Table 8.1. Dopaminergic Medications

Anti-Parkinsonism medication:
- Pramipexole (Mirapex)

Stimulant medications:
- Amphetamine (Adderall)
- Lisdexamphetamine (Vyvanse)
- Methylphenidate (Ritalin, Concerta, and others)

Stimulant alternatives
- Modafinil (Provigil)
- Armodafinil (Nuvigil)

Pramipexole (Mirapex)

This medication, approved for the treatment of Parkinson's disease, has been studied since the early 2000s for the treatment of bipolar depression and as of this writing is the dopaminergic medication that has been the most extensively researched. A 2019 review of five different studies with a total of more than five hundred volunteers found that nearly two-thirds of patients had at least some benefit from pramipexole.[2] These studies included volunteers with unipolar as well as bipolar depression, but another review published in 2013 that looked at trials in only bipolar patients found similar results.[3] In most of these studies, pramipexole was an add-on medication, taken along with other medications. The main side-effect problem is nausea, which can be minimized by starting at a low dose and increasing slowly.

STIMULANT AND STIMULANT-LIKE MEDICATIONS

Another class of dopaminergic drugs, usually referred to as *stimulant* medications, was first developed in the 1930s. The effects of these medications include an improvement in concentration and attention, which is why they are used to treat attention-deficit hyperactivity disorder. They also increase energy level and combat fatigue. This latter effect prompted psychiatrists to prescribe stimulants to depressed patients almost as soon as they became available. However, while the stimulants indeed help with energy and motivation, they appear to have little effect on mood.

Researching New Treatment Approaches: The Tyranny of the Marketplace

After reading about the benefits of pramipexole for bipolar depression, you may be wondering why you don't see commercials for it on TV, like you do with other medications for bipolar disorder. After all, it's effective, safe, and, because it is an older drug, inexpensive.

The reason that you don't see commercials for pramipexole is captured in that last word—*inexpensive*. It's the same reason why no pharmaceutical company representative will be paying a visit to your doctor to tell her about the advantages of pramipexol so that she'll start prescribing it.

Because the patent for pramipexole expired years ago, several generic pharmaceutical companies manufacture it, and the competition among them has the effect of making the drug so inexpensive and the profit margin so slim that promoting the drug is just not worth it.

The efficacy of ketamine for the treatment of bipolar depression was discovered at the National Institutes of Health several decades before Spravato became available for patients. It was only when Johnson & Johnson was able to chemically tweak ketamine a bit and develop a new intranasal delivery system that they were able to patent Spravato and, without competition from other companies, provide it at a price acceptable to shareholders.

The vast majority of research on medications is done by pharmaceutical companies, for whom profit is a significant factor—some may argue, the only important factor. This was not always the case—much of the research on lithium was done without industry support. But I think it's fair to say that if its benefits had been discovered in today's funding environment, lithium might never have reached patients at all.

Some of the slack in drug research is taken up by private nonprofit foundations, such as the Stanley Medical Research Foundation (www.stanley research.org/) and the Brain and Behavior Research Foundation (www.bbrfoundation.org/), which award grants to study interventions that don't necessarily promise big profits.

But only "Big Pharma" has the resources to invest the tens of millions of dollars required to get FDA approval and bring a new treatment to market, meaning that only if a drug or device can be patented—and priced accordingly—is that intervention likely to become widely available.

A related group of drugs that share some of the characteristics of the original stimulant medications and have some of the same effects on concentration and energy were developed in the 1980s and of these, modafinil has been studied the most for the treatment of depression. Several studies have been published on modafinil for patients with bipolar depression and showed promising results.

KETAMINE/ESKETAMINE (SPRAVATO)

In the mid-1990s, neuroscientists who were attempting to unravel the mysteries of how antidepressants work discovered that most of them, regardless of whether they work through serotonin, norepinephrine, or other neurotransmitters, all decrease activity in another chemical system in the brain, a circuit that uses glutamate as its chemical messenger, specifically, a subset of glutamate receptors called NMDA (N-methyl-D-aspartate) receptors. This suggested that a molecule that blocked NMDA receptors might have antidepressant effects. Just such a molecule happened to be available in the form of *ketamine*, a drug that had been developed as an anesthetic in the 1960s and used safely as a surgical anesthetic for several decades. In 2000, research scientists at Yale administered ketamine intravenously to four volunteers suffering from depression, and the results were remarkable: volunteers experienced a dramatic decrease in their symptoms of depression *within several hours of getting the infusion*.

Fast forward nearly two decades to 2019, when a form of ketamine called esketamine (Spravato) that is administered by a nasal spray was approved by the FDA to treat patients with depression who had failed to respond to antidepressants.

Although not currently labeled by the FDA for the treatment of bipolar depression, several small studies using the parent compound, ketamine, showed positive results, and research is proceeding apace to determine whether esketamine is also effective in treating bipolar depression.

Several features separate ketamine and esketamine from any other available treatments for bipolar disorder. First, they appear to work through a mechanism that is entirely different from those of currently available treatments; many patients with major depression who did not benefit from available medications for treating their depression have gotten significantly better with this treatment, and there is every reason to hope that the same will be true for patients with bipolar depression. Second, the benefits of these drugs become apparent to patients within hours, not weeks.

This raises the possibility of using ketamine or esketamine as a first-line treatment that provides almost immediate relief from symptoms of severe depression as patients start another medication, such as lithium or lamotrigine, to keep symptoms from returning.

These drugs are so new for the treatment of mood disorders that how to prescribe them (To which patients? When? Alone or with other drugs?) are questions yet to be answered. One thing is clear, however: ketamine and esketamine are very likely to become very important drugs for the treatment of bipolar depression.

Old Drugs, New Uses

Pramipexole and ketamine are only two of numerous older pharmaceuticals that are being repurposed for the treatment of mood disorders. Several preparations of the cough suppressant dextromethorphan are being tested for the treatment of major depression. Neudexta, a combination of dextromethorphan and quinidine (a drug used to treat irregular heartbeat) was approved by the FDA in 2011 to treat a neurological condition called pseudobulbar affective disorder. Dextromethorphan had the same effects on a subset of neuronal receptors as ketamine and, like that drug, has been found to have fast-acting antidepressant effects. As of this writing, another dextromethorphan-containing combination, this time with the antidepressant bupropion, is being trialed by Axsome Therapeutics.

There are indications that inflammatory processes may be illness-sustaining factors in some cases of mood disorders, and a variety of anti-inflammatory drugs are being researched. These include celecoxib (Celebrex) and infliximab (Remicade and Inflectra). Drugs that reduce inflammation indirectly, such as cholesterol-lowering drugs and insulin-enhancing agents, are being investigated as well.

Infusions of scopolamine, an anti–motion sickness agent, showed rapid-onset antidepressant effects in several studies.

Only time will tell if the right combination of efficacy and profitability will bring any of these interventions to patients with bipolar disorder.*

*M. E. Ebada, "Drug Repurposing May Generate Novel Approaches to Treating Depression," *Journal of Pharmacy and Pharmacology* 69, no. 11 (2017): 1428–36.

THE PROMISE OF NEUROSTEROIDS

You are likely familiar with the term *steroids* but probably for all the wrong reasons. Yes, some athletes and body-builders abuse steroid compounds related to the natural male hormone testosterone to increase muscle mass, but the term *steroid* refers to a large group of hormones that are important regulators of a variety of bodily functions ranging from glucose (blood sugar) metabolism to the body's salt balance, immune system regulation, and sexual functioning.

FIGURE 8.1. Chemical structure of the neurosteroid allopregnanolone

Note the four rings in the molecular structure, a feature shared by all steroid compounds.

A subcategory of steroids, called the *neurosteroids*, is found only in the brain and has important functions there, including mood-regulating functions. Research at the National Institute of Mental Health in the 1990s showed that the level of one of the neurosteroids, *brexanolone*, increases in the brain during pregnancy but then drops after birth, triggering depression symptoms in some women. Researchers hypothesized that giving brexanolone to women suffering from *postpartum depression* might treat this disorder, and clinical studies quickly bore this out. Now available as Zulresso, a pharmaceutical version developed by Sage Therapeutics, brexanolone is given as an intravenous infusion over several days. Similar to the antidepressant effect of ketamine, depressed volunteers who received brexanolone reported a significant improvement in mood within hours.[4] Brexanolone has been approved only for the treatment of postpartum depression by the FDA. However, its success story has triggered research on other neurosteroids and the development of other new neurosteroid medications, several of which are being evaluated for the treatment of bipolar depression.

Results of a small 2014 study using another neurosteroid, pregnenolone, to treat bipolar depression showed promising results.[5] In 2018, the same company that developed brexanolone for postpartum depression announced that it was evaluating a synthetic neurosteroid that it developed, zuranolone, for the treatment of bipolar depression in both bipolar I and bipolar II patients.[6]

Like ketamine and esketamine, the neurosteroids are an entirely new group of drugs, and they appear to treat mood disorders through a mechanism that is completely different from that of any of the pharmaceuticals that have been available up until now. The few clinical trials on their efficacy in bipolar disorder have been quite encouraging.

In 2012, a paper titled "GABAergic Neuroactive Steroids: A New Frontier in Bipolar Disorders?" was published and concluded optimistically, "Current evidence suggests that the investigation of neuroactive steroids on mental disorders might open new frontiers in the investigation of the etiology and treatment of mood disorders, particularly bipolar disorder."[7]

LOOKING AHEAD

In the past decade, science has made almost unbelievable progress in understanding the intricate workings of the human brain. This new understanding means that, for the very first time, pharmaceuticals are being developed based on how they interact with specific biological systems in the brain. Thanks to work in the fields of genetics and neuroscience, molecular pathways have been identified that seem to be involved in the development of the symptoms of mood disorders. Many new pharmaceutical agents now being tested have been selected because they are known to have certain molecular effects, drugs that, for now at least, bear only the code names assigned to them by pharmaceutical companies, names like MRK-016 and SAGE-217. In some cases, clinical trials are being carried out on older medications that have been used for decades to treat other medical problems. No one suspected that these pharmaceuticals might help persons with bipolar disorder, but they are substances that are known to work through some particular biochemical process that we now know can go awry in mood-disorder patients.

The days of accidentally stumbling upon effective treatments for bipolar disorder, as in the case of lithium, are coming to an end. Older drugs are being redeployed, and entirely new drugs are being developed based on knowledge of the biochemistry of bipolar disorder. After decades of nearly aimless searching in the dark for new treatments, bright lights are indeed on the horizon.

────────────────── KEY TAKEAWAYS ──────────────────

▶ Thanks to recent discoveries in genetics and neuroscience, new medication approaches to treating bipolar disorder are being developed based on a better understanding of its causes.

▶ The discovery of the importance of the brain's dopamine system for mood regulation has led to the use of several old medications, for example, pramipexole and stimulant medications, for bipolar depression.

▶ Ketamine and esketamine (Spravato), an old and a new medication, have been found to be very helpful for treatment-resistant depression and may find a use in the treatment of bipolar depression as well.

▶ The neurosteroids are a new group of compounds being tested in bipolar patients, with promising early results.

CHAPTER 9

More Medications, Hormones, and Dietary Supplements

M any other pharmaceutical agents have proved helpful in the treat-ment of bipolar disorder. Some are *symptomatic treatments*, mean-ing that they treat symptoms rather than the underlying disorder and therefore are usually used for only a short time. Others are medications that affect functioning in another body system that is important for normal mood regulation.

Sleeplessness and anxiety are common problems for persons with mood disorders. As we will see in chapter 15, sleep deprivation is often acutely destabilizing for persons with mood disorders. Anxiety raises the levels of stress hormones like cortisol in the body, and therefore keeping this un-comfortable symptom in check is an important part of staying well.

MEDICATIONS FOR ANXIETY AND SLEEP DISTURBANCES

Benzodiazepine Medications

The benzodiazepine medications represented a major advance in the treatment of psychiatric symptoms when they were first developed, and they continue to be widely prescribed (table 9.1). They often have a place in the treatment of bipolar disorder because they are highly effective for the treatment of anxiety and insomnia and, in higher doses, are safe and effective sedatives. If this sounds too good to be true and you're wonder-ing if there's a hidden drawback, there is. These medications can be mis-used; it's possible to become psychologically dependent on them and even physically addicted to them. (Withdrawal symptoms in persons taking high doses of these medications can include serious problems such as seizures.)

Moreover, their sedating effects decrease over time, and after several weeks of use, their effectiveness as tranquilizers decreases. For these reasons benzodiazepines are best thought of as temporary measures. Nevertheless, there are patients who benefit from and can safely take these medications over the longer term.

Benzodiazepines really have two main uses in treating bipolar disorder: they are used to treat patients who are very sick and to treat patients who are doing very well. The explanation for this seeming contradiction is in the doses used and how the medications are combined with other medications. In acutely manic patients, the short-acting benzodiazepine lorazepam (Ativan) can be an effective short-term tranquilizer, especially in combination with a typical antipsychotic medication like haloperidol (Haldol). This combination is familiar to psychiatrists working in emergency settings, because it works quickly and effectively in calming even the most agitated patients. An acutely ill manic patient, perhaps delusional and agitated, who hasn't slept for days can be asleep less than an hour after receiving this combination, especially by injection. The longer-acting benzodiazepine clonazepam (Klonopin) has also been used and extensively studied in the treatment of acute manic symptoms, and it appears to be another effective adjunct medication.

These medications are not mood stabilizers and are not effective in treating hallucinations or delusions, but as antianxiety medications they are unsurpassed. Remember that before effective psychiatric medications became available, patients with severe mania died of the physical stress of the manic state. By simply slowing manic patients down for a few hours or days until antipsychotic medications and mood-stabilizing medications start working, benzodiazepines can be literally lifesaving.

TABLE 9.1. **Benzodiazepine medications**

Pharmaceutical name	Brand name
Alprazolam	Xanax
Chlordiazepoxide	Librium
Clonazepam	Klonopin
Clorazepate	Tranxene
Diazepam	Valium
Lorazepam	Ativan

Note: These medications are best thought of as temporary agents and are frequently prescribed for occasional "as-needed" use.

At the other end of the spectrum of illness severity, patients who are not having severe mood symptoms can safely take these medications for anxiety symptoms and insomnia. During periods of unavoidable psychological stress, such as after the death of a loved one, benzodiazepine medications can help with insomnia and lessen the psychological tension that may bring on mood symptoms in bipolar patients. It's important to emphasize here that these medications should *not* be used as substitutes for making changes to chronically stressful situations. A person who finds that he feels the need to take a sedative to deal with everyday situations is well on his way to psychological dependence on tranquilizers, medication abuse, and addiction. We'll discuss this in more depth in chapter 19.

Another way these medications are used is to treat patients who have anxiety disorders. Anxiety disorders (such as recurrent panic attacks) are effectively treated with benzodiazepines. The connections between mood disorders and anxiety disorders are poorly understood, but there are certainly some people who need treatment for both. The treatment of panic disorder and other severe anxiety disorders sometimes involves taking benzodiazepine medications on a longer-term basis, but prolonged use of benzodiazepines is the exception rather than the rule in treating bipolar disorders.[1]

Most people can take these medications safely, but a minority get into serious trouble with them. When taken longer term, they can produce *tolerance*: needing higher doses to get the same effect, and escalating doses can very quickly lead to psychological and physical addiction.

The elderly are especially prone to problems with these medications, which increase the risk of memory problems, falls, hip fractures, and motor vehicle accidents.

Benzodiazepine medications are usually safe and effective, especially in the short term, but there are significant risks, especially when they are taken for prolonged periods or in high doses.

Novel Anxiety Medications

Two medications developed as treatments for epilepsy have proved to be helpful in patients with anxiety problems. Both are active in a neuroreceptor system that is known to be involved with anxiety, the GABA pathway (for gamma aminobutyric acid), and their names reflect this: *gaba*pentin (Neurontin) and pre*gaba*lin (Lyrica). These medications have several advantages for treating the anxiety that can be associated with bipolar disorder. The first is that there is little or no risk of developing a psychological dependence on them. Gabapentin is not a "controlled substance" in FDA parlance, and although pregabalin is, it has been assigned the lowest possible risk rating, schedule V (other schedule V drugs include cough preparations with small amounts of codeine). Also, gabapentin and pregabalin can be taken over the longer term without losing effectiveness. For these reasons, they can be helpful for persons with prolonged anxiety problems that have no clear precipitant, a pattern that is often called *generalized anxiety*.[2]

"Z-drugs"

This group of medications gets its name from the fact that several start with the letter *z*. Zolpidem was the first of these medications, introduced in 1992, and zaleplon followed soon after. Zopiclone is another (it is not available in the United States).

The Z-drugs were derived from the benzodiazepines and share many of their features. However, they are more specific to sleep circuitry than are the benzodiazepines. These medications are prescribed almost exclusively for insomnia because they are absorbed rapidly and are quickly metabolized by the body. This makes them nearly ideal sleep medications, as they work fast and don't stay around too long, meaning that a next-morning "hangover" feeling is uncommon. The Z-drugs are somewhat less likely than benzodiazepines to cause rebound insomnia when patients stop taking them and therefore are less likely to cause dependence. They are also less likely to lose their effectiveness over time (tolerance).[3]

Like benzodiazepines, however, they can be misused, and it is possible for people to become addicted to them, though this is rare unless they are taken in much higher doses than recommended.

The elderly are more sensitive to these medications, and, as with benzodiazepines, they increase the risk of falls, hip fractures, and motor vehicle accidents.

TABLE 9.2. Z-drugs (non-benzodiazepines)

Pharmaceutical name	Brand name
Eszopiclone	Lunesta
Zaleplon	Sonata
Zopiclone*	Imovane, Zimovane
Zolpidem	Ambien, Ambien CR, Intermezzo, and others

*Not commercially available in the United States.

Melatonin

Melatonin can be thought of as a sleep hormone. Most of the body's melatonin is produced in and released into the bloodstream from the pineal gland, a small organ located deep within the brain. It also happens to be synthesized by a variety of plants and is found in the seeds of sunflowers and coriander.

Although melatonin can be quite helpful in treating sleep problems, it is not a sedative or "sleeping pill," meaning that it doesn't put you sleep by tamping down brain functioning like the benzodiazepines and Z-drugs do. Instead, melatonin tells the sleep center of the brain that it's time to start the sleep process. Interestingly, in animals that are active at night, such as the rat, melatonin has the opposite effect, essentially giving a "wake up!" signal. Thus, melatonin should be considered a sleep *regulator*. In addition to regulating the sleep cycle, it also regulates several other bodily processes that operate on a twenty-four-hour cycle, or to use the scientific term, processes that show a *circadian rhythm*. The word *circadian* derives from the Latin words *circa* (about) and *dies* (day).

Taking melatonin essentially boosts the brain's "go to sleep" signal— and in a very natural way, as it is the same molecule that the body produces. Taking melatonin has been shown to synchronize the circadian rhythm and improve the onset, duration, and quality of sleep.[4] I often recommend melatonin as the first thing to try for sleep problems, as it has none of the problems associated with benzodiazepines and the Z-drugs. Melatonin does not cause tolerance, dependence, or adverse effects on alertness or mood the following day (the hangover effect). Most sleep experts suggest taking 1 to 3 mg of immediate-release melatonin (i.e., avoiding slow-release preparations) two hours before bedtime for insomnia, because this dose and timing appears to best mimic the normal physiological cycle of the body.[5]

There is a pharmaceutical that mimics the effects of melatonin called *ramelteon* (Rozerem). Ramelteon has been shown to be "modestly effective" in improving sleep parameters, but whether it is superior to melatonin has not been tested.[6]

Melatonin: The Brain's "Go to Sleep" Hormone

The pineal gland releases its hormone, melatonin, into the bloodstream in a daily cycle that follows the light/dark cycle. The timing of this cycle is transmitted to the pineal gland from a collection of brain cells called the *suprachismatic nuclei* (SCN) that functions as the body's internal clock. The SCN has been called the brain's *Zeitgeber*, a German word meaning "time-giver," and is responsible for signaling the time of day to the brain and other organs. The SCN, in turn, is reset in the morning when bright daytime light falls on the light-sensitive cells of the eye.

As bedtime approaches, the SCN signals the pineal gland to increase its release of melatonin, and the level rises in the bloodstream. This rise signals other areas of the brain involved with sleep to initiate the sleep process. The melatonin level then starts falling at about 4 a.m. and stays low as long as bright light falls on the retina. The first light of the day resets the *Zeitgeber*, and the cycle starts again.

FIGURE 9.1. Melatonin levels in the bloodstream

The evening rise of the level of melatonin in the bloodstream signals the brain to initiate sleep. The level then falls through the night and is lowest during the daylight hours.

Illustration by Jenna Macfarlane

THYROID HORMONES

In several sections of this book, I'm going to talk about the interrelationships of mood and hormones. The pulsing daily rhythms of melatonin from the pineal gland that may be involved with the mood changes of seasonal affective disorder (SAD), the mood fluctuations that can follow changing levels of female reproductive hormones (important in understanding postpartum mood symptoms and premenstrual syndromes), the stress hormones secreted by the adrenal gland—all these hormonal changes seem to be important in the regulation of mood. But perhaps the most important hormones in this respect are the thyroid hormones.

The thyroid gland plays a major role in the body's energy regulation. Too little thyroid gland activity leads to sluggishness and weight gain, and too much leads to metabolic overdrive—rapid pulse, nervous energy, and anxiety. While the precise role of thyroid hormones in the regulation of mood remains unclear, it's clear that normal thyroid functioning is essential for effective treatment of mood disorders. Put another way, if a patient's mood symptoms don't respond to the usual treatments or if a treatment that has been effective seems to lose its effectiveness, a thyroid problem, especially abnormally low thyroid functioning (hypothyroidism), should be suspected.

Several studies have shown that hypothyroidism is surprisingly common in patients with rapid-cycling bipolar disorder. When one group of scientists tested for thyroid abnormalities in stored blood samples from almost four thousand patients who had been hospitalized for psychiatric problems over a period of four years, they found a high association between thyroid abnormalities and a diagnosis of rapid-cycling bipolar disorder.[7]

But it is also clear that some patients with bipolar disorder whose thyroid hormone levels are in the "normal range" when blood tests are done can nevertheless benefit from treatment with thyroid medications. Studies have demonstrated that many patients with bipolar depression symptoms that are not responding to treatment have thyroid function that is "normal" by the usual criteria, but blood tests show them to be in what might be called the "low normal" or even "barely normal" range.[8] It may be that depressed individuals need a higher level of thyroid hormones than do those who are not depressed. Perhaps the extra thyroid hormone somehow makes these patients more responsive to other treatments. Patients who have a partial response to lithium or other mood stabilizers may have better control of their mood symptoms when a small dose of thyroid replacement hormone is added, even if their thyroid hormone levels are normal. As a paper on treating rapid-cycling bipolar disorder put it, "Normal thyroid [blood test results] should not discourage the clinician from pursuing thyroid supplementation" in bipolar patients.[9]

Notice that I haven't used the term *thyroid medication* in this discussion. That is because it has been possible for many years to synthetically produce the exact same molecules that the thyroid gland itself naturally produces. (Hence the brand name, Synthroid, of the most commonly prescribed brand of levothyroxine.)[10] What dose of hormone to prescribe is determined by measuring hormone levels in the blood, something that should be done several times a year for anyone who takes a thyroid hormone replacement.

HERBAL PREPARATIONS AND NUTRITIONAL SUPPLEMENTS

There are some nutrients that we must include in our diet to remain healthy. These are compounds that our body cannot manufacture but are nevertheless necessary for normal cellular functioning. The most familiar of these are, of course, the *vitamins*, compounds manufactured by some plants and animals but not by humans. Their name, from the Latin word *vita* meaning "life," indicates just how important to health they are. Unless we eat foods that contain the vitamins we need, serious illness results. Scurvy, beriberi, and pellagra are three illnesses—now, thankfully, unfamiliar—that result from deficiencies of vitamin C, vitamin B1, and niacin, respectively. All these illnesses have significant central nervous system symptoms, especially B1 deficiency, which causes severe central nervous system degeneration.

There are other naturally occurring substances that our bodies are not very good at producing but that are important for health. These are substances that modern diets, as opposed to ancient human diets, tend not to include in the amounts that some believe are necessary for optimal health. A good example of these substances are the *essential fatty acids*, a collection of complex fat molecules that are found in some vegetables and other plant sources (such as flaxseed) and in large amounts in some fish. Nutritionists have long touted the health benefits of diets rich in seafood, and the lower incidence of breast cancer and heart disease in the Japanese population has been attributed to such a diet.

Botanicals are plant-derived naturally occurring substances that have pharmaceutical effects in the body; that is, although they have no nutritional value, they interact with some biological system in the body so as to treat a symptom or an illness. A good example of this group is *digitalis*, derived from the foxglove plant (*Digitalis purpura*), which happens to be an effective treatment for heart failure. It is thought that foxglove produces this chemical in its tissues as protection against animals and insects. Digitalis is fatal in high doses, but tiny amounts have beneficial effects. Similar plant "toxins" form the basis of many modern pharmaceuticals, for example, pain medications from the opium poppy and the antimalaria drug quinine from the bark of the cinchona tree.

The FDA tends to be reluctant to regulate naturally occurring substances as pharmaceuticals. Instead, they are considered "nutritional supplements" and are regulated as foods, even if the manufacturing process takes place in a pharmaceutical manufacturing facility and doesn't involve food or plants or anything one would think of as "natural."

OMEGA-3 FATTY ACIDS AND FISH OIL

Some evidence suggests that essential fatty acids, especially a subgroup called *omega-3 fatty acids*, may be useful in the treatment of mood disorders, especially bipolar disorder. The particular compounds thought to have the most health benefits have tongue-twisting names typical of complex organic compounds: eicosapentaenoic acid (EPA) and docosahexaenoic acid (DHA).

Numerous studies have indicated that omega-3 fatty acids, taken as fish-oil capsules, are beneficial for individuals with mood disorders. A review article that analyzed five studies in persons with bipolar depression concluded that there is "strong evidence that bipolar depression may be improved by the adjunctive use of omega-3."[11] Studies of omega-3 in mania have not shown any benefit.

Omega-3 fatty acids are incorporated into cell membranes in association with molecules that are known to be involved in cell signaling. They seem to be active at some of the same points in cellular signaling mechanisms where lithium and valproate are thought to work. Since valproate is, after all, a *synthetic* fatty acid, the idea that natural fatty acids might have benefits in mood disorders shouldn't seem strange at all. Other circumstantial evidence has been cited to support the importance of omega-3 fatty acids for good mental health. Archaeological and epidemiological studies suggest that modern humans consume much less food that is rich in fatty acids than ancient peoples did and that we may be deficient in these important compounds compared with our ancestors. This fact, combined with evidence that the prevalence of depression is increasing and the age of onset of mood disorders is decreasing, has been cited as further evidence of a link between these important compounds and mental health. Omega-3 fatty acid therapy is an adjunctive treatment, added to other agents such as lithium; it should *not* be substituted for proven treatments. However, given the apparent low risk of these compounds, supplementation of standard treatments for mood disorders with omega-3 preparations under the supervision of one's physician is an option some patients will want to explore.

N-ACETYL CYSTEINE

The health benefits of foods that are high in *antioxidants* are well known. Sales of green tea, which is high in naturally occurring antioxidants, for example, have soared in recent years, and green tea has been studied as an adjunctive treatment for everything from diabetes to cancer.

So just what are antioxidants? Although oxygen is a vital ingredient for biological functioning, it is highly reactive chemically, combining with just about anything in a reaction called oxygenation, often with untoward results. When oxygen rapidly combines with the organic compounds in gasoline, we call it "fire." When oxygen combines with various molecules in the body, a much less dramatic but still damaging process called *oxidative damage* can occur. Plants and animals all have substances, the antioxidants, molecules that essentially prowl about scooping up these damaging oxygen-containing molecules when they occur. You can think of oxidative stress as a kind of biological overheating, requiring antioxidants to step in and cool things down.

In humans, the main antioxidant in the brain is a substance called *glutathione*, which the body manufactures by combining several ingredients, including N-acetyl cysteine. High levels of oxidative stress deplete glutathione in the brain, but since glutathione is not well absorbed from the gut, the best way to increase levels is to take in the more easily absorbed NAC. Intravenous NAC is routinely used to halt the oxidative damage to the liver caused by overdoses of acetaminophen (Tylenol) as well as in other situations when the antioxidants of the body are overwhelmed.

A placebo-controlled study of adjunctive NAC (that is, as an add-on to standard medications such as lithium) in bipolar depression found a significant benefit, and a follow-up study in which all the subjects took NAC for another two months showed continued benefit.[12] Like omega-3, NAC is clearly an adjunctive medication, the benefits of which should be considered promising rather than firmly established. Nevertheless, it is an option some may wish to explore—again, with the guidance of their physician.

ST. JOHN'S WORT

Hypericum perforatum, commonly known as St. John's wort, is one of about three hundred species of shrubby perennial plants of the genus *Hypericum* with bright yellow flowers; the plants grow in most of the temperate regions of the world. Teas and other extracts of St. John's wort have been recommended by herbalists for centuries to treat everything from insomnia to the painful viral skin infection called shingles. In the late 1980s hypericum (*H. perforatum*) was investigated as a possible treatment for HIV infection when it was found to have activity against retroviruses, but its activity unfortunately did not translate into clinical usefulness for this disease.

A 1996 article in the *British Medical Journal* that systematically reviewed twenty-three studies involving a total of 1,757 patients concluded that "extracts of hypericum are more effective than placebo for the treatment of mild to moderately severe depressive disorders."[13] More recent studies have been less encouraging. When St. John's wort was compared with a placebo in two hundred patients who had been rigorously evaluated and diagnosed with major depression, the herbal preparation was no better than the placebo in treating depression. This study concluded that "the results do not support significant antidepressant or antianxiety effects for St. John's wort when compared to placebo in a clinical sample of depressed patients" and that "persons with major depression should not be treated with St. John's wort, given the morbidity and mortality risks of untreated or ineffectively treated major depression."[14] In a follow-up study, the same researchers reported that when the individuals who had not responded to St. John's wort were given standard antidepressants, most of them improved, suggesting that the herbal preparation had failed not because these were "treatment-resistant" patients but simply because St. John's wort wasn't effective against their depression.[15]

Questions about the effectiveness of St. John's wort are one thing, but reports of it making things worse are unfortunately not hard to find:

A 53-year-old man without prior psychiatric treatment presented to our clinic with depression. His history was significant for hypomania cycling into depression every June and December for 20 years, consistent with a diagnosis of bipolar II disorder. . . . Of note, his 18-year-old son is treated for bipolar I disorder with lithium. He had no medical history and had never been prescribed psychotropics, although in May 1998, he bought a bottle of St. John's wort with the hope that it could improve his mood.

Shortly after taking St. John's wort 900 mg/day, he noticed a surge in self-esteem. His thoughts raced, he was more talkative, his sleep decreased, his sex drive increased, he spent money excessively, and he drove faster than usual. Two months later, his behavior changed dramatically. He missed work because he just "didn't care," he angrily lashed out at his wife, he shoplifted from the supermarket, and he surfed the Internet for romantic intrigue. He communicated with many women by e-mail, later met these women, and engaged in unprotected sexual relationships with as many as four women in 1 week. He regarded these affairs as a "hobby," lacking any appreciation for their impact on his marriage. He had visual illusions and believed that people at work were trying to undermine him. Although he had experienced mood elevations in the past, he explained that this episode was particularly long and severe and admits that he was doing things which "didn't make sense."

Subsequently, he reduced his SJW to 300 mg/day, and his depression recurred. His treatment team discontinued the SJW and initiated lithium [and] he reports steady improvement in mood.[16]

I think it's fair to say that St. John's wort isn't good enough as an antidepressant to help persons with bipolar disorder, but it's enough of an antidepressant to cause problems for them and so is best avoided, except perhaps in the garden.

—————————————— KEY TAKEAWAYS ——————————————

▶ Benzodiazepines and Z-drugs are often prescribed to individuals with bipolar disorder to treat insomnia and anxiety. Although effective, there are risks associated with them, especially if used longer term.

▶ Melatonin is the body's sleep hormone and can be effective for insomnia.

▶ Robust thyroid functioning is necessary for mood disorder treatments to be effective; this sometimes means taking thyroid hormones.

▶ A number of nutraceuticals and botanicals have been shown to help patients with bipolar disorder as add-ons to medications. St. John's wort, however, should be avoided, as it has been reported to trigger manic symptoms.

CHAPTER 10

Brain-Stimulation
Treatments

I f you're unfamiliar with the term *brain-stimulation treatments*, you're not alone. It's a relatively new term for a variety of treatment techniques, one of which has been around for many decades but several of which are quite new. These techniques involve using tiny electrical impulses to stimulate areas of the brain. The oldest of these is electroconvulsive therapy, in which an electrical current is applied directly to the scalp while the patient is under general anesthesia. Newer techniques use much smaller electrical impulses and require no anesthesia. The details of how these treatments work are still far from certain, but they all appear to treat mood disorders by affecting the levels of electrical activity in certain areas of the brain, areas that are underactive or overactive during episodes of abnormal mood. They bring activity levels into a more normal balance, in much the same way that tiny electrical impulses are used to reregulate heart rhythms in individuals who have a cardiac pacemaker.

ELECTROCONVULSIVE THERAPY (ECT)

Although the effectiveness of electroconvulsive therapy (ECT) in mood disorders was not a completely accidental discovery, its original theoretical basis has since been shown to have no validity, so the development of modern ECT, like so many other treatments in psychiatry, was serendipitous. In the early 1930s the Hungarian physician Joseph Ladislas von Meduna proposed that there was a mutual antagonism between epilepsy and schizophrenia: patients who suffered from epilepsy did not suffer from schizophrenia and vice versa. Modern research has shown that this is not the case, but von Meduna was convinced of the truth of this assertion on the basis of his microscopic postmortem examination of the brains of persons with the two conditions. He conducted animal experiments attempting to find a way to produce seizure activity artificially. In 1935 he published a paper reporting a dramatic improvement in symptoms after artificially inducing seizures in several patients who suffered from what he thought to be schizophrenia (in retrospect, it's probable that at least some had severe mood disorders with psychotic symptoms). Von Meduna used injections to produce seizures, but several years later two Italian psychiatrists reported that seizures could be produced by briefly passing a low-voltage electrical current through the skull by means of electrodes applied to the scalp. Ugo Cerletti and Lucio Bini first developed their technique in animals and then tried it on several patients with "schizophrenia," and they also reported remarkable success.

Although patients with schizophrenia do indeed often show improvement in some of their symptoms after these treatments (catatonia is one), it quickly became apparent that it was the severely depressed patients who showed the most dramatic improvement—improvement that was little short of miraculous.

The Ups and Downs of ECT: Why the Bad Rap?

In his famous textbook of psychiatry, Emil Kraepelin described patients in a catatonic state from psychotic depression: "The patients lie in bed taking no interest in anything. They betray no pronounced emotion; they are mute, inaccessible; they pass their [bowel movements] under them; they stare straight in front of them with [a] vacant expression . . . like a mask and with wide open eyes."* In the 1940s, after receiving "electroshock" treatments, psychiatrists observed that these patients recovered completely from their symptoms within a matter of days. The most recent major breakthrough in the treatment of psychiatric problems—the discovery of the Wassermann test for syphilis in 1906—now seemed almost insignificant compared with this astonishing, even miraculous new therapeutic technique. Naturally, interest in ECT spread quickly around the globe.

But ECT's success was also nearly its downfall. Like many other seemingly miraculous treatments, it was overprescribed at first and probably was administered to many hundreds of persons it had little chance of helping. It's important to remember, however, that those were desperate times in psychiatry. With the discovery of antipsychotic medications nearly a decade and the discovery of antidepressants nearly two decades into the future, "little chance" of helping was better than no chance at all. Since, as we shall see,

(continued)

*Emil Kraepelin, *Manic-Depressive Insanity and Paranoia*, trans. R. M. Barclay, ed. G. M. Robertson (1921; reprint, New York: Arno Press, 1976), 97.

ECT is a highly effective treatment for mania, some institutions were inclined to use it for any highly agitated patients and sometimes on merely uncooperative ones (a misuse that was dramatized—with many inaccuracies unfortunately thrown in—in the film *One Flew Over the Cuckoo's Nest*). Another negative factor was that in the first decade or so after its development, ECT could have some very serious complications. An epileptic seizure is a violent event: all the muscles of the body contract simultaneously for a few moments, sometimes with such force that broken bones result. Breathing stops as well, and heart-rhythm irregularities can occur.

The nearly indiscriminate overprescription of a therapy with serious potential side effects unsurprisingly led to a backlash. By the late 1960s and 1970s, although modern anesthetic techniques were making ECT safer and more careful research was being done to determine which psychiatric disorders the treatment helped with and which it did not, the damage to ECT's reputation had already been done. (That *Cuckoo's Nest*, awarded the Oscar for best movie in 1975, depicted ECT as it would have been administered circa 1945 certainly didn't help.) State hospitals drew up regulations sharply curtailing its use, and legislation was in effect briefly in California banning the procedure completely.

Fortunately, the pendulum has swung back to center. ECT is now safer than most surgical procedures, side effects are minimal, and guidelines for when it should be used have been clarified. A 1980 survey of 166 ECT patients reported that about half thought a trip to the dentist was more unpleasant than an electroconvulsive treatment.†

†C. Freeman and R. E. Kendell, "ECT I: Patients' Experiences and Attitudes," *British Journal of Psychiatry* 137 (1980): 8–16.

Modern ECT

Since its introduction decades ago, there have been many improvements in ECT technique that have dramatically reduced side effects and adverse events. There have been changes in the way the electrical stimulus is used to minimize the electrical energy that is delivered, and, perhaps even more importantly, modern anesthesia essentially eliminates most physical symptoms.

About the only patients who absolutely must not receive ECT are the few individuals with medical conditions so severe that even ten to fifteen minutes of general anesthesia is too dangerous—people with severe cardiac or lung diseases, for example. ECT is safe in elderly persons and during pregnancy.

The Experience of ECT

Most psychiatric hospitals have specialized treatment suites for ECT; in general hospitals, ECT is often administered in the recovery room of the hospital's surgical suite (the area where patients waking up from surgery are taken for observation).

An ECT treatment lasts only about sixty seconds; most of the "treatment" time is the ten minutes or so it takes to administer general anesthesia before the actual treatment and another ten minutes for the patient to awaken from it.

The crucial anesthetic advance for ECT was the introduction in the 1950s of agents called *muscle relaxants*, or more properly *neuromuscular blocking agents*, which temporarily paralyze the patient by blocking nerve-fiber signals to the muscles. These medications prevent the violent muscle contractions during seizures that characterized early ECT use.

After an intravenous medication is given to put the patient to sleep, the neuromuscular blocking agent is given so that the patient's muscles are temporarily paralyzed. Electrode disks similar to those used for cardiac defibrillation are applied to the scalp. Modern ECT equipment designed for the purpose delivers a precisely timed and measured electrical stimulus. In *bilateral* treatments, an electrode is applied over each temple. In *unilateral* treatments, wherein the object is to stimulate only half of the brain, one electrode is placed in the middle of the forehead or the crown of the head and the other at the temple. (Unilateral treatment causes less post-ECT confusion and memory problems and is now used almost exclusively, although patients for whom unilateral treatments are ineffective often switch to bilateral treatments.)

The electrical stimulus is applied for two to eight seconds, triggering seizure activity in the brain. Because of the muscle relaxant, the "seizure" in modern ECT is pretty much an electrical event only, with few or no jerking movements such as those that usually characterize seizures, and thus what ECT causes is usually called a *modified seizure*.

The ECT equipment also records an electroencephalogram (a measurement of the electrical activity of the brain), allowing the physician to monitor the seizure activity, which usually lasts less than a minute. There might be some muscle contractions observed during this time, but the muscle relaxant keeps the patient nearly motionless. Usually a quickening of the heart rate and an increase of blood pressure occur, which also signal that the "seizure" has taken place. The anesthetist uses a face-mask breathing device to deliver oxygen until the patient wakes up five or ten minutes later, and the treatment is over.

(continued)

During the years when I was part of the Brain Stimulation Center at Johns Hopkins, I often saw medical students on their psychiatry rotation assigned to a morning of observing ECT enter the suite apprehensively, not knowing what to expect but looking like they're expecting the worst. What they see is an anesthesiologist inducing general sedation, the placement of the electrodes, a bit of toe-wriggling during the actual "seizure," and the patient emerging from anesthesia a bit groggy. The students' reaction is uniformly something like, "Was that it?" said in an almost disappointed manner. *Cuckoo's Nest* it's not!

Patients awakening from anesthesia after ECT are a bit groggy, of course, and many are also slightly fuzzy headed and feel "spacey" for another hour or so. This effect is probably related to the treatments themselves, not just the anesthesia, and it resembles the mild post-seizure confusion that patients with true epilepsy often experience. Occasionally, a more prolonged period of confusion called *delirium* is seen, especially after bilateral treatments and especially toward the end of a course of treatments. Sedatives can treat this problem, but when it occurs, consideration should be given to stopping the treatments or giving them less often.

The most troublesome possible side effects of ECT relate to its effect on memory: about two-thirds of ECT patients report memory loss, at least temporarily. The most common memory problem is with *visuo-spatial* memory, the type needed to get places and find things. In a famous article in the *British Journal of Psychiatry*, a practicing psychiatrist who received a course of ECT to treat depression wrote of his experiences and noted that afterward, he could no longer remember how to get where he needed to go using the London Underground.[1] He suddenly found that he had forgotten where the different lines went and needed to consult maps even for routine trips that he had taken for years. After a time, everything became familiar again, and he was knowledgeable enough about what was going on to find the whole thing amusing rather than worrisome (or at least that's what he wrote in the article). If patients are not prepared to expect this possible side effect, they can be quite alarmed when they return home and find their house oddly unfamiliar or that they can't put their hands on their favorite frying pan or remember where in the world those darn hedge clippers are. Getting lost going to the supermarket? Not at all uncommon—at least for a few weeks. The experience of the English psychiatrist is a reminder that being forewarned and prepared for these potential problems is important so that if and when they occur, they are not so frightening.

Another type of memory loss sometimes seen with ECT affects the memory of events occurring during the several weeks when the patient is receiving ECT. Since treatments are typically given three times a week and a patient usually needs six to twelve treatments for complete recovery, a course of ECT will last two to four weeks. Patients not infrequently lose the memory of some events that occurred during those weeks. Patients sometimes also suffer *retrograde amnesia* as well: memory loss of the period of time before they actually started ECT. This is thought to occur because ECT somehow disrupts the process by which shorter-term memories become incorporated into longer-term memory. (If you've ever lost an hour's worth of computer work because you failed to save your work before something untoward "froze" your computer, you get the idea of what retrograde amnesia is. The short-term memories that are still in the brain's memory "buffer" are lost because of the ECT.) Patients who have successfully completed a course of ECT may say they don't remember checking in to the hospital, or they might not recollect a home visit or a trip they took with their family during the treatments. This problem seems to be worst just after a patient receives ECT. In a study of forty-three patients who were interviewed about their memory a few weeks after completing ECT, some reported difficulty remembering events for a period up to two years before their ECT. But when these patients were tested again seven *months* after their treatment, the more distant memories had been almost completely recovered.[2]

As you might suspect, these kinds of memory problems are almost impossible to pick up on tests, and so despite many years of memory research on ECT patients, it has been difficult to quantify precisely the effect of ECT on long-term memories. Another factor that confuses the issue is the effect that severe depression has on memory. Several studies indicate that complaints of memory problems after ECT correlate better with the severity of the patient's depression than with how they do on memory tests.[3]

ECT for Bipolar Disorder

Electroconvulsive therapy can be thought of as a symptomatic treatment for both phases of bipolar disorder: although it can quickly interrupt an episode of depression or mania, it does not have a long-term effect as a mood stabilizer (a *symptomatic* treatment treats *symptoms* but not the underlying disease). Medication treatment will still be necessary to sustain the benefit of ECT and to keep the patient's mood state stable after the treatments are finished.

Typically, when the decision is made to give a course of ECT, medications are stopped, or their doses are reduced. (Sedative medications often shorten and otherwise interfere with the ECT "seizure," and so do the anti-convulsant mood stabilizers—they are anticonvulsants, after all. Lithium seems to make patients more prone to episodes of confusion after their treatments.)

ECT is generally considered to be the most effective antidepressant treatment available. Naturally, it should be a treatment consideration whenever a bipolar patient continues to be severely depressed despite antidepressant medication treatment. It is also *rapidly* effective. Often, patients dramatically improve after just three or four treatments—that is, after five to seven days. Severely suicidal patients or those who have stopped eating and drinking and are in danger of malnutrition and dehydration—any patients for whom profound depression has become an imminently life-threatening illness—are candidates for ECT. Pregnancy is also considered to be an indication for use of ECT to treat serious bipolar depression because of the risk many mood-stabilizing medications pose to the fetus.[4] Because depression can be highly resistant to antidepressant medications and also risky in some elderly patients, ECT is frequently rec-ommended as a first-line treatment for severe depression in older people as well. Depressed bipolar patients who receive ECT can become slightly hypomanic. When this occurs, obviously it's time to stop the treatments. Unlike the antidepressants, ECT does not seem to increase the cycling of the illness.[5]

ECT is also a highly effective treatment for mania. A 1994 review of fifty years' experience of the use of ECT for treating mania found that it pro-vided complete symptom remission or marked improvement in 80 percent of the manic patients studied. Many of the patients in these studies failed to respond to many other available treatments—making this success rate all the more impressive.[6] ECT seems to work more quickly in mania than in depression. One study found that patients recovered after an average of six treatments, about half the usual requirement for the treatment of depres-sion.[7] Severely manic patients whose highly agitated state becomes phys-ically dangerous are obvious candidates for ECT, as are pregnant manic patients.

ECT is a valuable therapeutic tool for any bipolar patient who is ex-tremely sick and seems to be getting sicker despite aggressive treatment with medication. It is perhaps the most effective treatment there is for severe depression and severe mania, and it often works more quickly than medications.[8]

TRANSCRANIAL MAGNETIC STIMULATION (TMS)

Transcranial magnetic stimulation (TMS) is a new therapeutic technique in some ways similar to ECT that is effective in treating mood disorders. The great advantage of TMS over ECT is that TMS is much simpler to administer: no seizure activity is induced by the treatment, and therefore no anesthesia is necessary. Even more advantageous is that there are almost no side effects.

This novel technique takes advantage of a principle of electromagnetism called *induction* to deliver an electrical stimulus to the brain without applying electrical energy to the scalp (as in ECT). During TMS treatments, a magnetic coil is held against the scalp, and the magnetic field that develops in the coil causes electrical current to flow through nearby neurons within the skull. No electricity passes through the skull, as in ECT; rather, the magnetic field "induces" a tiny electrical current in the underlying brain tissue. Since the electrical current that is generated in the brain tissue by TMS is miniscule, no seizure occurs; thus, no anesthesia is needed. Pulses of magnetic energy are delivered over a period of about twenty to forty minutes while the patient simply sits in a chair, awake and alert throughout the whole procedure. Other than some soreness from muscle stimulation, there appear to be no side effects of any kind.[9]

There are now several FDA approved TMS devices. Most closely resemble a dentist's office setup: a comfortable reclining chair with a headrest for the patient and above the chair an articulated instrument "arm." Instead of a dentist's drill at the end of the arm, there is a case about the size of your hand that houses the coil. A few straps hold the coil in place. One device houses the coil in a helmet-like case reminiscent of the hooded hair driers used in beauty salons.

It is possible to give a placebo TMS treatment, facilitating valid research on the efficacy of TMS in depression. (A true placebo-controlled study of ECT would require giving two groups of patients anesthesia but giving the electrical stimulus only to patients in one of the groups. Risking anesthesia to receive a fake ECT treatment is something few people would volunteer for, and ethically it is rather dubious.) When the TMS coil is applied to the scalp at a slightly different angle from that normally used to give treatments, it does not cause electrical current to flow through the brain tissue and thus does not have the usual TMS effect. However, because stimulation of the muscles still occurs, the slight muscle soreness associated with the treatment occurs as well, and so research subjects have no way of knowing whether they are getting a placebo treatment or the real thing. This made the all-important double-blind placebo-controlled studies fairly easy to do.

As we shall see in chapter 14, various studies indicate that the left pre-frontal lobes of the brain are less active than normal in depression. This finding has led researchers to try TMS treatments on depressed patients by

Magnetic Induction: You're Probably Using It at Home

If you use an electric toothbrush, you may have wondered why the base that charges it doesn't have any visible metal parts. How does electricity get from the base to the toothbrush without any metal conductor to carry it? The answer is *electromagnetic induction.* The phenomenon was discovered by Michael Faraday in 1831, who found that passing a bar magnet back and forth through a wire coil caused a current to flow through it. A change in magnetic flux (the moving magnet) causes a current to flow in any adjacent conductor. Your toothbrush charger has a tiny spinning magnet that induces enough current in the adjacent toothbrush to charge its battery. Induction cooking uses the same principle, as does the charging pad you may use to charge your mobile phone.

In TMS, the magnetic flux is produced in a coil inside the part of the TMS that is held against the appropriate scalp area. The nearby brain tissue is the "conductor" where a tiny electrical current is generated.

FIGURE 10.1. Electromagnetic induction

Passing a bar magnet back and forth through a coiled wire causes a current to flow through the wire. This phenomenon is the basis of transcranial magnetic stimulation.

Illustration by Jenna Macfarlane

stimulating the left prefrontal lobes. One of the first studies on TMS in the treatment of depression appeared in the *American Journal of Psychiatry* in 1997.[10] In this study from the National Institute of Mental Health, twelve patients received active or placebo TMS stimulations over a period of twenty minutes every weekday for two weeks. There was a statistically significant mood improvement in these patients after the real TMS treatments but not after the placebo treatments. Several patients continued TMS after the completion of the study and experienced further clinical improvement in their depressive symptoms. The FDA approved the first TMS device in 2008 and another device in 2013 for the treatment of major depression.

Over the past ten years or so, TMS has continued to evolve. It has become clear that more magnetic pulses per session are more effective, but psychiatrists are still learning how best to administer them. The strength of the magnetic stimulation that is most beneficial, the exact placement of the coil, the number of magnetic impulses delivered per treatment session, the total number of treatments, and the duration of therapy are all under investigation at various centers around the world.[11]

Further developments include *theta burst stimulation TMS* (TBS) which combines high-frequency and low-frequency pulses during TMS treatments. TBS treatments last only about five minutes as opposed to the twenty to forty-five minutes required for regular TMS treatments. Another new variation is *synchronized TMS* (sTMS), in which the magnetic bursts are delivered in sync with the patient's brain waves. Both of these investigational treatments use less magnetic energy and appear to be more comfortable for patients.[12]

Although as of this writing, most insurance companies will not cover TMS for patients with bipolar disorder, this may soon change as data are accumulating that TMS is also effective for the treatment of bipolar depression.

TMS has been a promising development in the treatment of mood disorders and is already opening up a whole new array of treatment options.

VAGAL NERVE STIMULATION (VNS)

Another approach for treating depression is vagal nerve stimulation (VNS), approved by the FDA for treatment-resistant major depression in 2005.

The vagal nerve (or *vagus*) is a long nerve that emerges from the base of the brain and travels down the neck and into the chest and abdomen. It regulates some vital bodily functions such as digestion and heart rate. Its connections in the brain occur through important centers thought to be involved with emotional regulation and specifically with mood regulation. VNS is done by means of a pacemaker-like device that must be surgically implanted; it is connected to the vagus nerve as it travels through the neck and delivers tiny electrical signals. Because the connection is made where the nerve travels through the neck, it is a simple surgical procedure that is usually done on an outpatient basis.

Animal studies done as early as the 1930s demonstrated that electrical stimulation of the vagal nerve produced changes in the electrical activity of the brain, and studies in the 1980s demonstrated that VNS could control epileptic seizures in dogs.

In the 1990s VNS became available for the treatment of intractable epilepsy in humans, first in Europe and then in the United States. By the end of 2000, about six thousand patients worldwide had received VNS, almost all for the treatment of epilepsy. As with antiepileptic medications that later turned out to be effective mood stabilizers, VNS was noted to have beneficial effects on mood in several patients who had received it to treat their seizures. Some had substantial antidepressant effects from VNS, even though the treatment didn't improve their seizure control.

In one of the first studies of the VNS treatment of depression, thirty adults received VNS for severe treatment-resistant depression; nine had a diagnosis of bipolar I or bipolar II disorder. Some of these patients had taken dozens of different medications and undergone ECT, with little benefit. About half of the patients benefited from VNS.[13] In a follow-up study, most of the patients who had shown a response were continuing to do well, and several were found to have experienced continued improvement when they were evaluated after one year of VNS treatment.[14]

The time line for improvement with VNS is much longer than with other treatments. Although some patients notice improvement in weeks, in others, benefit slowly accrues over months or even years. A five-year observational study found that patients with unipolar and bipolar depression who received VNS in addition to medications did better than patients who received medications only.[15]

Unfortunately, as of this writing, there is virtually no insurance coverage for VNS, and accessing this treatment will usually mean participating in a clinical research trial.

EMERGING TECHNOLOGIES

Several other methods of delivering small electrical stimuli to areas of the brain are being investigated as possible treatments for mood disorders. One of these is *deep brain stimulation* (DBS), a technique that has been used since the mid-1990s to treat Parkinson's disease, tremor, chronic pain, and other neurological conditions. Like vagal nerve stimulation, DBS uses electrodes powered by a pacemaker-like device in the chest wall. Unlike VNS, however, the wires from that device travel into the skull, and the electrodes are implanted directly into deep brain centers. An invasive neurosurgical procedure is required, and so DBS has been investigated in only a small number of patients with the most treatment-resistant mood disorders, including some with bipolar disorder, but the results have been very promising.

Another investigational treatment is *transcranial direct current stimulation* (tDCS), in which a small electrical current is delivered over a period of time by means of electrodes applied to the surface of the scalp. This technique resembles electroconvulsive therapy in that an electrical current is passed directly through the skull, but the current is much smaller. Whereas the current delivered by an ECT device is usually 800 mA, tDCS devices deliver only 2 mA. As with transcranial magnetic stimulation, the patient can remain awake, simply sitting in a chair during the treatments, and no anesthesia is required. These treatments, like TMS, last about twenty minutes and are repeated daily for several weeks. A big advantage of tDCS over TMS is that the equipment is much simpler and hence less expensive. Several studies of tDCS have been published, and the results have been encouraging.

One of these studies was a placebo-controlled clinical trial in which volunteers with unipolar and bipolar depression received either active treatment using a 2.5 mA current for twenty minutes or placebo treatments. The placebo (control) group volunteers received a 1mA current for ten seconds that then dropped to one-third of a mA for the rest of the treatment except for another one minute of 0.5 mA about halfway through the twenty-minute session. The researchers were surprised to find that both groups showed significant improvement in depression scores and suggested that what they thought would be sham treatments delivered enough electrical stimulation to be helpful.[16]

In reviewing the studies that have been done so far on tDCS for this section, I was reminded of the studies done in the 1990s on TMS. In those early studies, results of individual studies tended to be somewhat unimpressive, but taken all together, it was difficult not to conclude that these research-ers were on to something and that further work might well pay off—and it certainly did. I suspect the same will be true for tDCS, and refinements in treatment techniques may well lead to a valuable new intervention.

─────────────── KEY TAKEAWAYS ───────────────

▶ Brain stimulation treatments consist of several therapeutic techniques that use electrical energy to stimulate areas of the brain.

▶ Electroconvulsive therapy (ECT) has been around the longest, is the most studied, and may be the most effective. ECT requires general anesthesia and often causes temporary memory problems.

▶ Several newer types of brain stimulation treatment (TMS and tDCS) use much smaller amounts of electrical energy to stimulate the brain and can be more precisely targeted to affected areas than ECT can. Whether these treatments are as effective as ECT remains to be confirmed, but results so far are very encouraging.

CHAPTER 11

Counseling and Psychotherapy

Although medical treatments such as pharmaceuticals are the foundation of the treatment of bipolar disorder, counseling and psychotherapy are important, perhaps indispensable, additional therapeutic interventions. Some people still picture psychotherapy as something that happens in a richly paneled, dimly lit office where a bearded psychiatrist sits taking notes in a high-backed leather chair behind a patient lying on a couch who is trying to remember what she dreamed about last night. Or perhaps they think of talk-radio therapists, dispensing sound-bite-sized advice to the lovelorn and lonely between car commercials on the AM dial. All of this is psychotherapy of a sort, but the practice of psychotherapy is a serious and well-studied clinical intervention for individuals in psychological distress that requires years of training and experience to master.

There are many types of counseling and therapy that are enormously helpful in bipolar disorder. By reading this book to this point, you've already received several hours of a kind of therapy. You've allowed an objective but sympathetic individual with knowledge and experience about mental illness and psychological processes (that's me) to present facts about bipolar disorder to increase your understanding of the illness. This understanding has, I hope, helped you make sense of your thoughts and feelings about this problem as it affects you. There's even a name for just this sort of treatment: *psychoeducation*, and it has been shown in research studies to reduce illness recurrences, decrease the number and duration of hospitalizations, increase the time to illness relapse, and lead to reduced stigma.[1]

This is, in large measure, what psychotherapy is all about: not interpreting dreams, not simply doling out advice, and certainly not supplying all the answers, but providing good, objective information.

BRAIN AND MIND

In chapter 4, I described how manic-depressive illness came to be called a "functional" psychiatric illness in the early twentieth century. After the discovery of the biological causes of mental illnesses, such as general paresis (central nervous system syphilis) and cretinism (intellectual disability caused by thyroid deficiency), psychiatric illnesses came to be divided into two categories: *organic* and *functional*. Organic psychiatric illnesses were "real" illnesses, caused by germs or abnormal hormone levels or something else that could be seen under a microscope or measured by a blood test. In functional illnesses, on the contrary, it was assumed that there wasn't anything wrong with the person's brain functioning in a physical sense. Patients with manic-depressive illness or schizophrenia were thought to be having some kind of abnormal reaction to life events.

The question then became, why do some people have these abnormal reactions while others with nearly identical backgrounds and experiences do not? It was at this point that the attempt to understand and treat these illnesses turned away from medicine and toward psychology. Sigmund Freud spent his lifetime treating and trying to understand patients who were unhappy in their relationships, disappointed in themselves for the choices they made, perhaps confused and anxious about decisions they were facing. Freud and his followers developed a large and sophisticated system for understanding human behavior based on understanding childhood development. Their treatments in essence consisted of helping patients understand themselves better; let go of grudges, resentments, and fears rooted in their past; and learn better, more mature strategies to cope with life's challenges. This approach has come to be called *dynamic* psychology or psychiatry, and it is based on the belief that mental life is best understood as a dynamic interplay between emotions and intellect, present circumstances and unconscious memories of past experiences, and many other psychological factors.

Although this approach was extremely successful in helping people with a wide variety of problems and symptoms, practitioners of dynamic psychotherapy soon discovered that it didn't make much of an impact on the symptoms of illnesses like schizophrenia or bipolar disorder. Psychological theories arose to explain their symptoms, but these patients were simply considered too intrinsically disturbed or too psychologically stunted or their families too dysfunctional for them to benefit from therapy. This was a dark time for patients with mental illnesses and their families, who in effect were blamed for causing these terrible illnesses in the first place.

Then a revolution occurred: lithium, chlorpromazine, and other effective medications for "functional" illnesses came along. In the 1970s, persons with bipolar disorder and schizophrenia left therapists behind and made tracks for a new kind of doctor: the *biological* psychiatrist, a *pharmacotherapist*, someone who would treat them like real people dealing with a "real" illness. For a time there was a kind of schism in American psychiatry between those who believed that dynamic psychology best explained mental illnesses and those who believed that biology was the key that would unlock the mysteries of psychiatric disorders.

When I was interviewing for psychiatric training programs in the mid-1970s, this biological psychiatry/dynamic psychiatry split was at its most pronounced. Many university medical center departments of psychiatry proudly identified themselves to me as either "biological" or "psychodynamic" in their approach. Usually each camp denigrated the other: psychodynamic psychiatry was "touchy-feely" soft science based more on nineteenth-century literary theory than on medicine; biological psychiatrists were "pill-pushers" who didn't even talk to their patients and had no appreciation for the human experience. But a few departments of psychiatry—Johns Hopkins's was one—were teaching their residents that mental experiences were neither a series of chemical reactions nor simply a collection of dynamically interrelated thoughts and feelings but both. We learned at Hopkins that people with bipolar disorder are still people, still subject to disappointments and loss, to relationship problems and blows to their self-esteem. To regard their moods as just the expression of so many chemicals to be fine-tuned with more chemicals was to do them a great disservice. Fortunately, this schism has now healed for the most part, and even the most ardent biological psychiatrists realize that psychodynamic understanding of the patient is *always* important. Perhaps the most important development has been the conclusion, now supported by decades of research, that the most effective treatment for persons with mood disorders (and, indeed, most other psychiatric illness) combines *both* therapeutic approaches, which are now understood to be complementary rather than competing.

The variety of available psychological treatments has broadened tremendously in the past twenty-five years or so. Sophisticated techniques have been developed that work for particular kinds of problems. Some involve individual sessions with a therapist, others a group setting. Some are focused on a particular problem, such as marital or family difficulties or addiction; others on a particular symptom, such as depression or panic attacks. Some are designed to last only a few sessions; others are more open ended. Some are not "therapy" in the traditional sense at all: support groups, made up of individuals who offer guidance and support to each other, don't even include a "therapist." Moreover, a lot of research has been done to determine which psychological treatments work best for which problems. The prescription of a particular kind of counseling or therapy for a particular kind of problem is often backed up by as much research as is the prescription of a particular medication.

WHAT CAN THERAPY DO?

No one today would even think of recommending counseling or therapy as the only treatment for bipolar disorder; to do so would constitute malpractice. But because we have highly effective medications for this illness, some doctors, and perhaps many more patients, want to turn away from counseling and therapy altogether and approach the illness as a purely "chemical" problem that has a purely "chemical" solution. This is a mistake, for several reasons.

First of all, the diagnosis of bipolar disorder is almost always a traumatic event, not only for patients but for their family members as well. In addition to the emotional turmoil that is the symptom of the illness itself, there is an emotional reeling that results from coming face to face with fears about how this diagnosis will affect one's life. Vaguely familiar terms like *manic depression* and all-too-familiar terms like *mental illness* conjure up all sorts of confused and confusing ideas and feelings. "Why has this happened to me?" (or perhaps "This *can't* be happening to me!") and "My life will never be the same" and "Whose fault is this?" are only some of the thoughts and questions that start spinning through the minds of people affected by this diagnosis.

Remember that I described therapy as "providing good information, objective feedback, and solid encouragement in a supportive, confidential setting." It becomes obvious, doesn't it, that this kind of psychological treatment is going to be necessary and helpful? Some research suggests that the first year after a diagnosis of bipolar disorder is a crucial time for persons with the disorder and that the education, support, and encouragement that psychotherapy provides are vital in making treatment successful in the long term.[2]

Another traumatic event that persons with bipolar disorder face all too frequently is relapse. The management of bipolar disorder is still far from perfect, and despite everyone's best efforts, relapse can and does occur. Many patients feel like they're "back to square one"; they blame themselves or their medication or their doctor; they become angry, disappointed, discouraged, and confused about what to do next. Again, counseling helps the person put things back into perspective, get over the setback, and move on. I shall discuss individual therapy in more detail later in this chapter.

There are many different approaches to helping persons with bipolar disorder through psychotherapy.

GROUP PSYCHOTHERAPY

Psychotherapy can be very effective in a group setting. The worry I often hear expressed by patients for whom group therapy is recommended is that they don't want to "sit around listening to other people's problems" week after week. But no group therapist worth his salt is going to let the group deteriorate into a "pity party"; instead, he will guide the group members onto the track of learning from, and helping solve, one another's problems—not just ventilating about them. An excellent way to become a better problem solver is to see how other people are solving, or failing to solve, their own problems. By observing and being asked to objectively react to another person's problems, group members learn how to think more objectively, and less emotionally, about their own.

In traditional group psychotherapy, groups are usually made up of persons with a variety of problems. In the treatment of bipolar disorder, however, *homogeneous* groups (composed exclusively of persons with bipolar disorder) have been studied more and have been shown to be effective. Several studies show that bipolar-disorder patients in group therapy have fewer relapses and improved productivity at work or school.[3] The research suggests that the shared aspect of the problems seems to be integral to the therapeutic experience. Persons with bipolar disorder who are in groups with other bipolar-disorder patients report that the practical advice they receive about living with the illness is extremely helpful. Their understanding of the disorder, of how it affects their relationships and self-attitudes, is enhanced, and the guidance they receive from group members is perceived as invaluable.[4] This aspect of group therapy—sharing and learning from one another—is the basis of another type of "therapy," one that doesn't require a therapist: peer support groups. We shall discuss this helping format in chapter 22.

I've already mentioned a kind of therapy called psychoeducation. This type of treatment is especially suited to the group setting. A *psychoeducational group* can be thought of as combining more traditional group therapy with a didactic, instructional approach and often includes reading materials and discussion questions about bipolar disorder. These may include information about symptoms, about the warning signs of relapse, and about how to better communicate with family members, employers, and coworkers regarding the illness, among other topics. A presentation of facts about the illness or techniques for dealing with it becomes a taking-off point for a discussion of the individual's experiences and using new knowledge to feel better and function more effectively. A study of patients who were "minimally symptomatic" compared how effective attending a psychoeducational group was, compared to receiving individual therapy. The researchers found that each treatment improved the patients' functional level and residual symptoms—and the group treatment was much less expensive. For this and other reasons, this approach is gaining favor. There is even a psychoeducational treatment program called *Facilitated Integrated Mood Management* that can be completed in only five sessions.[5] Numerous studies have shown psychoeducation to be a valuable adjunct to other treatment approaches to bipolar disorder.

COGNITIVE BEHAVIORAL THERAPY (CBT)

As we saw in earlier chapters, available pharmaceutical treatments for the depressed phase of bipolar disorder are less than perfect by a long shot. The mood stabilizers are not completely effective as antidepressants for some patients, and antidepressant medications carry the risk of precipitating mania or accelerating the frequency of cycles. But psychotherapy has a proven track record in helping with depression and, as far as we can tell, has no risk of precipitating mania or of accelerating the course of bipolar disorder.

In the 1960s Dr. Aaron Beck and his colleagues developed a theory of depression and psychotherapeutic treatment for it called *cognitive behavioral therapy*, or CBT for short. This type of psychotherapy has been researched more thoroughly than have most others, and it has a proven track record in helping with symptoms of depression; in some studies—though not in others—it has been found to work as well as antidepressant medication for some patients, or even better.[6] Beck originally called CBT simply "cognitive therapy." Psychologist Donald Meichenbaum, who has written extensively on Beck's cognitive therapy as well as on other types of therapy that use the techniques of behavioral psychology to help change thinking patterns (cognition), is perhaps most responsible for creating the broader category we now call "cognitive behavioral therapy." Although some researchers and theoreticians will describe subtle differences between the terms *cognitive therapy* and *cognitive behavioral therapy*, they now seem to be used interchangeably by most clinical psychologists and by researchers as well.

The theory of cognitive therapy maintains that people who are chronically or frequently depressed have developed a distorted view of themselves and of the world and have adopted certain patterns of thinking and reacting to challenges that perpetuate their problems. This emphasis on thinking, or *cognition*, lends the theory and the therapy its name. As we saw in chapter 1, depressed persons tend (1) to think negatively about themselves, (2) to interpret their experiences in a negative way, and (3) to have a pessimistic view of the future. Cognitive theory calls this the *cognitive triad*. The theory further proposes that all this negative thinking causes a person to develop a repertoire of mental habits called *schemas* or *negative automatic thoughts* that spring into action and reinforce the negative thinking.

John is a thirty-two-year-old computer specialist whose idea for a new project has just been turned down by his company. He comes to his therapy session and brings along a lengthy handwritten critique of the project that the senior vice president of his division, Ms. Kaiser, left behind after coming by John's cubicle to tell him that the project had been turned down.

"You see, I should have known better than to take on that big a project. The senior vice president, no less, comes by with the bad news. 'Better luck next time,' she said. Now I'm never going to move up in this company."

"Why do you say that?" I asked.

"If someone that high up thinks I'm incompetent, I'm done for. That's the last time I bother trying something I'm not cut out for."

"Did she say she thought you were incompetent?"

"Well, no, of course not."

"I see. This vice president doesn't tell people what she thinks."

"Oh, no, that's not true at all. She's got a reputation for coming right out with her opinions about things."

"But she treats you differently from everyone else?"

John began to get a little annoyed. "Well, I wouldn't think so, but how should I know? I'd never talked with her before."

"What do you make of that?" I asked. "The fact that she came in person to give you the news about your proposal?"

"Well, I did think it was unusual."

"Could it mean she was impressed with some aspects of your proposal and wanted to meet you?"

"Well, I suppose that's possible."

I continued reinterpreting John's negative assumptions: "And how about the handwritten critique?"

"It was really negative," John went on glumly. "She went through every point and shot them down one by one."

"When had you sent the proposal to Ms. Kaiser? How long did she have to look at it?"

"Oh, I didn't send it to Kaiser; she's over the whole division. I sent it to Bob Rodney, my team leader. I guess he sent it up to her, but I don't know how long she spent with it."

"Well, she must have spent several hours with it if she gave you back such a carefully organized critique. Don't you think?"

"Yeah, I guess she wouldn't have taken all that time and trouble if she had thought it was worthless."

"And your team leader must have thought it had some potential if he sent the proposal to his boss. Have you asked him for some feedback?"

"No, I assumed he'd be down on me for it, too."

"But do you see how your negative assumption stopped you from checking in with your team leader and prevented you from getting what could have been positive feedback and encouragement from him?"

"I see what you mean. If I hadn't jumped to conclusions, I might have gotten some positive strokes."

John is down on his talents and assumes everybody else is, too. In situations that can be interpreted many different ways, both positive and negative, he tends to go for the negative rather than seek alternative positive explanations. This in turn sometimes causes him to do things that reinforce his negative thinking, and the vicious cycle repeats itself. This might seem to be a trivial example, but it's not difficult to come up with several negative schemas that people with bipolar disorder are prone to:

Negative: "I got manic even though I was taking my lithium. It doesn't matter what I do. What's the use?"

Realistic: "Relapses occur even with medication. It might have been much worse and lasted much longer if I hadn't been on medication. Perhaps this new medication will be more effective for me."

Negative: "Everyone will avoid me when I go back to work. No one wants to work with a mentally ill person."

Realistic: "Some people might avoid me at work, perhaps many at first. But when they see that I'm the same old me, they'll come around. And those who don't are people I don't want as friends anyway."

Cognitive therapy techniques more specifically focused on bipolar disorder have also been developed. Part of the treatment deals with the negative automatic thoughts that interfere with treatment by medication. For example, if a person with bipolar disorder is troubled by the negative automatic thought "Taking mood-stabilizing medication is a sign of personal weakness" every time she takes a dose of lithium, she might be more likely to skip doses or stop taking the medication altogether. Cognitive therapy works on the psychological barriers to proper treatment by replacing automatic negative thoughts with realistic ones.

SPECIALIZED CBT

There are several subtypes of CBT that deserve mention.

Dialectical behavioral therapy (DBT) is a form of CBT that was developed for the treatment of borderline personality (more about this diagnosis in chapter 20). In addition to working on distorted thinking, patients receiving DBT also focus on modulating their emotional reactions to stressful situations and learn how to cope better with suicidal thinking and nonsuicidal self-harming behaviors like cutting or burning themselves. The emphasis of DBT is on defusing intensifying emotional situations, coping with uncomfortable feelings, and being prepared for crises. A group of researchers at the University of Pittsburgh developed and tested a form of DBT specially tailored to adolescents with bipolar disorder. They compared this form of DBT to treatment as usual in a small group of adolescents with bipolar disorder. The volunteers were described as "relatively ill youth who had early illness onset, psychiatric hospitalizations, and poor functioning." At the end of the study, the adolescents in the DBT group "demonstrated significantly less severe depressive symptoms . . . and were nearly three times more likely to demonstrate improvement in suicidal ideation."[7]

Mindfulness-based cognitive therapy (MBCT) is another variation on CBT. As its name suggests, it teaches the patient to become more aware of thinking patterns and emotional states by noticing and observing mood fluctuations and changes in symptoms. The focus is to observe these changes in a nonjudgmental way and to respond to these signals in a regulated, preplanned manner. Meditation is also a component. In a study on twenty-three volunteers with bipolar disorder who were treated for eight weeks, MBCT reduced anxiety and enhanced mindfulness, emotional regulation, and a cognitive skill called *executive functioning*, which can be loosely defined as "thinking before acting."[8] The volunteers in this study also had a functional MRI scan before and after their treatment. This is a specialized brain imaging technique that shows activity levels in different parts of the brain. Compared to before their course of MBCT, the bipolar volunteers' scans showed a return toward normal in areas of the brain known to be underactive in persons with depression. Of note, these volunteers were either in a normal mood state or having only mild symptoms, indicating that even these relatively well persons with bipolar disorder benefited from MBCT.

FAMILY-FOCUSED THERAPY (FFT)

Family-based psychotherapies for bipolar disorder take into account not only the symptoms and experiences of the person with bipolar disorder but also the extent to which the emotional experiences of bipolar disorder affect the patient's family members. It also considers how the patient's family, their attitudes, and their behaviors can affect the course of the disorder in their loved one. One such family therapy is *family-focused therapy* (FFT), and Dr. David Miklowitz at UCLA has spent more than twenty years developing, fine-tuning, and evaluating this intervention.

Basically, FFT aims to reduce stress in the home environment through psychoeducation for the patient and the family, enhancing communication skills among family members, and problem-solving training.

To some extent this model grew out of research showing that patients with schizophrenia had more illness relapses if there were conflicts and stresses at home and within the family. This therapy works hard at family support. Educating the patient and her family members about the symptoms of bipolar disorder and its treatments is a priority, emphasizing that bipolar disorder is indeed an illness and that its symptoms are not under voluntary control. Family sessions are held to identify difficulties and conflicts within the family unit—whether caused by the illness or by other, perhaps preexisting, factors or situations. Conflict resolution and problem-solving techniques are presented and practiced, and healthy communication skills are developed through role playing and rehearsals.

In a study comparing the benefit of FFT for adolescents who had recently recovered from a mood episode to that of psychoeducation sessions alone (both groups also were on medication), Dr. Miklowitz and his colleagues found that FFT-treated patients recovered more quickly from whatever depressive symptoms they had at the start of the study and they spent fewer weeks in depressive episodes. Perhaps not surprisingly, patients whose families were having more conflicts at the start of the study benefitted the most.[9]

"TRADITIONAL" INDIVIDUAL PSYCHOTHERAPY

I hope I haven't given you the impression that traditional psychotherapy isn't useful for patients with bipolar disorder. Quite the contrary. Kay Redfield Jamison has written, "At this point in my existence, I cannot imagine leading a normal life without both taking lithium and having had the benefits of psychotherapy. Lithium prevents my seductive but disastrous highs, diminishes my depressions . . . and makes psychotherapy possible. But, ineffably, psychotherapy *heals*. It makes some sense of the confusion, reins in the terrifying thoughts and feelings, returns some control and hope and possibility of learning from it all."[10]

So far in this chapter I've talked about treatments that focus on helping patients deal with the acute stresses of diagnosis, hospitalization, reintegration back into their job, or other specific issues related to an episode of illness. I've discussed CBT and its variations that focus on chronic or smoldering depressive symptoms that medication alone doesn't seem to quite take care of, as well as being more alert to emotional states and triggers.

What, then, of traditional psychotherapy? By *traditional psychotherapy* I mean individual meetings with a therapist, usually over an extended period (months or years), in which the person in treatment discusses his past and present experiences and feelings with the goal of self-understanding, self-acceptance, and personal growth. (*Dynamic* or *insight-oriented psychotherapy* is the same thing.) Disappointments and accomplishments, affections and enmities, fears, inspirations, passions, and worries—all are "grist for the mill" of therapy, as psychotherapists are fond of saying. The patient and the therapist will, of course, talk about symptoms like sadness and anxiety too, but traditional therapy sees symptoms as indicators of underlying psychological conflicts rather than as the focus of treatment in and of themselves. Traditional psychotherapy emphasizes exploring the *meaning* of symptoms and the development of self-awareness and maturity.

So when would we recommend traditional psychotherapy to a person with bipolar disorder? For what types of problems would it be helpful?

Basically, for the same types of problems that people without bipolar disorder go to therapists for: dealing with psychological traumas and setbacks—past and present—that, understandably, cause feelings of sadness, anger, or anxiety, or thought patterns, self-attitudes, and interpersonal styles that disrupt a person's ability to be happy in relationships, effective at work, carefree in play, and confident in making decisions about the future. Sounds like a tall order, doesn't it? Well, of course it is. That is why psychotherapists

---

Sigmund Freud and Psychoanalysis

Sigmund Freud (1856–1939), considered by many to be the founder of modern psychotherapy, graduated from the University of Vienna with an MD degree in 1881. Although he trained as a neurologist, a three-month fellowship in Paris where he studied and worked under Jean-Martin Charcot, an internationally renowned neurologist, proved to be his turning point. At the time, Charcot was studying patients with what was then called *hysteria*, a condition in which patients have neurological symptoms such a blindness or paralysis that cannot be neurologically explained. Charcot had come to believe that these patients' symptoms were caused by psychological traumas, and he was attempting to treat them using hypnosis. Freud was so impressed that upon his return to Vienna, he quit his job as a hospital neurologist and opened a private practice to treat "nervous disorders."

As he developed his treatment techniques by seeing patients, Freud wrote extensively, publishing in-depth case studies of patients with phobias, depression, and other psychological symptoms, eventually developing a theory of mental life as well as a treatment technique that he called *psychoanalysis*.

Freud was dissatisfied with hypnosis as a technique to access patient's deepest fears and memories and quickly abandoned it in favor of simply getting patients talk freely about themselves. He soon was having them lie comfortably on a couch during sessions and eventually started sitting out of sight behind them so as not to influence what they said with his own reactions or facial expressions—the famous "analytic couch" was born.

Although the analytic couch has virtually disappeared in current practice, along with many other aspects of Freudian theory, Freud's fundamental insights continue to form the basis for the practice of psychotherapy. Thanks to Freud, we now take for granted that psychological traumas can cause debilitating symptoms like panic attacks, severe depression, and flashbacks and can be effectively treated by talking about traumatic experiences in a safe, confidential setting with a knowledgeable and supportive professional, an approach that is directly attributable to him.

COUNSELING AND PSYCHOTHERAPY **169**

often study and train in their profession for as many years as physicians train in theirs. That is why people are sometimes in therapy for months or even for years at a time. That is why psychotherapy is such an intense, powerful experience and the therapeutic relationship between patient and therapist a unique one.

Bipolar patients often have had more than their share of setbacks and psychological traumas—both past and present. Persons with bipolar disorder, because it is a genetic illness, often have had difficult, even traumatic, childhoods. Perhaps a parent was afflicted with the illness, perhaps the parent could not or would not receive proper treatment, and the child may have suffered disruptions to family life, periods of poverty or homelessness, or even physical or emotional abuse. Psychotherapy can be enormously beneficial in helping people face and work through their difficult pasts; let go of the anger, resentment, and fear that often comes out of these experiences; and move on with their lives.

The fact that a person has bipolar disorder can make ordinary life decisions seem complex and overwhelming. There is no better way of dealing with these sorts of anxieties and apprehensions than traditional psychotherapy. I remember a young woman who came to see me for a routine medication-monitoring appointment when I was working in the hectic medication clinic of a community mental-health center, a clinical setting in which patients were scheduled every twenty minutes. "I've been dating a man for several months now, and I think he might ask me to marry him," she told me. She looked worried. "I haven't told him about my illness. I don't know what to tell him. How do you think I should handle this?" I stared at her helplessly for a moment and panicked just a little when I heard the nurse slipping the chart of the next patient into the bin outside the interviewing-room door. I hope I didn't sound as rushed as I felt when I tried to convince her that the situation raised an enormous number of complex issues. Adequately dealing with the questions of how, when, where, why, and with whom she discussed her diagnosis was going to need much more than one—or a dozen—twenty-minute appointments with me.

I doubt very much that this was the first time this young woman had been confused about what to tell someone about her diagnosis. Perhaps she muddled through other situations at work, at church, or in her neighborhood, maybe saying nothing about her diagnosis because of feelings of shame or maybe blurting out too much about herself and then feeling vulnerable and exposed. Perhaps being diagnosed with bipolar disorder reactivated feelings she had struggled with in childhood or adolescence about being teased for being too fat or too skinny—or perhaps more likely in a bipolar patient, for being "hyper" or "weird." I was sure that since we had discussed the fact that bipolar disorder is a genetic illness, a possible marriage proposal raised questions in her mind about having children who might be affected by the disorder. How had the diagnosis affected her identity as a potential parent, as a woman? Or perhaps none of these issues needed to be explored but instead other, completely different ones. Well, all these issues are what good old-fashioned once-a-week "How do you feel about that?" psychotherapy is all about.

PSYCHOTHERAPY IN BIPOLAR DISORDER: IS IT REALLY NECESSARY?

All the psychiatrists I know talk about how much time they spend trying to persuade their bipolar patients to supplement their medication treatment with some form of therapy. There are many reasons why persons with bipolar disorder are reluctant to do so. Some patients have made uneasy peace with taking medication for a psychiatric illness (or, as they might say to themselves, for a "chemical imbalance"), but they see going to psychotherapy as confirmation of the "mental" aspect of their "mental illness." But if you think about it, the treatment of even the most "medical" of medical illnesses—heart disease, say, or a ruptured lumbar disk—usually requires nonmedical interventions, and sometimes these turn out to be just as important as the pharmaceutical or even surgical treatments prescribed by the doctor. The patient with diabetes would hardly regard staying on a healthy diet and watching her weight as unnecessary adjuncts to the insulin injections she receives. The recovering coronary bypass surgery patient wouldn't ignore the physician's recommendation for a cardiac-hardening exercise program. Would anyone have an operation for lumbar disk problems and skip the physical therapy sessions afterward? I don't think so.

We know that chronic psychological stresses make a whole variety of physical illnesses more difficult to treat: asthma, high blood pressure, irritable bowel syndrome. Psychological stresses will make mood-disorder symptoms more difficult to control as well.

A 2018 review paper analyzed more than thirty clinical trials of psychotherapeutic interventions for bipolar disorder, including psychoeducation groups, CBT, DBT, MBCT, FFT, and several others. The authors' happy conclusion was that "psychotherapy interventions for the treatment of bipolar disorder have substantial evidence for efficacy."[11]

If a particular type of therapy or counseling is available, is affordable, and has been recommended by the physician or treatment team, persons with bipolar disorder owe it to themselves to take advantage of the unique healing powers of these marvelous therapeutic techniques.

There are many forms of psychotherapy because some work better than others for particular patients; thus, it may take several tries to find the best match for an individual patient.

THE PSYCHIATRIST-PSYCHOTHERAPIST: AN EXTINCT SPECIES?

You have probably noticed that I have been referring to the psychiatrist and the psychotherapist as two different individuals. Unfortunately, most patients in America do not find one person serving both functions. It would, of course, be preferable for all sorts of reasons for the person prescribing medication and the person doing psychotherapy to be one and the same individual. But for a variety of complicated reasons, most people with bipolar disorder will see a psychiatrist for medication management and a nonphysician therapist—often a social worker or psychologist—for therapy. Some of the reasons for this state of affairs are the changes in medication management of bipolar disorder that have come about with the development of new medications; there are now so many different pharmaceuticals used in psychiatry that staying skilled in their use has become more and more time-consuming. Perhaps even more significantly, as more and more effective medications become available for more psychiatric problems, more and more patients want (and need) to see a psychiatrist for their treatment. There simply aren't enough psychiatrists to do both medication management and therapy, especially in busy clinics. Since medical school and psychiatric training take longer and cost more than the training required to become a psychotherapist, psychiatrists are usually more expensive than other professionals. When the administrator of a busy clinic or health maintenance organization (HMO) is looking to staff the organization's mental-health program, "split" treatment—psychiatric treatment split between a psychiatrist for medication management and a nonphysician therapist for psychotherapy or counseling—means more cost-effective treatment for patients.

The superior cost effectiveness of split treatment allows so many more patients to receive psychiatric treatment so much more cheaply that it's difficult to envision a return to the days when psychiatrists did therapy and prescribed medications, too. Fortunately, there are excellent training programs for clinical social workers, psychologists, and counseling professionals that are producing superb psychotherapists. And as we have seen in this chapter, psychotherapy is becoming more specialized, too. It has become nearly impossible to be an expert therapist and at the same time an expert psychopharmacologist. For all of these reasons, the medication management and the therapy of the person with bipolar disorder will usually be handled by two professionals rather than one.

--------------------- KEY TAKEAWAYS ---------------------

▶ Psychotherapy should be considered an integral part of the treatment of bipolar disorder, as important for patients with this illness as diet and exercise are for a patient with diabetes.

▶ A large body of clinical research has established that many forms of psychotherapy, including several that were developed especially to treat bipolar disorder, are effective in reducing symptoms and promoting improved functioning.

CHAPTER 12

Treatment Approaches in Bipolar Disorder

The causes of bipolar disorder remain for the most part unknown. Treatment approaches have been stumbled upon largely by accident—for example, the discovery of the therapeutic effects of lithium—and although they have been refined by decades of experience, they are still largely what physicians call *empirical*. This means that the treatment is based on accumulated clinical experience rather than on a true understanding of the mechanism of the disease or symptom in question.[1]

THERAPEUTIC RESULTS AS A GUIDE TO TREATMENT

Although we have a tremendous amount of experience in the use of pharmaceuticals to treat bipolar disorder and have data on their effectiveness in large groups of patients, the treatment of individual patients with the illness is often guided by treatment results rather than by the kinds of hard data physicians use to treat other illnesses. What do I mean by this? Let me explain by looking at a very different kind of illness, pneumonia.

A young man is rushed to the emergency room with a high fever, a pain in his chest, difficulty breathing, and a congested cough. The young man's chest x-ray shows that one of the lobes of his right lung is filled with fluid. A specimen of the young man's sputum is rushed off to the laboratory and examined under the microscope. Microscopic examination reveals that his lung is loaded with bacteria, specifically, pneumococcus. The diagnosis is clear: pneumococcal pneumonia. The doctor starts the young man on penicillin, an antibiotic known to be effective against most strains of pneumococcus, and within eight hours his fever is dropping. The dose of penicillin and the length of time the young man will need to take it have been determined by years of experience, calculated to the milligram and to the hour.

In a day or so the lab reports that the young man's pneumonia is not caused by a penicillin-resistant bug. Thus, his speedy recovery is assured.

The doctor treating this young man had quite a bit of hard data on which to base her treatment decisions. The appearance of the x-ray indicated that this was probably a typical bacterial lobar pneumonia rather than viral pneumonia, tuberculosis, or any of the various other conditions with similar symptoms but that look different on x-ray images. Also—and crucial for prognostic purposes—the x-ray showed that only one lobe was involved. The microscope provided the likely identity of the bacterial culprit within minutes, allowing the quick choice of a drug known to be effective most of the time against this type of germ. The identity of the bacterial culprit was solidly confirmed several days later when it grew in the culture dish and could be further tested. Most important, the lab results showed exactly which drugs work against the germ causing the problem in this particular patient. Contrast this scenario with one in which a patient with manic symptoms comes into the ER. There are no tests to order—just the eyes and ears and experience of the psychiatrist.

Fortunately, or perhaps unfortunately, full-blown mania often leads to an unmistakable diagnosis, and effective antimanic drugs are readily available. But what of the person who comes to the office and says, "I'm depressed" or complains of "mood swings." There are many more diagnostic possibilities. We know that antidepressant medications can sometimes make a patient with bipolar symptoms worse. How is a physician to know whether a person who comes in with symptoms of depression will turn out to have a bipolar illness? There are hints, of course, such as family history, but wouldn't it be fantastic if we could order a test for bipolar disorder before considering an antidepressant for a person who is having symptoms of depression? But we can't, at least not yet.

And once the acute symptoms of mania have been controlled? Emil Kraepelin described some patients who had remission of their bipolar symptoms that lasted for decades (it was apparently quite rare for this to happen, but he observed them, nevertheless). Do we prescribe a mood stabilizer for a patient who might not get sick again for ten or even twenty years? Wouldn't it be great if we could stop the medication after a period of time and have the patient come in every couple of months for some kind of scan that could pick up changes in brain functioning before symptoms become apparent? That way the patient would take medication only as it becomes necessary. Sometimes patients respond to one mood stabilizer but not another, or to a combination of two mood stabilizers but not to either one used alone. How to choose? Wouldn't it be fantastic if we could take a blood sample and look for some kind of chemical reaction around little paper disks soaked with lithium or Prozac in a petri dish to help choose effective medications for a particular patient?

At the present moment, we don't have any blood tests, scans, or other laboratory tests to make the treatment approach to bipolar disorder nearly as informed and logical as our approach can be in many other illnesses, although fortunately, as you will read later in this chapter, this is beginning to change.

Because we do not yet understand the causes of bipolar disorder, the medical approach to the treatment of the illness can be discussed only in general terms. Patients are started on one of the medications that have proved effective in many other patients with similar symptoms, and if these patients' symptoms are not effectively treated, other interventions are tried. We can't yet pick from among similar medications knowing beforehand which will work best. There is unfortunately a lot of "trial and error" and "wait and see" when it comes to prescribing medications for a specific patient. This can be tremendously frustrating for all involved—for the patient, of course, and for family members and, yes, for the physician, too.

But the good news is that more and better medications are becoming available all the time. Forty years ago there was only one mood-stabilizing medication, lithium. Twenty years ago there were three. Now we have at least five and several more on the way. There are easily twice as many antidepressants on the market as there were only fifteen years ago. The newer antipsychotic medications have fewer side effects and also have mood-stabilizing properties that the older agents lacked. As of this writing, medications and other treatments are becoming available that have entirely different mechanisms of action than older medications. Even more options are on the horizon.

Electroconvulsive therapy is one of the most effective treatments for mood disorders and one of the safest medical procedures available—and it is probably underutilized in bipolar disorder. Transcranial magnetic stimulation and other brain-stimulation treatments may come to replace ECT (and perhaps even medications) if they are able to deliver what they seem to be promising.

Don't forget counseling and psychotherapy. Research has proved how very important this unique treatment is in controlling the symptoms of mood disorders. More effective therapy programs for bipolar disorder are being refined by researchers with studies that are as rigorous as those used to evaluate any pharmaceutical.

And I haven't even talked about light therapy and sleep manipulation yet (those are coming in chapter 15). Researchers have discovered that exposure to bright light and changes in sleep patterns can help regulate mood and perhaps help medications work better and faster.

While we should be grateful for the many options that have come along, the growing number of available treatments is accompanied by one big problem: how to choose among them.

PHARMACOGENOMICS: A VERY BIG WORD FOR A VERY SIMPLE CONCEPT

It's a word made from two elements: *pharma*, referring to pharmaceuticals, and *genomics*, referring to the study of heredity and genes. Simply put, pharmacogenomics involves using information about people's genetic makeup, their genes, to help with selecting and dosing medication for them. It's a component of *personalized medicine*, a rather new approach in medical treatment that attempts to individualize treatment by taking factors that are unique to the individual into consideration when planning a treatment intervention.

As you will see in chapter 16, the search for genes associated with the risk of developing bipolar disorder ("risk genes") has been pretty disappointing. Studies of thousands of people looking for genes common to individuals with bipolar disorder have picked up a number of genetic signals, but the results of quite a few studies have not been replicated; that is, when geneticists have repeated studies in other groups of patients, rather than confirming what had been reported, new and different signals were found.

At this point, geneticists have concluded that there are many, many genes involved in developing bipolar disorder and that any one of them may only increase a person's risk of developing the illness by a few percentage points. This is why there is no reliable genetic test that will "diagnose" bipolar disorder in an individual. A test that showed that a person had a 2 percent greater risk of developing an illness would be pretty useless in any practical sense.

So instead, rather than searching for risk genes, a lot of genetic research is taking a different approach: looking for genes that predict how an individual will respond to and tolerate a medication.

The most exciting development in this area for persons with bipolar disorder is the ongoing research into lithium response. The International Consortium on Lithium Genetics (ConLiGen) has been working for about a decade to find genes that are involved in a person's response to lithium.

Can Genetic Tests Lead to Better Treatment?

You can divide the genes that pharmacogenomic test panels evaluate into two groups: pharmaco*dynamic* genes and pharmaco*kinetic* genes.

Pharmacodynamic testing (PD) looks at genes that affect how a medication works in the brain. PD testing is in its infancy, but it holds perhaps the most promise for patients: the promise of being able to know which drug(s) will be effective for a particular person. As of this writing, there is only one gene that can be tested that is thought to make a prediction about effectiveness of medications, a gene involved in serotonin signaling called *SLC6A4*.

As you might expect, this gene is involved in the mechanism of action of the selective serotonin reuptake inhibitor antidepressants (SSRIs). You may remember that these medications block the neurons' *serotonin transporters*, the "pumps" that scoop up serotonin and transport it back into the neuron that released it. This effectively increases the amount of serotonin available for signaling. In persons who have certain versions of this gene, SSRI antidepressants don't interact with the serotonin transporters as they should, making them less effective. These patients will often respond to an antidepressant with a different mechanism of action, such as vortioxetine (Trintellix), which works directly on the serotonin *receptor*, essentially bypassing the "broken" serotonin transporters. See figure 13.1.

We know that some individuals with bipolar disorder respond dramatically to lithium, which acts as a "silver bullet" for them. In these patients, lithium is the necessary and sufficient treatment; it completely controls their symptoms all by itself—and they don't respond nearly as well to any other medication approach. ConLiGen published a paper in 2016 that identified two stretches of DNA that appear to be involved. Both are *noncoding DNA*. These areas of DNA, which make up most of our DNA molecules, don't code for proteins and were therefore called "junk DNA" for many years. It is now known that many stretches of "junk" DNA actually are important for turning genes "on" and "off" or otherwise regulating gene activity, but the functions of these particular stretches are not known. Nevertheless, it's only a matter of time before this mystery is unraveled, bringing us that much closer to a test for lithium response that can identify which patients with bipolar disorder should take it.

In the meantime, these genetic tests have been shown to be effective in improving outcomes for patients with depression, mainly by helping prescribers select medications that patients will tolerate more easily and adjust doses based on genetic results.

> ### What Dose Is Right for Me?
>
> Pharmaco*kinetic* genes affect how the body handles (metabolizes) medications. Most medications are broken down in the liver, whose job it is to get rid of any molecules in the bloodstream that don't look like food. This is why most medications need to be taken every day. As soon as certain medications are taken and absorbed by the gut into the bloodstream, the liver starts eliminating them.*
>
> Some individuals are *slow metabolizers* of certain medications, meaning that their body processes these medications much more slowly than most. This means that taking the usual dose of a medication will cause it to build up quickly in their body and reach higher than usual levels, causing side-effect problems and even toxicity. Other individuals are *rapid* or even *ultrarapid metabolizers*. This means that their body is so efficient at processing and getting rid of certain medications that normal doses of these medications are ineffective for them. Their body breaks down the medication so quickly that it never has a chance to build up a high enough level to be effective.
>
> Most psychiatric medications are broken down by a group of enzymes in the liver called *cytochrome enzymes*, and most pharmacogenomic panels test for a half dozen or so of them. By analyzing the genes that code for cytochrome enzymes, predictions can be made about how an individual will process a medication, allowing individualized dosing.
>
> *Some medications are processed by the kidneys rather than by the liver. This includes many antibiotics and also lithium.

SOME PRINCIPLES OF TREATMENT

Now and then, one of the medical journals publishes a "treatment algorithm" for an illness or disorder. An algorithm is a step-by-step procedure for solving a specified problem with mathematical precision.

Figure 12.2 gives you an idea of what the start of a treatment algorithm for treating manic symptoms might look like.

In the late 1990s, a group of experts in bipolar disorder developed and published just such a treatment algorithm for treating bipolar disorder, a project that took years to complete.[2] It was developed by convening a series of meetings of the experts, asking them what they would do in certain situations, and recording consensus recommendations. While the results were somewhat helpful, at least for a time, it turns out that there are a lot of

What Is an Algorithm?

An algorithm is a set of step-by-step instructions to achieve a certain goal. Perhaps the most familiar example of algorithms are kitchen recipes. An algorithm for the goal of making brownies might start with "Preheat your oven to 350 degrees," and then continue with "Line a 9 × 9 inch baking dish with parchment paper," and so on.

Algorithms can be developed to solve problems, too. Here's one for dealing with a misbehaving table lamp (Figure 12.1):

FIGURE 12.1. An algorithm for fixing a lamp that won't turn on

```
→ TURN LAMP SWITCH TO "ON"

    LAMP
  ILLUMINATED?  ────────→   YES (END)
       │
       ▼
    LAMP       YES      BULB          NO      REPAIR
  PLUGGED IN? ──────→ BURNED OUT? ────────→    LAMP
       │                   │
   NO  ▼              YES  ▼
  PLUG LAMP             REPLACE
  INTO SOCKET            BULB
```

Illustration by Jenna Macfarlane

problems with treatment algorithms. An obvious one is that they go out of date rather quickly as new medications or other treatments are introduced. Another is that they never include all the treatment options, only those that a particular group of experts know about and can agree on. But the big problem with treatment algorithms is that their "if this happens, then do that" approach never captures the myriad manifestations of bipolar disorder, the inevitable twists and turns of the world of real treatment and real patients, not to mention the specific situations and needs of the individual. The field of pharmacogenomics promises to take at least some of the guesswork out of selecting and dosing medications, but for now, there's nearly as much art as science involved in doing it well.

Between 1999 and 2005, a major clinical trial that included more than four thousand patients attempted to address these complexities. Although it did include an algorithm (several of them, in fact), one of the

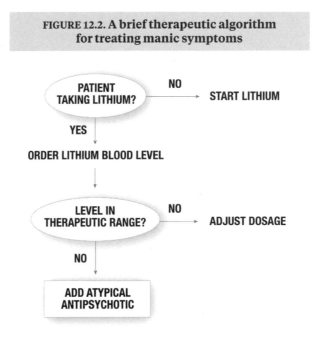

FIGURE 12.2. A brief therapeutic algorithm for treating manic symptoms

Illustration by Jenna Macfarlane

main purposes of the study was to investigate how "real-world" patients, as opposed to carefully selected patients with uncomplicated illness, do when given treatment based on using "best practice" evidence-based approaches. This was the Systematic Treatment Enhancement Program for Bipolar Disorder.[3] The STEP-BD generated more than sixty scientific papers on every aspect of the treatment of bipolar disorder and also on the course of the illness, common complications, the prognosis, and even genetics. It confirmed the effectiveness of many accepted approaches to the treatment of bipolar disorder but also called into question some equally accepted approaches (the most important of these being the significant doubt that it cast on the effectiveness of antidepressant medications in treating bipolar patients). Much of this chapter is based on findings of the STEP-BD; I will review some of the principles of treatment that serve patients (and their physicians) well.

Tincture of Time

With so many powerful and effective medications available in psychiatry now, it's easy to become impatient when symptoms don't subside as quickly as one would wish. But in the treatment of mood disorders, a crucial principle to remember is to *take the long view.*

The medications we use to treat mood disorders usually take at least two to four weeks to even begin helping, and sometimes much longer to have their full effect. One of my mentors, to drive home just this point, is fond of telling his patients, "The *second* year on lithium is always better than the first." When treating an episode of bipolar disorder, it simply doesn't make sense to change medications quickly. Even hospitalized patients are rarely well served by adding too many medications too quickly—patients simply wind up taking more medications than they need and at higher doses than may be necessary.

When a diagnosis of bipolar II or cyclothymic disorder is being considered, the time line should stretch out even more. The mood changes in these variations of bipolar disorder can sometimes be much more subtle than those of bipolar I. It may take three to six months of taking a mood stabilizer for its beneficial effects on a subtly unstable mood to become apparent.

I saw Craig about two weeks after he had been discharged from a hospital in another city. He had been on a business trip and started to have fairly severe manic symptoms: insomnia, racing thoughts, angry irritability. He had been having good control of his symptoms on a mood stabilizer, but a series of high-stress job interviews in several different cities, jet lag, worry, and poor sleep had activated his illness, and he soon found himself hospitalized in a city several hundred miles from home.

He pulled a fistful of medication bottles out of his pocket and put them on the desk in my office. "I brought all these new medicines, but I have to admit, I've only been taking the lithium."

I picked up the bottles one by one: lithium, valproate, an antipsychotic, an antianxiety agent, and a sleeping pill.

"How long were you in the hospital?" I asked.

"Eight days."

"And you were discharged on all *this?"*

"That's right. I can't believe I really need all this. I was so drugged when my wife came to pick me up, I couldn't work for another week and a half. I think this is the first day I've felt safe to drive."

Craig's illness had always been well controlled on his medications; it was hard for me to believe that all these medications had really been necessary. How had this happened?

When I asked Craig about his treatment in the hospital, a sadly familiar story emerged: a new medication had been added to the mix almost every other day while he was there. He was started on the antipsychotic medication as soon as he was admitted. Well, that wasn't unreasonable; I might have recommended that myself—for a while, at least. But when he didn't sleep well the next night, a sleeping pill was added. A few days later, when he mentioned that he had been worried about his finances lately, an antianxiety medication was added. After a week he told his doctor he was feeling less hyper but still not back to his usual self—so the valproate was added to the lithium. By the time he left the hospital, he wasn't complaining of mood problems anymore because he was too sedated to know what kind of mood he was in.

"Craig, you know I want you to call the clinic before you make any changes in your medication on your own," I said with a smile. "But I have to admit, in the end you did exactly what I would have recommended that you do. You certainly don't need all this."

Craig smiled back.

In Craig's case it was the doctor who forgot to take the long view, but I think it's probably just as easy for patients or their family members to fall into the trap of expecting results too quickly.

"Cindy's still having mood swings, Doctor," Jim said as he sat down beside his wife in the office. "The Lamictal isn't working. Is there something else we can try?"

Jim and Cindy were a couple in their thirties. They had two small children, and Cindy usually cared for her attorney sister's little boy during the day as well as her own children.

Cindy was tense and quiet as her husband continued. "She's been on this medication for weeks now, and things are no different. She started arguing with me about the television being too loud the other night, and when I tried to reason with her, she picked up the remote control and threw it at me. This has got to stop."

"What do you think, Cindy?" I asked. "Do you think the medication has helped any?"

"Well, I'm not sure, but I think maybe it has."

"Well, I'm sure it hasn't," said Jim. "The night before the remote incident she—"

"Jim," I said, "it's much too early to be sure about anything yet. I know Cindy's been taking the Lamictal for over a month, but she's been at a full therapeutic dose for less than one week." I turned to Cindy. "What have you noticed that makes you think the Lamictal might be helping?"

"Well, Jim was out of town for a few days last week, and so was my sister. I had the three kids twenty-four hours a day the whole time again. You know how keyed up I got the last time that happened."

In fact, it had been a similar situation that had brought Cindy into treatment in the first place. About three weeks before our first meeting, Cindy had been with the three boys, six, five, and three years old, because of coinciding business trips taken by Jim and her sister. She had needed to call Jim and get him to fly back home because she was becoming more and more irritable with the children, snapping at them, slamming doors, starting to feel out of control.

The next week she came to see me, and as we talked about her history, it emerged that she had experienced episodes of depression after both of her children were born, that she had had these "hyper" episodes about once a year since college, and that her mother had suffered from "mood swings" and alcoholism. A diagnosis of bipolar II or perhaps a "soft" bipolar disorder seemed likely, and we decided on a trial of a mood stabilizer.

"The kids just didn't get to me this time," Cindy continued. "First, I thought they were being on their best behavior because of what had happened that last time, and maybe they were for an hour or so. But by evening I realized that they were really about as active as they usually are, and that there was something different about me. I wasn't as, you know, sensitive. Several times now I've noticed that I can handle things better."

"Not the other night," Jim chimed in. "I'm not noticing much difference."

"Well, maybe Jim's right," Cindy went on. "Maybe you could give me something for the times when I'm feeling really stressed? Some Valium or Xanax? I never used . . . I don't know what to call them—nerve pills? And I'm sure I wouldn't need them often."

"I don't think we should add more medication until we're sure you're getting the maximum benefit from the one you're on. And from what you're telling me, I think that's beginning to happen," I said. "The fact that you've never felt the need for tranquilizers before makes me think that the bipolar disorder explains all your symptoms and needs to be the focus of our attention. It's absolutely too early to expect the Lamictal to have had its full effect. Let's talk about this a bit more."

Cindy and Jim were very anxious for Cindy's symptoms to stop. Who could blame them? But to give up on a mood stabilizer because it hasn't completely controlled every symptom so soon is foolish. It's unlikely that another would work any faster—and it might not even work as well, in which case Cindy would be right back to square one after another couple of weeks.

Diagnosis, Diagnosis, Diagnosis

If the three most important words in the real estate business are *location, location, location,* then the three most important words in medicine are *diagnosis, diagnosis, diagnosis.* There was a tendency at one time in psychiatry to see medications as *symptomatic treatments.* This means picking a medication and making the decision to use it based on identification of *symptoms,* not underlying *diagnoses.* Cindy wanted to try another medication for "stress"—that is, for feeling tense and irritable. But the symptoms of our working diagnosis, bipolar disorder, include periods of tension and irritability. If Cindy's poor stress tolerance were a symptom of her mood disorder and she took an antianxiety medication to cover it up rather than getting more intensive treatment of the mood disorder, she'd end up taking a medication she didn't really need for a symptom that wasn't going to get much better because the underlying problem, bipolar disorder, wasn't being properly treated. Insomnia is a similar symptom, very commonly a symptom of the mood disorder but all too often treated with sleeping medications as if it were an isolated symptom.

Every once in a while, I see a patient with bipolar disorder who has read an internet article about attention-deficit hyperactivity disorder and requests medication for ADHD. Some of its symptoms—like impulsivity; impatience; fast, disorganized thinking; and poor concentration—are, of course, also seen in bipolar patients. These are distressing symptoms that deserve attention, but they deserve the right kind of attention. If they are an expression of the mood changes of bipolar disorder, then medication for ADHD won't help. (In fact, the medications used to treat ADHD, stimulants and antidepressants, can make things worse.)

Making a diagnosis is the process of identifying the one disease that can explain all the patient's symptoms. This is a variation of the scientific principle called Occam's razor, named after William of Occam (or Ockham), the medieval theologian-philosopher credited with coining this principle: the simplest explanation for a phenomenon is always preferable to a more complex one and is most likely to be correct. Obviously, a patient may have two different disorders that require two different treatment approaches. But if all the patient's symptoms can be understood as expressions of *one* disorder, treating that one will likely alleviate all the symptoms.

I see this problem of multiple diagnoses and symptomatic treatments even more commonly in depressed patients. In depression, anxiety and insomnia can be thorny and uncomfortable expressions of the mood disorder—and physical symptoms can be as well, especially in the elderly.

I have seen elderly patients taking antidepressant medications (often at an inadequate dose) who are also taking sleeping pills, tranquilizers, anti-inflammatory and pain medications for arthritis, stool softeners and laxatives for constipation, and sometimes vitamins and tonics thrown in for good measure (perhaps because of complaints of "low energy"). All these problems are symptoms of depression (even the arthritis pain, because depressed patients become more distressed by pain), but sometimes it's hard to see the forest for the trees. Before you know it, the patient is taking a dozen or so different medications for all the different symptoms of depression, and the disease that underlies them all, a mood disorder, has been missed.

What Is the Role of Antidepressants in Bipolar Disorder?

Perhaps the most unexpected finding to come out of the STEP-BD was the surprising lack of evidence that antidepressant medications are helpful in treating bipolar disorder. One of the studies within the STEP-BD compared depressed patients treated with a mood stabilizer plus an antidepressant (either sertraline or bupropion) with patients treated with a mood stabilizer and a placebo. The main patient-outcome goal for this part of the study was "durable recovery" from depression, defined as maintaining a normal mood for at least eight weeks. Using this standard, antidepressants were no more effective in these bipolar patients than the placebo (the patients taking the antidepressant with their mood stabilizer did no better than those who took only a mood stabilizer). Not only that: when some secondary measures were assessed, the results suggested that the patients on the mood stabilizer alone did somewhat *better* than the patients who took an antidepressant, for example, depressed patients with bipolar II disorder. Furthermore, as a follow-up to the placebo-controlled study, the patients who *did* recover and who were taking the antidepressant with their mood stabilizer were divided into two groups: one group continued on both medications, and the other group stopped taking the antidepressant. Again, the group that stopped taking the antidepressant did just as well as those who did not: taking an antidepressant did not keep patients well longer and did not delay a relapse, compared with taking a mood stabilizer alone. Although it did not reach the level of statistical significance, the data suggested that patients who had rapid-cycling symptoms (several episodes of mania or depression in a year) had a relapse of depression *sooner* than those who stopped taking the antidepressant: that is, continuing on an antidepressant increased the risk of getting depressed. Talk about counterintuitive!

It has been known for many years that antidepressants can trigger manic or mixed symptoms in bipolar patients. Clinicians have also long suspected that antidepressant medications increase cycling in bipolar patients, causing them to have more episodes of depression and manic or mixed symptoms. The STEP-BD appears to reinforce both of these impressions. However, every psychiatrist who cares for patients with bipolar disorder treats some who can safely take an antidepressant and who require it to stay well.

So what should we conclude about the use of antidepressant medications in bipolar patients? I think it's fair to say that antidepressants should be used with extreme caution in patients with bipolar disorder, and that an antidepressant should be discontinued as soon as possible over the longer term of treatment. Antidepressants should be stopped immediately if the patient develops insomnia or feels overactivated or "wired" after she starts taking an it. I have had patients describe this as feeling "anxious," and while it may be a feeling that is similar to anxiety, when I see a bipolar patient taking an antidepressant who reports severe "anxiety," I have a low threshold for stopping it.

Sometimes there don't seem to be any immediate untoward effects from starting an antidepressant, but it may become clear over time that the patient is cycling more often. If, in the months (or even years) after a patient starts taking an antidepressant, he notices *new* mood symptoms, such as mixed symptoms or problems with "rages" for the first time, the continued use of the antidepressant should be seriously questioned.

Don't Forget Psychotherapy

Finally, I can't stress enough that *every bipolar patient needs psychotherapy* at one point or another. Several weeks or months of counseling are absolutely essential after the diagnosis and initiation of treatment for bipolar disorder. Just as a person with diabetes needs to follow dietary recommendations to get the best control of her glucose levels and a hip-fracture patient needs physical therapy for optimal functioning, persons with bipolar disorder need psychotherapy at times to have the best possible control of their mood symptoms.

Psychotherapy is one intervention for the depression of bipolar disorder that I can confidently state does *not* have any risk of triggering manic symptoms or increased cycling. Many persons with bipolar disorder go through a period of depression after they recover from a period of mania or hypomania. It can be tempting to think about using an antidepressant to deal with this problem. For the reasons noted above, however, this is not usually a good idea. During some periods of bipolar depression, the intervention that needs to be started, or given at a higher "dose" (by seeing a therapist more often), is psychotherapy.

KEY TAKEAWAYS

▶ Bipolar disorder is complicated—and so is its treatment. What works for one patient may not work for another, and some trial and error is inevitable.

▶ Patience is a virtue! Most treatments take weeks to become fully effective; changing or adding medications too soon often creates problems.

▶ Beware of antidepressants. They can make bad things (like depression) worse (like increasing cycling and triggering mixed states).

▶ Genetic testing is improving the ability of prescribers to individualize selecting and dosing medications, a field called *pharmacogenetics.*

▶ Don't forget psychotherapy—it's a powerful treatment in its own right.

PART III

What Causes
Bipolar Disorder?

Physicians have theorized about the causes of bipolar disorder for centuries. The ancient Greeks blamed depression on an excess of "black bile" in the body (the word *melancholia* comes from the Greek words for "black" and "bile"). In the mid-twentieth century, following on discoveries of changes in brain chemistry that could be detected when antidepressant drugs were administered to experimental animals, deficiencies and excesses of brain chemicals like serotonin and norepinephrine were thought to be at the root of this complex disorder, and the term *chemical imbalance* found its way into the media.

Starting in the late 1990s, however, attention turned away from "chemical imbalances" and started to focus on aspects of brain functioning that are altogether different from these ideas. The change started with the discovery that, in a sense, the brain never stops developing. Neuroscientists had thought that by time we are eighteen months old or so, we had all the brain cells we would ever have and the "hard wiring" of the brain, like the hardware of a computer, was a finished product. We now know that this is not the case; in many of its areas, the brain is continuously rewiring itself as it adapts to changes in the environment. The prerequisite for this process is the brain's *neuroplasticity*.

The original meaning of the word *plastic* is "capable of being easily shaped or molded," and we now know that mood disorders are caused by problems with this prerequisite. Normally, the brain is continuously rewiring and reprogramming itself; in persons with mood disorders, however, this process is slowed and becomes inefficient. Connecting the dots between impairments in neuroplasticity and symptoms of bipolar disorder such as low mood or grandiose delusions is a long way off, but it is clear that the treatments that help persons with bipolar disorder all have something in common: they enhance neuroplasticity. Some do so by changing the chemical environment of the brain in such a way as to protect neurons so they can better function and adapt (lithium and valproate); others boost the processes by which stem cells* in the brain become new brain cells.

After the foregoing paragraphs, some readers will have read all they really care to know about the causes of bipolar disorder; others will want more of the details. If you are one of the former, you can skip the rest of this section, and I won't be offended in the least. If you're one of the latter, read on.

Stem cells are immature, general-purpose cells that lie dormant in many organs in the body. They can be triggered to develop into whatever kind of cell the body happens to need, from liver cells to heart muscle cells to neurons.

CHAPTER 13

The Brain Is Like the Internet

Many people imagine that the human brain is a kind of wonderful computer. Although this is a vast oversimplification of the true capabilities of the brain, it's a good place to start in trying to understand how this fantastic organ of the mind works.

Like the computer that I'm using to write these words, a human brain receives input, processes the information it receives, and then delivers output. Like a computer, it stores information and often uses this stored information to help process further input. The human brain receives its input from the sense organs—the eyes, ears, taste buds, touch receptors, and so forth—and delivers output in terms of behavior.

You may know that a computer computes by means of many thousands of microscopic switches embedded in its processing chip. The pattern of "on" and "off" in the switches is what stores information; processing is the control of the flow of signals through these switches. The human brain contains about eleven billion nerve cells, or *neurons*—but as powerful as a computer with eleven billion switches might be, our brain is many orders of magnitude more impressive than that. This is because each neuron is not just a switch but rather is an impressive microprocessor in its own right. Each neuron receives input from many other neurons, processes this information, and sends output to many others. The brain, then, is not like a computer with billions of switches; it is more like the internet: a network of billions of computers, all capable of being individually programmed. Each neuron in the brain may receive input and then transmit signals to up to fifty thousand other neurons. The number of all the possible connections in the human brain is incomprehensibly large, a hyper-astronomical number on the order of the number of molecules in the universe.

As mentioned in the introduction to this section, there is a lot of evidence that bipolar disorder (and perhaps all mood disorders, as well as anxiety disorders) is caused by some defect in the mechanisms by which the individual neurons are programmed. As I mentioned, neurons have the ability to be "reprogrammed" in response to various situations (stress is one), a capability called *neuroplasticity* (remember that the original meaning of *plastic* refers to a material that can be shaped and reshaped, like modeling clay). But before we get to that, we need to talk about neurotransmitters.

Although the human nervous system uses electrical signals to do much of its work, it uses chemical signals as well; molecules called *neurotransmitters* are the means by which nerve cells communicate with each other. Neurons send these chemical signals to each other at the *synapse*, an area where two neurons nearly touch. The first neuron releases neurotransmitters, which flow across this narrow space to link up with targets called *receptors* on the next neuron (figure 13.1). When enough of the receptors are occupied by neurotransmitter molecules, which fit into the receptors like keys fit into locks, the recipient nerve cell is activated and fires off its own signal. There needs to be some mechanism for this signaling system to be turned off and reset, of course. After neurotransmitter molecules link up with receptors across the synapse, they must somehow be removed in preparation for the next batch. This happens in a variety of ways in different cells, but one of the most important mechanisms is by reuptake into the neuron that released them. A *reuptake pump* on this neuron removes neurotransmitter molecules from the synapse and transports them back into the interior of the cell, where they can be repackaged for rerelease.

Neurons are continually communicating with each other. Neurotransmitter molecules passing from one neuron to another across synapses maintain a steady tone of chemical signals, with the signal getting stronger, or pulsing up, at times and the neuron detecting and reacting to these pulses. Thus, as I noted earlier, neurons are not just switches that can only be set to "on" or "off" but rather are tiny information-processing units that are constantly communicating with other neurons to which they are functionally linked.

Soon after Roland Kuhn discovered that G 22355 was an effective antidepressant (see chapter 4), neuroscientists started to investigate the effect of this pharmaceutical on brain chemistry. They discovered that imipramine is a powerful inhibitor of one type of reuptake pump, blocking the reuptake of a group of neurotransmitters called *neurogenic amines* (or *neuroamines*). Remember that neurons turn off their chemical signals ("turn down" is probably more accurate) by scooping up neurotransmitter molecules from the synapse and repackaging them. Just as partly closing the drain in a bathtub while the water is running will cause the tub to begin to fill, if you block the reuptake of neurotransmitter molecules into cells, the net effect will be an increase of neurotransmitters in the synapse. Neuroscientists

FIGURE 13.1. The neuron

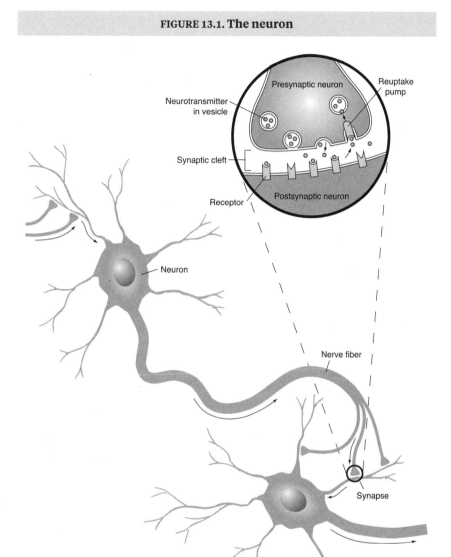

found that nearly all the medications that are effective antidepressants cause a blockade of neurotransmitter reuptake in brain cells. This observation led to the "amine hypothesis" of the mood disorders. This theory stated that depression is caused by an abnormally low level of the neurotransmitter *norepinephrine* and that mania is caused by too high a level. (This may be where the unfortunate term *chemical imbalance* had its origins.)

Further work soon indicated, however, that too little norepinephrine was too simplistic an explanation. As more antidepressant medications were discovered, researchers found that some effective ones seemed to have little effect on norepinephrine. Fluoxetine (Prozac) is one of a family of pharmaceuticals that are powerful inhibitors of the reuptake of a different neurotransmitter, *serotonin*; they have almost no direct effect on norepinephrine. Other antidepressants seem to affect yet other neurotransmitters.

Another argument against a simplistic theory involving too much or too little norepinephrine comes from an observation about the time course of these chemical changes in the brain. Antidepressant-induced changes in neurotransmitter levels at the synapse occur almost immediately after the drug is taken—in a matter of hours. But, as is well known, it takes several weeks for these agents to start alleviating the symptoms of depression. If the problem were simply too little neurotransmitter in the synapses of certain brain circuits, why would it take several weeks after the drug raised neurotransmitter levels at the synapse for the symptoms of depression to improve? We now believe that antidepressant treatment, by artificially changing levels of neurotransmitters in the brain, triggers some reaction in neurons that enhances neuroplasticity, a reaction that takes weeks to occur.

We now know what that reaction is. It has been shown in animal studies that after several weeks of exposure to an antidepressant drug, there is an increase in the process by which stem cells in the brain develop into mature neurons. These new neurons must then integrate themselves into brain circuits. The reason antidepressant medications take several weeks to work is that it simply takes time for these cellular processes to play out. This effect is the most dramatic in an area of the brain called the *hippocampus*, a brain center known to be important in the regulation of emotions.

Antidepressants change neurotransmitter levels in the brain, but that is just a first step, the trigger for more complicated changes that involve the growth of new neurons and the sprouting of new connections between nerve cells.

Because of the unique therapeutic effects of lithium in bipolar disorder, there has naturally been a lot of effort to figure out where this medication is active in the brain and what its effect is on brain chemistry. Lithium doesn't seem to affect neurotransmitter levels in the synapse and doesn't interact with neurotransmitter receptors or affect the reuptake pumps. In fact, it has none of the types of direct effects on cells that the antidepressants have. Only in the past few years has the probable site of lithium action been found, and it's not at the synapse at all. Lithium (and perhaps the newer mood stabilizers as well) seems to work at a different cellular level: *inside* the neuron. Several small molecules inside the neuron, with odd names like

BDNF (for brain-derived neurotrophic factor) and CREB (for cAMP response element binding protein), are thought to be key to maintaining neuroplasticity. Lithium has been found to have dramatic effects on the levels of these molecules in neurons.

There is also increasing interest in another neurotransmitter, *glutamate*, which doesn't seem to be affected by antidepressants at all, although it is affected by lamotrigine (Lamictal) and other mood stabilizers; glutamate also seems to be crucial to neuroplasticity.

One way to think about neuroplasticity is that it underlies the brain's responsiveness to the environment and its ability to react to change and stress. Neuroplasticity is also thought to be involved in memory and learning. If you consider the symptoms of bipolar disorder, which include thinking and concentration problems in addition to mood changes, and consider how episodes of the illness can be triggered by stresses of various types, this idea that neuroplasticity is disrupted in bipolar disorder begins to make sense. Neuroplasticity may be a necessary part of maintaining mood within a normal range, somehow "tuning" the responsiveness of our mood state to experiences and environment, allowing us to react to and then recover from stresses.

There is strong evidence that chronic stress impairs neuroplasticity. This last finding is extremely interesting because it may explain why stress triggers mood episodes in persons with mood disorders. (Much more on stress and bipolar disorder is to come in chapter 18.)

Taken together, these findings on the importance of cell plasticity and growth explain why medications that help with symptoms of bipolar disorder, especially bipolar depression, take several weeks to do so.

It may be a while before we understand how all the molecular and cellular pieces of this complicated story fit together, but the work to unravel the basic cause (or causes) of bipolar disorder is proceeding apace. And when we understand exactly what is "broken" in bipolar disorder, the job of fixing it will become much easier.

───────────────── KEY TAKEAWAYS ─────────────────

▶ The brain is not just a computer but more like the internet, with billions of brain cells (neurons) that are actually independent processing units.

▶ Areas of the brain are constantly remodeling themselves in response to changes in the environment; the brain's capacity to do this is called *neuroplasticity*.

▶ Although early research focused on neurotransmitters, which are the chemical messengers of the brain, it is now known that problems with neuroplasticity underlie bipolar disorder and probably other psychiatric illnesses as well.

▶ We know this because almost every treatment that helps persons with bipolar disorder has been shown to enhance neuroplasticity in some way.

▶ Some treatments do this by protecting the neurons that are already present (lithium) and some by triggering new neurons to develop from stem cells in the brain (antidepressants).

CHAPTER 14

More Bipolar Biology

There are several more topics in the realm of biology that tell us a lot about bipolar disorder. A common theme, it seems, is to show that staying well with bipolar disorder depends quite a lot on taking care of one's general health. In part IV of the book (chapters 20–23), I will discuss some of the lifestyle changes that are vital in helping persons with bipolar disorder stay well. Many of these changes are such things as getting a good night's sleep, exercising regularly, and eating a healthful diet. Now I know some readers (surely not you) will read through that list and say to themselves, "Right, a good night's sleep, exercising, blah, blah, blah. I know all that stuff. Tell me something *important*." Well, this next section, on stress, explains exactly why these things are important and why stress is *not* good for your brain.

HOW THE BODY HANDLES STRESS

The most dramatic bodily response to stress is the familiar "fight or flight" response. If you are hiking along the Appalachian Trail and suddenly encounter a bear twice your size, some dramatic physical changes take place in the body, changes that prepare you to face combat with the creature ("fight") or, perhaps more likely, run as fast and as far as you can ("flight"). There is a hormonally triggered flood of energy-containing glucose, fat molecules, and proteins into your bloodstream; your heart rate and blood pressure go up to get these energy molecules to the muscles as quickly as possible; and your breathing becomes faster and deeper to provide the oxygen needed to turn the energy molecules into power. Simultaneously, body systems that are not involved in fighting or fleeing shift down: digestion slows, cellular growth and tissue repair grind to a halt, and even the immune system temporarily goes into hibernation. The stress response is really a brilliantly orchestrated symphony of physiological responses in many organ systems that prepares the body for intense physical exertion.

All of this is terrific in a physical emergency, but if this hyperactive physiology goes on for too long, bad things begin to happen.

In other animals, the stress response is either active or inactive; the system is either "on" or "off." But in humans (and the animals most closely related to them), elements of the stress response can be active for much longer periods of time. Neuroscientist Robert Sapolsky highlighted this difference between humans and other animals in a book about the role of stress in health and disease that he called *Why Zebras Don't Get Ulcers*. The title refers to the fact that when a grazing zebra spots a lion on the edge of the jungle, its stress response kicks in at full force and the animal bounds off at breakneck speed, but then, if it's been fast enough and lucky enough, the zebra escapes the hungry lion and simply resumes eating, as calm and placid as if nothing had happened, with bodily functions quickly returning to baseline. Other than the sight of a lion, there isn't much that brings on the stress response in zebras, because zebras don't have the cognitive capacity to worry. But we are quite different: "We humans can be stressed by things that simply make no sense to zebras. . . . It is not a general mammalian trait to become anxious about mortgages or the Internal Revenue Service, about public speaking or fears of what you say in a job interview, about the inevitability of death."[1] Nevertheless, these very un-zebralike sources of stress activate many of the same physiological responses in the human body as a zebra's sighting of the lion or a hiker's encounter with the bear activates.

The main hormones responsible for the stress response are the *glucocorticoids*, a group of hormones produced by the adrenal glands, and the most important of these is *cortisol*. You can think of cortisol as responsible for controlling the bodily changes that are part of the stress response: the release of glucose into the bloodstream, the damping down of the immune system, and the suppression of cellular growth. It is this last feature of cortisol that is most relevant to persons with bipolar disorder.

As you may remember from the previous chapter, our mood-regulation system depends on the constant active remodeling of networks of neurons in the brain, especially in an area of the brain called the hippocampus. The cells in the hippocampus are always busy, sprouting new connections and disconnecting and reconnecting with other neurons, and new neurons are constantly needed to replenish the ones that simply wear out from all this work. It's easy to see, then, how too much cortisol damping down cellular growth over too long a time can have a very deleterious effect on the mood system. The damaging effect of high levels of cortisol on the brain has been abundantly demonstrated in animal studies.

FIGURE 14.1. The effects of chronic stress on hippocampal neurons

A is a representative neuron from a control animal, and *B* is from an animal that was subjected to chronic stress for several hours daily for ten consecutive days.

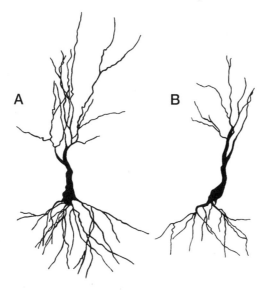

Source: A. Vyas, R. Mitra, B. Rao, and S. Chattarji, "Chronic Stress Induces Contrasting Patterns of Dendritic Remodeling in Hippocampal and Amygdaloid Neurons," *Journal of Neuroscience* 22 (2002): 6810–18.

Mice, for example, are timid little creatures. They scurry around their environment, not being still for long except to eat, and they prefer darkness. A relatively humane way to subject mice to stress is to confine them to a Lucite tube in a well-lit environment for several hours, an experimental technique known as "chronic immobilization stress." If you do this day after day, the mice will exhibit changes in their behavior that resemble depression in humans: they don't eat as much, and they lose weight. Sleep is disrupted, and sexual activity reduced. They are less active; they spend less time running on the wheels in their cages. Tests of object recognition and memory show that their cognitive functioning suffers as well. When the blood level of corticosterone, the mouse equivalent of cortisol, is measured, it is found to be elevated. But the most striking findings involve changes in neurons in the hippocampus. As figure 14.1 shows, when the hippocampal neurons of mice subjected to chronic stress are compared to those of control mice, the difference is unmistakable.

The neurons of the stressed animals look shrunken and stunted compared to those of the non-stressed animals. Most importantly, research has shown that it is cortisol that is responsible for these changes. Injecting corticosterone into rodents not subjected to chronic stress produces exactly the same effect: shrunken brain cells in the hippocampus, the area of the brain thought to be the most important in mood regulation.[2]

But here's the most impressive thing of all: stress-caused damage to brain cells in the hippocampus can be *prevented* by lithium. Scientists at Rockefeller University, along with colleagues at other institutions, designed an experiment to investigate whether lithium might protect neurons in the hippocampus from the effects of stress. Some experimental mice were divided into two groups. One group was given lithium for two weeks and the other was not; then both groups were subjected to chronic stress. Figure 14.2 is one of those pictures worth a thousand words.

The first cell is from a control animal that was not subjected to stress; it shows a normally developed cell (*A*). Cell *B* is a representative neuron from a stressed mouse, showing, as expected, a stunted and shrunken cell. *C* is a cell from the hippocampus of a mouse that received lithium for two weeks before being subjected to stress and continued on lithium through the period of stress. You don't need to be a neuroscientist to see that the cell from the lithium-treated mouse (*C*) was protected from the effects of stress and looks just as healthy as the one from the control animal (*A*).

FIGURE 14.2. Protecting hippocampal neurons from the damaging effects of chronic stress with lithium

A is a representative hippocampal neuron from a control animal, *B* is from an animal subjected to twenty-one days of immobilization stress, and *C* is from a stressed animal that had been pretreated with lithium for two weeks before experiencing the stress.

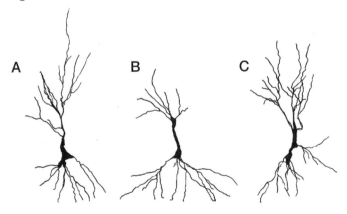

Source: G. Wood, L. Young, L. Reagan, B. Chen, and B. McEwan, "Stress-Induced Structural Remodeling in the Hippocampus: Prevention by Lithium Treatment," *Proceedings of the National Academy of Sciences* 101 (2004): 3973-78.SS. Copyright 2004 National Academy of Sciences, USA.

So what should we conclude from all this? First of all, stress is *not* good for your brain. Stress raises the levels of steroid hormones in the bloodstream, and cortisol, the most important of these hormones, is practically toxic to neurons in the most important mood-regulation center of the brain, the hippocampus. So, it follows rather obviously that persons with bipolar disorder should avoid the kinds of stress that increase their cortisol levels. And what are those stresses? They are all those things that your doctor (and probably your mother) told you to avoid: an unhealthful diet, not exercising, smoking, drinking alcohol, not getting a good night's sleep—well, you get the idea. And although zebras don't worry about financial problems, deadlines, or relationship conflicts, humans do. Those things increase cortisol levels as well. In the chapters of part IV, I'll talk about how to put this knowledge into practice.

Stress Management: Act More Like a Zebra!

Why Zebra's Don't Get Ulcers, Dr. Robert Sapolski's book on the biology of stress, is filled with scientific evidence on how bad stress is for our body—which includes our brain. Having studied the topic for decades, he has several recommendations for the sorts of lifestyle changes and other factors that protect against the effects of stress by helping to keep your stress-response system appropriately "tuned" and levels of stress hormones low.

- *Exercise*: How much? Most experts recommend twenty to thirty minutes at least three times a week.

- *Meditation*: Numerous studies have shown that various types meditation lower cortisol and resting adrenalin levels, which in turn lowers blood pressure.

- *Social support*: A supportive network of family and friends and feeling part of a community have been shown to improve physical and mental health outcomes and increase longevity.

- *"Pick your battles"*: In his book, Sapolsky shares a Quaker aphorism:

  > In the face of strong winds, let me be a blade of grass.
  > In the face of strong walls, let me be a gale of wind.

  He then adds, "Sometimes, coping with stress consists of blowing down walls. But sometimes it consists of being a blade of grass, buffeted and bent by the wind but still standing when the wind is long gone."*

*Robert M. Sapolsky, *Why Zebras Don't Get Ulcers* (New York: Holt, 2004), 416, Kindle edition.

BIPOLAR DISORDER AND HORMONAL SYSTEMS

By far the most important hormone systems in the regulation of mood are the thyroid hormones and the adrenal hormones. We've already discussed both of these systems a bit, but a brief review will help.

The thyroid gland, located just below the larynx (the "voice box") at the base of the neck, secretes several hormones into the blood. These hormones are central to the body's regulation of energy. Thyroid hormones help control the rate of calorie consumption by the body, known as *metabolism*, and the rate at which calories are converted to and stored as fat. If the thyroid gland secretes an excess of its hormones (*hyper*thyroidism), the person's metabolism speeds up; if not enough is secreted (*hypo*thyroidism), the metabolism slows down. This "speeding up" or "slowing down" affects emotions and behavior as well and can cause symptoms mimicking a mood disorder even in persons who otherwise don't seem to have mood problems (table 14.1).

When a person is suffering from *severe* hyper- or hypothyroidism, the clinical picture is pretty unmistakable. But in mild thyroid problems, changes in mood and activity level can be the *only* symptoms. Not only can thyroid disease cause mood symptoms directly; it can also make the symptoms of a preexisting mood disorder more difficult to treat. We have already discussed the link between rapid-cycling bipolar disorder and thyroid disease. Mood disorders can be resistant to treatment if there is even the slightest thyroid problem. These are more reasons why it is necessary to pay attention to this hormonal system and to test for thyroid hormone levels in persons with mood disorders.

The adrenal glands sit atop the kidneys in the lower back and secrete several hormones, the most important of which are the corticosteroids. We've discussed one of these, cortisol, in some detail. In addition to their role in the stress response, the corticosteroid hormones are critical to the regulation of metabolism.

Corticosteroids are potent anti-inflammatory agents, and many pharmaceutical products, such as cortisone and prednisone, are artificial versions of these adrenal hormones. These drugs are a component in some creams used to treat allergic skin reactions, but corticosteroids are also given orally and intravenously to treat inflammatory conditions such as rheumatoid arthritis, asthma, and inflammatory bowel disease, and they are often given as a treatment for acute pain, especially back pain.

On one hand, excessive corticosteroids from adrenal tumors can cause symptoms of agitated depression with suicidal thinking. On the other hand,

TABLE 14.1. Psychiatric symptoms of thyroid disease	
Hyperthyroidism	*Hypothyroidism*
Irritability	Depressed mood
Insomnia	Drowsiness
Restlessness	Lethargy
Hyperactivity	Poor concentration
Paranoia	Slowed thinking
Poor concentration	Apathy and social withdrawal
Delusional thinking	Hallucinations

hypomanic symptoms seem to be more common in patients being treated with artificial corticosteroids for medical conditions. Persons with bipolar disorder need to be cautious when taking these drugs for medical conditions and should ask about alternatives when such treatment is being considered. (Steroid creams do not cause psychiatric symptoms. The creams are formulated so that the medication affects only the tissue it comes into direct contact with. Only minute amounts of the active ingredient are absorbed into the bloodstream.)

Another hormonal system affecting the course of bipolar disorder is the female reproductive hormonal cycle. Substantial changes in the levels of the female reproductive hormones *estrogen* and *progesterone* occur during the menstrual cycle, during pregnancy and after childbirth, and at menopause These fluctuations can have dramatic effects on mood in some women. This important topic will be discussed in its own chapter in part IV.

PICTURING BIPOLAR DISORDER IN THE BRAIN

For decades clinical scientists have searched for a way to test for bipolar disorder. As we have developed more sophisticated methods of probing the workings of the brain, we have been able to measure subtle differences in brain functioning in mood-disorder patients, and although none of these observations has led to the development of reliable tests yet, we are nevertheless learning a great deal about the disorder with these techniques.

As we saw in chapter 4, early researchers who dissected the brains of deceased people who had had bipolar disorder or examined their brain tissues under a microscope found no abnormalities of brain structure and questioned whether bipolar disorder was really a brain disease at all. We now know that it is—but that's because we have learned how to look for and measure abnormalities of brain *chemistry*. Looking at the *structure* of the brain, whether with the naked eye, the microscope, or the x-ray machine, has been unrevealing until quite recently. But now two new imaging techniques are beginning to allow us to picture bipolar disorder in the brain.

The first of these techniques is *magnetic resonance imaging,* or *MRI.* MRI is based on the discovery that the atoms of objects placed in a powerful magnetic field absorb energy or "resonate" at characteristic frequencies that can be measured with the proper equipment. In medical MRI scans, the patient lies encircled by a large doughnut-shaped instrument that generates a powerful magnetic field. Sensitive instrumentation measures the different resonances of different tissues: bone, muscle, fat, blood, and so forth, and the signals from each are assembled by computer into a picture. MRI is a very sensitive technique, and even small and subtle tissue differences show up with astonishing clarity.

A number of studies have demonstrated that the brains of persons with bipolar disorder have an increased number of unusual MRI findings called *T2 hyperintensities.* These are small areas of high MRI signal intensity thought to indicate changes of water content in brain tissue. MRI scans of persons with blood-vessel diseases of the brain and several other brain diseases also indicate T2 hyperintensities, and they seem to increase with the normal aging process. But although T2 hyperintensities are not unique findings in bipolar disorder, they are found in higher numbers in this cohort than in control subjects matched for age, and there is an especially strong association with later-onset bipolar disorder (over the age of sixty).[3]

It's not clear exactly what is represented by these signal differences on the MRI images of persons with bipolar disorder. Most of the other conditions in which T2 hyperintensities are found involve loss of neurons and other brain cells and also the pathological process called *demyelination,* the loss of the fatty insulating material of nerve fibers. For many years, it was thought that T2 hyperintensities were the result rather than the cause of bipolar disorder, the tiny "scars" of past episodes. Some have proposed, however, that they are markers for underlying cerebrovascular disease, which may cause bipolar disorder to develop in some individuals with a genetic predisposition.[4]

More recently, another form of MRI imaging has been developed that has revolutionized the field of brain imaging. *Functional* MRI (fMRI) is a technique in which the MRI instrument is adjusted so that it can measure the amount of oxygen in areas of the brain in exquisite detail. In this way, not only is the structure of the brain revealed, but variations in the level of metabolic activity of brain areas can be visualized. Functional MRI scans can pinpoint changes in activity in brain areas only a few cubic millimeters in size that last only a second or two.

While these are early days in using this approach to understand bipolar disorder, various basic facts are emerging. As might be expected, several centers deep in the oldest part of the brain that are already known to be important in strong emotions such as fear and anger (a set of structures known collectively as the *limbic system*) show differences in activity in bipolar patients compared to healthy controls. In addition, however, it has been found that areas of the prefrontal lobes also show patterns of activity that are different in individuals with bipolar disorder; these are areas of the brain where advanced intellectual processing takes place. One of the most consistent findings in fMRI studies of mood disorders is a decrease in metabolic rate in an area of the left prefrontal lobe in depressed patients, a finding that led to the development of transcranial magnetic stimulation, one of the brain-stimulation treatments discussed previously. Some neuroimaging studies of bipolar disorder have found a similar pattern of underactivity in this area, but others have not, suggesting that "unipolar" depression and bipolar disorder have different biological bases.

Yet another new form of MRI neuroimaging is called *diffusion* magnetic resonance imaging (dMRI). This technique visualizes water molecules as they move along brain connections and can reveal variation in the connections between different brain areas. Studies using this approach have found differences in the size of bundles of fibers connecting different centers of the limbic system in persons with bipolar disorder.

Neuroimaging in psychiatric illness is a relatively new field, but research in this area is booming. It's difficult to keep up with the development of new imaging techniques, let alone the new findings that emerge from their use. Unfortunately, the metabolic patterns seen in these studies are apparent only when groups of individuals are compared; most of the studies compare a dozen or so individuals with bipolar disorder to a similar number of healthy controls to detect differences. The differences are too small and the range of normal results too large for these approaches to be helpful for clinical purposes such as forming the basis for a reliable test for bipolar disorder—so far, at least. But these findings show conclusively that bipolar disorder is a brain disease with real physical changes in the function of areas that can be visualized and measured with the right equipment.

———————————— KEY TAKEAWAYS ————————————

▶ Stress, especially chronic stress, takes a toll on brain cells and has been implicated in triggering episodes and worsening the course of mood disorders.

▶ It is important that persons with mood disorders have a well-functioning thyroid gland. There is evidence that "almost normal" and even "low normal" thyroid hormone levels can interfere with treatments for mood disorders and that improving thyroid functioning with hormone supplementation can improve a person's response medications and other treatments.

▶ New techniques for visualizing the brain have already led to new treatments for mood disorders, such as TMS, and hold great promise for understanding the illness better.

CHAPTER 15

The Science of Cycles
Chronobiology

C hronobiology (from *khronos*, the Greek word for "time") is the science of bodily rhythms and biological clocks. Nearly every organism
on the planet lives in rhythm with the astronomical cycles of the earth, the
sun, and the moon. The activities of animals and the growth cycles of plants
harmonize with the daily rising and setting of the sun, the monthly ebb and
flow of ocean tides, and the annual cycle of the changing seasons.

Ancient peoples erected immense astronomical calculators and ob-
servatories to track these cycles at places like Stonehenge in England and
the monuments at Carnac in France, where rows of more than a thousand
stones stretch across the countryside. At these sacred places and others,
including the pyramids of the Mayans and the Incas, ancient astronomers
determined the dates and times of solstices, equinoxes, and eclipses. At
festivals like the Roman Saturnalia, our forebears celebrated the lengthening of the daylight hours that heralds the arrival of spring and the return of
the sun. Our modern midwinter holidays, Christmas and Hanukkah, recall
these sentiments with traditions centered on candles, lights, and greenery.

Once we humans learned how to predict eclipses, we were no longer
terrified by them. As we learned how to extend the daylight hours with fire
and gaslight and electricity, we depended less on the cycles of the sun to
structure our activities and felt more in control of time. We learned to warm
ourselves in winter and cool ourselves in summer. The changes of the seasons were still lovely to watch and interesting in the way they affected the
plants and animals around us, but they didn't really affect us very much
anymore—or so we thought.

But the changes of the seasons certainly *do* affect other creatures: we
know about the migration of birds, salmon, and whales; Arctic rabbits that
change color in winter; the astonishing changes in plant life that occur from
fall to winter to spring; and, of course, those hibernating bears. But humans
have evolved beyond all that, haven't we? Our cycles of activity, like sleeping

at night and being awake during the day, are just conventions set by our culture rather than expressions of our biology. We humans have severed our connections with the rhythms of the celestial bodies. Haven't we?

That's what many thought—until 1982, when a paper by researchers from the National Institute of Mental Health appeared in the *American Journal of Psychiatry*.[1] This paper, titled "Bright Artificial Light Treatment of a Manic-Depressive Patient with a Seasonal Mood Cycle," described a patient with bipolar disorder whose symptoms occurred in a pattern related to the seasons: depression in winter and mood elevation during the summer.

Seasonal patterns in bipolar disorder were described previously by astute clinicians, including (as you might expect) Emil Kraepelin, who observed, "Repeatedly in these cases, I saw moodiness set in in autumn and pass over in spring 'when the sap shoots in the trees,' to excitement."[2] But there was little organized research into the relationship between mood and the seasons. Then in the late 1970s, a group of researchers who were drawn together at NIMH by a mutual interest in seasonal mood changes started to look at these relationships.

Soon, mood-disorder patients with seasonal mood changes found out about the NIMH group and sought it out. One was a woman who experienced regular winter depressions characterized by low mood and the development of an intense craving for sweets and starches. She had made an important observation during the two winters before she came to NIMH: during both of those winters, she had taken vacations in the Virgin Islands. On both occasions, traveling south toward the equator—to a latitude where the winter days were significantly longer—resulted in a dramatic improvement in her mood. Furthermore, the improvement vanished abruptly when she returned to her colder—and darker—home up north. It was becoming obvious to the NIMH team that the crucial factor in seasonal mood changes was *light*.[3]

The word *photoperiod* refers to the length of daylight hours in the twenty-four-hour day. It has been known for many years that photoperiod has a profound effect on many living things. If you've ever put a poinsettia plant or Christmas cactus in a dark closet to coax it into bloom for the holidays, you've used photoperiod manipulation to influence the plant's physiology. The shortened photoperiod induces the plant to produce hormones that cause its flower buds to set.

One member of the NIMH team suggested trying to treat winter depressions by artificially lengthening the photoperiod. Several patients volunteered to sit in front of bright lights for several hours before dawn and several more after sunset. Within three days the first patient began to feel better. "The change was dramatic and unmistakable," Rosenthal later wrote.[4] Phototherapy was born.

CIRCADIAN RHYTHMS

We need to pause here and review an important concept in chronobiology, *circadian rhythms*. The term comes from the Latin words *circa*, meaning "around," and *diem*, meaning "day." It refers to rhythms in the body that have an approximately twenty-four-hour cycle, that is, the day-night cycle. It turns out that many bodily functions follow a circadian rhythm. Body temperature cycles daily, with the lowest body temperature occurring about 4:00 a.m. and the highest around 7:00 p.m. Blood pressure drops while we are asleep and jumps up about 7:00 a.m. in response to a surge in the adrenal hormone cortisol, which itself rises and falls in a twenty-four-hour cycle. The hormone melatonin, which is secreted by the pineal gland, located deep within the brain, has a circadian cycle and appears to be important in regulating sleep and wakefulness, as anyone who has used melatonin pills to help him sleep knows.

FIGURE 15.1. Circadian rhythms

A surge of cortisol in the early morning wakes us up, and then the level falls through the day. As evening approaches, a similar rise in the level of melatonin signals the brain that it's time for sleep.

Illustration by Jenna Macfarlane

Humans, like most animals, have an internal biological clock. It has been demonstrated under experimental conditions that this clock has a natural cycle of about twenty-*five* hours and needs to be reset every morning by environmental cues, primarily light, to stay in sync with the twenty-four-hour cycle of the day. Another fact about this internal clock, familiar to world travelers, is that this "reset" can shift by only about one or two hours per day. When we reset our watches for daylight saving time or travel to an adjacent time zone, we hardly notice the change. But when we travel across several time zones, it takes several days for our internal clock to become synchronized to the new time. During that time, we awaken and get sleepy at the wrong times for our new time zone and generally feel out of sorts, the phenomenon known as jet lag. Eventually, our internal clock adjusts, but the farther we've traveled, the longer it takes: about one day for each hour of time change. So what happens to people whose internal clocks are out of sync with their environment for prolonged periods?

English researchers set out to investigate this question in the late 1990s. They asked fourteen healthy young men and women to volunteer for a biological-clock experiment. Two or three at a time, the volunteers entered experimental living quarters where, for about a month, instead of a twenty-four-hour day, they lived on a thirty-hour day: twenty hours of wakefulness, ten hours of sleep. Every several hours while awake they took a ten-minute battery of psychological tests and rated their mood.

Since these individuals were forced to live on a thirty-hour cycle, their internal clocks could *never* catch up with their sleep-wake cycle. For them, this schedule was the equivalent of traveling through five time zones every day. During the experiment, the researchers had the volunteers take their temperature every few hours, and in this way they were able to determine what time it was for each person's biological clock. They found that the volunteers' internal clocks went in and out of synchronization with their artificially prolonged sleep-wake cycle and that the more out of synchronization the volunteers were, the worse their mood became. In fact, it was the *interaction* of the two cycles that seemed to make the most difference in their mood. They felt worst when their internal temperature clock was telling them it wasn't time to get up yet and their environmentally enforced sleep-wake cycle was telling them it was time to start winding down from a long day. The researchers proposed that "temporal alignment between the sleep-wake cycle and the [internal] circadian rhythms affects self-assessment of mood in healthy subjects."[5] Put more simply: when our sleep-wake cycle and our internal clock are out of synchronization, it has a deeply *negative* effect on our mood.

SEASONAL AFFECTIVE DISORDER (SAD)

Several theories for SAD involving circadian rhythms have been put forward, but none fits the experimental findings very well. It was proposed that people with SAD might have an abnormal delay in circadian rhythms. Early-morning bright light would be expected to correct this problem by advancing the cycle. Evening phototherapy would be expected to have the opposite effect and make things even worse. But research clearly shows that morning and evening phototherapy are equally helpful for SAD. It has also been suggested that SAD patients have lazy circadian rhythms and even that they are abnormally sensitive to light. But tests of these hypotheses have led to more confusion than clarity, and no one has come up with a theory that ties SAD to a particular circadian rhythm disturbance.

How One Researcher's "Winter Blues" Led to SAD

Sometimes, scientists are drawn to a particular line of research for a very personal reason. Dr. Norman Rosenthal, who was instrumental in our understanding of seasonal affective disorder is one such researcher.

For years, Rosenthal had noticed his own seasonal shifts of mood in his native South Africa, and he had seen these mood swings worsen when his psychiatric training brought him to New York—a city located much farther from the equator than his native Johannesburg was. In New York the summer days are much longer and the winter days much shorter than in South Africa. Rosenthal recalled his first autumn in New York this way:

> Daylight-saving time was over and the clocks were put back an hour. I left that first Monday after the time change and found the world in darkness. A cold wind blowing off the Hudson River filled me with foreboding. Winter came. My energy declined, and I wondered how I could have undertaken so many tasks the previous summer. Had I been crazy? Now there seemed to be no alternative but to hang in and try to keep everything afloat. . . . Finally, spring arrived. My energy level surged again, and I wondered why I had worried so over my workload.*

Dr. Rosenthal went on to do the seminal research that led to the identification of SAD and can be thought of as the "father" of bright-light therapy for mood disorders.

*Norman E. Rosenthal, *Winter Blues: Seasonal Affective Disorder, What It Is and How to Overcome It* (New York: Guilford Press, 1993), 6.

A research group from Columbia University attempted to discover the factors that predicted who would have a good response to photoperiod manipulation. They gave a course of phototherapy to 103 people who reported seasonal mood changes. Some of these individuals met the diagnostic criteria for bipolar I, some for bipolar II, and some had unipolar depressions—that is, they had never been manic or hypomanic.

The researchers found that it was not diagnosis (as bipolar I or II or nonbipolar depression) but a particular *pattern* of depressive symptoms that predicted a good response to phototherapy. The people helped by phototherapy tended to sleep more rather than less when they were depressed (hypersomnia) and to complain of low energy and fatigue. They noticed increased appetite during depressions, especially for sweets and starches ("carbohydrate craving"), and an accompanying weight gain. Finally, they had a striking diurnal variation in mood (a consistent pattern of change in mood through the day), but in a pattern that was the opposite of that usually seen in severe depression: instead of waking up early in the morning with the worst mood of the day and then feeling better as the day went on, these people felt better in the early part of the day but had an afternoon or evening "slump," a pattern called *reverse diurnal variation.*[6]

I've been talking about SAD as if it were a diagnostic category of its own, but it's not. SAD can refer to a bipolar I, bipolar II, or nonbipolar depressive illness that shows a seasonal pattern in its symptoms. But a lot of what we know about mood disorders suggests that bipolar I, bipolar II, and nonbipolar depressive illnesses are very *different* illnesses in course and causation. What does it mean that *each* can have a seasonal pattern? If it is not diagnosis but rather symptom pattern that predicts who gets better with light therapy, does this mean that our whole diagnostic classification system is called into question?

Don't throw out your *DSM* just yet. The bipolar-nonbipolar and bipolar I–bipolar II diagnostic divisions are still important for choosing treatments, and so is the "with seasonal pattern–without seasonal pattern" designation. It may just be a few more years before we figure out how all the classifications fit together.

In the meantime, patients with bipolar symptoms who notice a seasonal pattern should talk with their physician about phototherapy, especially if they have the typical SAD depressive symptom pattern: low energy, hypersomnia, carbohydrate craving, weight gain, and reverse diurnal variation of mood (afternoon or evening "slump").

Several years of research have found that bright blue–tinged light is the most effective for treating SAD, and there are now relatively inexpensive lights with this wavelength specifically designed for this application. The usual recommendation is that the patient use the light in the morning and start with an exposure of thirty minutes daily. A recent study suggests that reading while in front of the light is especially beneficial, because the light reflected from the page increases the total light exposure. The therapeutic effect of light therapy is sometimes evident within days, but as with antidepressants, several weeks of therapy may be needed to obtain good remission of symptoms. Side effects are minor: headaches and eyestrain, for example.[7] Too much light exposure can sometimes precipitate mild hypomanic symptoms: irritability, insomnia, feeling "hyper." Fortunately, this problem seems to respond quickly to decreased light exposure, and phototherapy doesn't seem to have the risks of mood destabilization that antidepressant medication does. Light therapy can be thought of as an adjunctive therapy for bipolar disorder with seasonal variation, an add-on treatment that works with medication and psychotherapy to regulate mood through a natural cycle of the body. There's another cycle that's also extremely important to pay attention to: the sleep-wake cycle.

THE SLEEP CYCLE AND BIPOLAR DISORDER

We're not finished with circadian rhythms yet. One of our most prominent circadian rhythms, the sleep-wake cycle, turns out to be significant in bipolar disorder. The study with our English volunteers demonstrated how important the sleep-wake cycle is in the regulation of mood in persons who do *not* have mood disorders. So it should come as no surprise that sleep-wake cycle manipulation has dramatic effects on persons with bipolar disorder. Clinical observations confirm this: sleep deprivation can be used therapeutically to treat the symptoms of depression, and it can also cause a switch into the manic state. To understand these observations, we need to take a closer look at normal sleep.

For quite a long time, sleep wasn't of much interest to experimental psychologists and psychiatrists. This may seem odd, especially considering Freud's and others' intense interest in dreams. Possibly because of a lack of investigative tools, interest in dreams never extended to interest in the process of dreaming, and so the physiology of sleep was a neglected area of research for many decades.

The change came in 1953, when a group of researchers used an electroencephalogram (EEG) machine on sleeping volunteers in a clinical laboratory to investigate the long-standing observation that people move their eyes beneath closed lids during some periods of sleep. When the researchers awakened the subjects during what came to be called *rapid eye movement (REM) sleep*, 90 percent reported that they had been dreaming. Further studies revealed that sleep is a complex process, with several different stages and rhythms of activity that together are now called *sleep architecture*.

As figure 15.2 indicates, after falling asleep, a person passes through lighter and then progressively deeper stages of sleep. Brain activity slows, and the heartbeat and blood pressure drop to the lowest levels of the twenty-four-hour day. The process is like a submarine descending into darker, quieter, deeper water. The deepest stage is called *slow-wave sleep* (SWS), because the EEG shows slow, synchronized rhythms in the electrical activity of the brain. SWS is thought to be the physically restorative part of sleep; experimental subjects who are awakened whenever they enter SWS but are allowed to experience the other stages complain of muscle aches and other symptoms of physical discomfort.

About ninety minutes after a person falls asleep, the sleep "submarine" begins to rise again. The EEG indicates a brain-activity pattern not much different from that seen in awake individuals. The EEG electrodes that track eye movements measure intense activity, and individuals awakened during this stage report dreaming: the sleeper has entered a period of REM sleep. After fifteen to twenty minutes of REM sleep, eye movement

FIGURE 15.2. **Normal sleep architecture**

Illustration by Jenna Macfarlane

ceases, and the sleeper drifts back down into the deeper stages again and has another period of SWS, which predominates during the first part of the night. As the night progresses, the sleeper spends more time in REM sleep and less in SWS. Toward dawn, sleep becomes lighter, and REM periods become longer, until finally the person wakes up. It is thought that REM sleep and body temperature are both tightly linked to the body's main circadian clock (often called the *strong oscillator*), because the lowest point of the body's temperature cycle coincides with the most intensive period of REM sleep.

When we look at EEG sleep studies done on depressed persons, the REM cycle seems to have shifted. Depressed individuals go into REM almost immediately after falling asleep, a phenomenon called *decreased REM latency*. Some slow-wave sleep still occurs in the later part of the night, but the overall amount of SWS is reduced. Some researchers have interpreted these findings as indicating that depressed individuals suffer from a *phase advance* of the REM cycle and that the rhythm of the strong oscillator has gotten out of phase with other bodily rhythms. We saw from the study on the English volunteers that when the strong oscillator (as measured by their temperature cycle) is out of synchronization with the sleep-wake cycle, dips in mood occur. In the few patients with bipolar disorder whose sleep architecture has been studied, striking shifts of the REM and temperature cycles were observed as the patients cycled in and out of depression and mania.[8]

These findings bring together a lot of what we know about the symptoms of depression and about circadian rhythms. The decreased amounts of SWS may explain the fatigue and bodily discomfort typical of depression. The shift of the usual period of REM from the early-morning hours to the early part of the sleep cycle may explain the early-morning awakening typically seen in depression.

These findings may also explain the therapeutic effects of sleep deprivation on symptoms of depression. Patients with the typical diurnal variation of mood seen in depression often report that they have their best mood of the day during the late evening, before they go to sleep, and feel their worst in the morning after they've slept. This and other observations led some researchers in the 1950s to experiment with sleep deprivation as a therapeutic technique for the treatment of depression. With the introduction of antidepressant medications, interest in sleep deprivation faded, but recently it has been growing again. This work shows that if patients are totally deprived of sleep—kept up all night—about 60 percent report a sometimes dramatic improvement in mood. Unfortunately, the effect is temporary; in most patients the benefits disappear after even a brief nap, making this interesting technique a not terribly useful one. But experiments with partial sleep deprivation indicate that waking patients up at about 2:00 a.m. and making sure that they do not sleep during the second half of the night is nearly as effective as total sleep deprivation. Advancing the sleep cycle by six hours, so that patients go to sleep at 6:00 p.m. and get up at 2:00 a.m., has also been found to have antidepressant effects.

Although the technique has not caught on in the United States, sleep deprivation and phase advance are popular in Europe as adjuncts to medication in the treatment of bipolar and nonbipolar depression. An Italian study published in 1997 compared the recovery time from depression in ten bipolar patients. All of them were treated with fluoxetine (Prozac), but five were also given several cycles of total sleep deprivation. The patients who had sleep deprivation got better faster on the medication than those who did not.[9]

The other relevant clinical observation about sleep in persons with bipolar disorder is that sleep deprivation can precipitate mania. This is a thoroughly documented finding, and for this reason my discussion of sleep deprivation as a treatment for depression comes with a "don't try this at home" warning: even one night of sleep deprivation can precipitate mania. There have been numerous reports of individuals with bipolar disorder becoming manic after transatlantic flights or after sleep deprivation caused by medical emergencies or family crises. Emotional upsets can, of course, lead to insomnia and poor sleep because of anxiety. It has been proposed that lack of sleep for *any* reason may be what tips the balance for many bipolar patients and brings on an episode of mania.[10]

All the work on chronobiology and biological clocks indicates that there are important links between bodily rhythms and mood, and we've barely scratched the surface of this fascinating area of study. So far we have only tantalizing hints about these links rather than clearly understood mechanisms and relationships. Nevertheless, studies of sleep and SAD point the way toward new and safer treatments for certain mood disorders—techniques like phototherapy and sleep phase advance. This work also indicates the importance of lifestyle regularity in controlling the symptoms of bipolar disorder, a topic we'll explore in more detail in chapter 22.

───────────── KEY TAKEAWAYS ─────────────

▶ Some patients with mood disorders have regular cycles of their mood that occur in rhythm with seasonal changes. Patients with this subtype of the illness, seasonal affective disorder (SAD), often benefit from bright-light therapy during the darker months of the year.

▶ Humans have a "biological clock" that regulates several hormonal cycles in the body. The melatonin cycle, which regulates sleep, is perhaps the most important.

▶ Sleep deprivation can be dangerously destabilizing for persons with bipolar disorder, and they need to carefully avoid it.

CHAPTER 16

The Genetics of Bipolar Disorder

I t has long been recognized that bipolar disorder exists in clusters within families. In *Manic-Depressive Insanity*, Emil Kraepelin wrote of one family in which "of the ten children of the same parents who were both probably manic-depressive by predisposition, no fewer than seven fell ill the same way; of the five descendants of the second generation, four have already fallen ill."[1]

For many years research on the genetics of bipolar disorder was hampered by foggy diagnostic criteria and a lack of laboratory methods to identify genes. But this state of affairs has changed dramatically. Not only have psychiatrists become more skilled in the diagnosis of bipolar disorder, but the biochemical methods available to locate and identify genes on the human chromosome have become tremendously more sophisticated. These developments will, sooner or later, lead to a better understanding of the genetic mechanisms of bipolar disorder, which will in turn lead to better diagnosis and treatment of the disorder.

A word of warning: this is perhaps the most "scientific" chapter in the book—genetics is hard! If the scientific details don't interest you or the going gets too tough, just skip to the "Takeaways" at the end of the chapter.

GENES, CHROMOSOMES, AND DNA

The patterns and rules of inheritance in living things were first described by Gregor Mendel, an Austrian monk who over many years performed elegantly planned and executed experiments with plants, mostly garden peas, in his monastery garden. Mendel discovered that traits are transmitted from parent to child in discrete bits of information, bits that we now call *genes*, the units of inheritance.

We now understand that genes are sets of instructions for building proteins. All plants and animals, from seaweed to snapdragons and from

DNA: The Most Famous Molecule on the Planet

For many years, geneticists were in the dark about how genes are transmitted from parent to offspring. Proteins were the favorite candidate molecules for decades, but by the mid-1940s, experiments with bacteria had shown that a family of biochemical compounds found in cells, called *nucleic acids*, contained genetic information. In 1953 James Watson, Francis Crick, and Rosalind Franklin published a series of papers in the British scientific journal *Nature* describing the structure of the most important of these compounds, deoxyribonucleic acid (DNA), and the modern age of genetics had begun.

DNA molecules are long spiral chains whose links consist of four simpler compounds called *nucleotides*. The four DNA nucleotides, adenine, cytosine, guanine, and thymine (usually abbreviated as A, C, G, and T), are the elements of an elegantly simple code. Just as you can write out a Morse code version of *Hamlet* using only dots and dashes, you can write out instructions for building hemoglobin, myosin, collagen, or any other protein using As, Cs, Gs, and Ts. That's what DNA does. You can think of the physical structure of a gene as the section on the DNA molecule that contains the code for one protein.

FIGURE 16.1. The DNA molecule

NUCLEOTIDES

A DNA MOLECULE IS AN UNRAVELED CHROMOSOME

Illustration by Jenna Macfarlane

(*continued*)

> When the DNA molecule is doing its work in the cell, it is unraveled and stretched out, surrounded by a whole retinue of ultramicroscopic attendants busily reading the coded instructions and making proteins. When it's time for the cell to divide, another set of attendants carefully coils the DNA molecule into a compact cylinder and surrounds it with protective proteins to form the threadlike structures you may have looked at under the microscope in high school biology: the chromosomes.

earthworms to elephants, are constructed of and operate by means of proteins. Myosin (muscle protein), hemoglobin (the oxygen-carrying protein of red blood cells), and collagen (the structural protein of skin and cartilage) are just a few examples. Even the nonprotein structural materials of the body, such as the calcium salts in our bones, depend on proteins. Proteins called enzymes direct the manufacture of bone from calcium salts by expediting certain chemical reactions. Many hormones are proteins (insulin, for example), and those that are not (for example, testosterone and cortisol) are manufactured by protein enzymes. All proteins are built according to specifications contained in genes.

GENETIC DISEASES

For some disorders, the links from a certain gene to a certain protein to a certain trait or disease are easy to follow. Sickle cell anemia is one such disease. When the blood of sickle cell patients is examined under the microscope, instead of seeing the normal saucer- or disk-shaped red blood cells, one sees abnormal crescent- or sickle-shaped cells. Once scientists had the biochemical methods that allowed them to look at the components of blood cells, they discovered that sickle cell patients had an abnormally shaped hemoglobin molecule (hemoglobin is the protein in red blood cells that transports oxygen). This abnormal hemoglobin tends to form abnormal chains within the cell, stretching the normally disk-shaped cells into the sickle shape characteristic of the disease.

Because hemoglobin is easily purified, it was one of the first proteins whose structure was completely described (a feat that earned Cambridge University biochemist Max Ferdinand Perutz the Nobel Prize in 1962). Researchers discovered that sickle cell hemoglobin (now called hemoglobin S) differs from normal hemoglobin by only one molecular element that is caused by a single misprint in the hemoglobin gene of persons with the disease. At one particular spot on the DNA molecule, there is an A instead of a T. An abnormal hemoglobin molecule results from the reading of these incorrect instructions, and the abnormal hemoglobin molecules cause the abnormally shaped red blood cells, which block blood vessels and result in the symptoms of the disease. The pathway from abnormal gene to abnormal protein to abnormal cells to symptoms has been completely described.

Genes have been identified and located in several other human diseases whose inheritance pattern indicates that they are single-gene illnesses, including cystic fibrosis, many forms of hemophilia, and Duchenne's muscular dystrophy.

It has become quite clear, however, that bipolar disorder is not one of these diseases.

WHAT WE KNOW

Despite nearly fifty years of research, geneticists have not been able to come up with a coherent scenario for the genetics of bipolar disorder. Unlike sickle cell anemia's clear pathway from gene to protein to abnormal cells, no such connecting of dots has occurred for bipolar disorder.

This state of affairs is not due to an inability to identify promising "candidate" risk genes for bipolar disorder. Ironically, the problem is that so *many* have been identified; a recent review of the genetics of bipolar disorder listed more than forty that have been identified as possible risk genes.[2]

Another complicating issue is that the genes encoded in our DNA are not the only mechanisms by which traits are passed from parent to offspring. The activity of genes can be modulated in cells in a number of different ways that are collectively referred to as *epigenetic* mechanisms, and these effects can be inherited as well—but only specialized molecular analysis can detect these effects.

Children of individuals with bipolar disorder have an increased risk of developing bipolar disorder themselves. Assigning a number to that risk is difficult, for some of the same reasons that the search for a bipolar gene has been so difficult. But the risk seems to be several times that of the general population, on the order of 10 percent. However, children of persons with bipolar disorder are also at a higher risk for unipolar (depression-only) illness, and when you add in this risk, the percentages go up into the high twenties. This means that the children of persons with bipolar disorder have about a one-in-four chance of developing some kind of mood disorder and about a one-in-ten chance of developing bipolar disorder.[3]

Genetics beyond DNA: The New Field of Epigenetics

Epigenetics is the study of patterns of inheritance that do not involve changes in the base-pair sequence of DNA. For the most part, epigenetic mechanisms involve attaching smaller molecules to the DNA of a gene, molecules that turn off, turn on, up regulate, or down regulate the activity of a gene. Perhaps the best-understood epigenetic mechanism is *methylation* of a gene, in which a small group of carbon and hydrogen atoms attach to a stretch of DNA. Another mechanism involves tiny snippets of RNA called microRNAs (miRNAs). The RNA molecule is usually part of the cell's protein-manufacturing process, but soon after miRNAs were discovered in cells, it was determined that at least some of them are involved in epigenetic effects that interfere with a cell's protein production.

Epigenetic effects appear to be heavily influenced by environmental factors. These effects are proposed to explain the multigenerational fallout of the Dutch Hunger Winter of 1944–1945. During the closing months of World War II, the Nazis halted shipments of food to the Netherlands, resulting in the starvation deaths of more than twenty thousand people. The offspring of women who were pregnant during those grim months were found to have increased rates of obesity and diabetes, abnormal triglyceride levels, and a shorter life expectancy. These individuals were also found to be at higher risk of developing schizophrenia than the general population was. Even more striking, the *grandchildren* of the Hunger mothers also show higher rates of these problems.

My colleague Dr. Kellie Tamashiro at Johns Hopkins has demonstrated these effects in rats, finding that changes to maternal diet can cause metabolic problems in offspring. Maternal stress has similar effects. She and members of her research team have demonstrated that maternal environmental factors can also affect offspring *behaviors*, including those in rats that are thought to be similar to anxiety and depression in humans.

It has been demonstrated that childhood trauma increases the risk of developing a number of psychiatric problems in adulthood, including depressive illness. It has long been known that genetics (i.e., DNA) interacts with environmental factors to trigger psychiatric illnesses, especially mood disorders. It may be that *epigenetic* mechanisms are the molecular "scars" of childhood adversity that increase the risk of developing a mood disorder.*

The discovery of these and other epigenetic effects on behavior will certainly advance our knowledge about the causes of bipolar disorder, but they also reveal just how complicated those causal factors are likely to be.

*G. J. Boersma, T. L. Bale, P. Casanello, H. E. Lara, A. B. Lucion , D. Suchecki, and K. L. Tamashiro, "Long-Term Impact of Early Life Events on Physiology and Behavior," *Journal of Neuroendocrinology* 26, no. 9 (2014): 587–602.

Individuals with bipolar disorder need to be alert to signs and symptoms of mood disorders in their children and to get them into treatment if such symptoms occur. Although we may be uncertain about the details of the inheritance of bipolar disorder, we are not at all uncertain about the importance of early diagnosis and treatment.

THE SEARCH CONTINUES

Several factors make scientists optimistic about eventually discovering genes for bipolar disorder. The explosive growth of technologies available to geneticists is perhaps the primary reason for optimism. The Human Genome Project was able to tackle the sequencing of the DNA in all forty-six human chromosomes only after automated technology to perform DNA sequencing became available in the 1990s and when supercomputers were developed that could analyze the literally astronomical amount of data that was generated. It is now possible to sequence the entire genome of an individual for a few hundred dollars, a fact that is all the more amazing when one learns that the budget of the investigation that resulted in the first whole-genome sequencing was in the tens of millions of dollars.

Even when genes and epigenetic factors are identified, however, predictions about who will develop symptoms will still be imprecise. It has become clear that many, perhaps dozens, of variant genes are likely involved in determining who develops the illness, and each one may increase the risk of developing bipolar disorder by just a few percentage points. Only when a "critical mass" of risk genes are present does an individual become ill.

Environmental factors acting through epigenetic mechanisms are also undoubtedly important (perhaps equally important) in determining who will and will not be affected; psychological and perhaps physical stresses and traumas appear to be paramount.

All this complexity means that there is as yet no reliable genetic test for bipolar disorder.

Finding risk genes may lead to new treatment approaches that will benefit everyone with mood disorders. Gene identification, as well as identification of the function of these genes or the gene products, will undoubtedly shed light on the biochemical basis of bipolar disorder. It may then be possible to design medications or other treatments based on knowledge about the causes of bipolar symptoms on a cellular or biochemical level—rather than stumbling upon treatments by accident, as has been the case so far. Genetics research is one of the most challenging but most promising areas of investigation of bipolar disorder, and it holds the promise of truly revolutionizing the treatment of this disease.

———————————— **KEY TAKEAWAYS** ————————————

▶ Bipolar disorder runs in families, and the children of persons with bipolar disorder are at significantly higher risk of themselves developing the illness.

▶ Children of persons with bipolar disorder have about a one-in-four chance of developing a mood disorder and about a one-in-ten chance of developing bipolar disorder. The number goes up if both parents are affected.

▶ The genetics of bipolar disorder are very complex: more than forty different risk genes have been identified, but which are most important, what combination is necessary, and how they all interact are all still unknown.

▶ There is no reliable genetic test for bipolar disorder.

PART IV

Bipolar Variations and Connections

I n this group of chapters, we'll explore several variations on the theme of bipolar disorder. We'll look first at how the course and symptoms of the illness can differ in children and adolescents and then note the differences in symptoms between men and women (with special attention to premenstrual mood symptoms, the challenge of postpartum mood disorders, and the dilemmas faced by women who have the illness during their childbearing years).

Chapter 19 deals with the complicated relationships between bipolar disorder and substance abuse. Individuals with bipolar disorder seem to be especially vulnerable to substance-abuse disorders, so much so that it's reasonable to think of chemical dependency as a complication of the illness. The symptoms of substance abuse and of bipolar disorder can become so intertwined that it is impossible to figure out which is which. We'll look for a way out of this confusion and discuss the treatment approaches that work in such cases. It's extremely important to confront chemical dependency head on, because research shows that alcoholism and drug abuse are often *fatal* complications of bipolar disorder.

In chapter 20, I'll give a brief overview of *borderline personality disorder*, a complex problem whose sufferers have severe problems in mood regulation. I'll discuss how these problems are both similar to and different from the mood problems of bipolar disorder—and to make it all the more complicated, note that these individuals more often than not have mood disorders in addition to problems more often thought of as part of "personality."

Then in chapter 21, for a complete change in perspective from the rest of the book, I'll examine some of the intriguing connections between bipolar illnesses and artistic genius and creativity.

CHAPTER 17

Bipolar Disorder in Children and Adolescents

For many years bipolar disorder was thought to be extremely rare in young people, even though research data on adults indicated that the first appearance of symptoms usually occurs before age twenty. (Emil Kraepelin found that the highest number of "first attacks" of manic-depressive illness occurred between the ages of fifteen and twenty.) Perhaps because of a reluctance to diagnose children with an illness known to be a lifelong problem and the unwillingness to prescribe for children the powerful medications used to treat its symptoms, bipolar disorder in young children received little attention from researchers until quite recently.

More recent research has shown unequivocally that bipolar disorder is much more common in young people than was previously recognized. In 2011 the World Health Organization estimated that pediatric bipolar disorder is the fourth-leading cause of disability in adolescents aged fifteen to nineteen worldwide, accounting for a total of 5 percent of disability in this age range.[1]

For a long time, the treatment of children and adolescents with bipolar symptoms consisted mostly of improvised variations on adult treatments. Fortunately, this too is changing; there is now quite a bit of research available to guide the clinician in crafting a treatment plan for young patients with bipolar disorder.

Even very young children can have bipolar symptoms. In one study that looked at such symptoms in the pediatric (under-eighteen) age range, nearly one-third of the patients were younger than twelve, and the average age of onset for these young bipolar patients was eight and a half.[2]

SYMPTOMS OF PEDIATRIC BIPOLAR DISORDER

Depression is comparatively easy to spot in children: the weepy, listless, and lethargic child is quickly recognized as a sick child. But how do you distinguish hypomanic or manic behavior in a child from the boisterousness and high energy typical in this age range? An even more difficult task is to differentiate manic symptoms from the hyperactivity and "can't sit still" picture of attention-deficit hyperactivity disorder.

The differentiation is possible if close attention is paid to changes in mood. Children with ADHD are hyperactive but don't have the expansive, grandiose mood of mania. The child with ADHD may disrupt a classroom with clowning around and restlessness, but a manic child may tell the teacher that the lessons are being taught incorrectly and try to take over the class. The manic child caught taking things that belong to someone else may say that it's wrong for other people to steal but not for her. The manic child may be convinced that he is destined for a brilliant career as a doctor or a lawyer despite failing nearly every subject in school. The manic child may believe that he is on the verge of becoming a rock star despite being unable to play a musical instrument.

All children, of course, fantasize in similar ways about their future, but most are able to separate their fantasies from reality and apply themselves to schoolwork and follow the rules at home. Manic children, convinced of the reality of their grandiose ideas, speak and act based on the belief that the usual rules and requirements don't apply to them.

Manic children jump from topic to topic in their speech patterns, are difficult to interrupt, and complain that their thoughts are moving too fast. Hypersexuality is a symptom in older children, who may become sexually promiscuous or masturbate excessively; they may suddenly start using sexual profanity or say that a teacher or a famous person is in love with them. Spending sprees may take the form of ordering items on the internet.

Very young children may have manic exaggerations of the normal magical thinking of childhood but will act on this thinking instead of using it as a basis for play. Many children may imagine that they can fly and may run through the backyard flapping their arms like the wings of a bird or making airplane noises. A manic child under the influence of the delusion that she has become an angel or a superhero may jump out of a window or off the roof of a house. The symptoms of bipolar disorder in children can be every bit as deadly as they are in adults.

As in adults, in younger patients the milder forms of bipolar disorder, "soft" bipolar disorders and cyclothymia, are common. However, younger patients with these symptom patterns are at high risk of developing more severe symptoms as they mature, that is, of turning out to have bipolar I or II disorder.

When a young person develops serious depression, how can we tell whether he might be having the first episode of what will turn out to be bipolar disorder? Although it's impossible to know for sure, there are some indicators that seem to be fairly reliable. In one study, researchers investigated a group of sixty adolescents, aged thirteen to sixteen years, who had been hospitalized for major depression over the course of three to four years; the purpose was to see whether any particular clinical variables might predict which of them would eventually develop a bipolar course of illness (20 percent of the group eventually did). Statistical analyses showed that bipolarity was predicted by a depressive symptom cluster that included rapid symptom onset; a slowed-down, "retarded" type of depression; and psychotic features (hallucinations or delusions). A family history of mood disorders (bipolar disorder or major depression) in many family members and through successive generations was also a predictor, as was a history of the adolescent developing hypomanic symptoms when she took antidepressant medications—a clinical indicator that turned out to be 100 percent accurate in predicting bipolar disorder in this group.[3]

BIPOLAR DISORDER AND ATTENTION-DEFICIT HYPERACTIVITY DISORDER (ADHD)

Psychiatrists use the term *comorbidity* to describe two separate conditions or illnesses that frequently occur together in the same patient. There is a high degree of comorbidity between ADHD and mood disorders. Although some studies have found this to be as high as 75 percent,[4] many of the studies looking at this question have used different methods and criteria for bipolar disorder, so precise numbers are lacking.

Distractibility, impulsivity, hyperactivity, and "mood swings" are symptoms of both ADHD and mania. For these reasons, the diagnosis of both mood disorders and ADHD is difficult in young people, and the relationships between the two diagnoses are, at this point, poorly understood.

Most experts agree that in children who have both bipolar disorder and ADHD, the ADHD symptoms can be safely treated with stimulant medications without worsening the course of their bipolar symptoms.

ADHD or Pediatric Bipolar Disorder?

Because the symptoms of these two conditions have so much overlap, it can be difficult to arrive at the correct diagnosis in children who show symptoms of both. Nevertheless, it is possible, as there are a number of indicators that a child with ADHD is suffering from bipolar disorder:*

- The ADHD symptoms show up later than usual, for example at age ten or older.
- Symptoms of ADHD appear abruptly in a child with no previous symptoms.
- ADHD medications appear to "stop working."
- ADHD symptoms are episodic and occur only during periods of elevated mood.
- A child with ADHD starts showing mood swings, manic symptoms such as grandiosity, and less need for sleep or symptoms of depression.

*Modified from B. Birmaher, "Bipolar Disorder in Children and Adolescents," *Child and Adolescent Mental Health* 18, no. 3 (2013): 140–48.

TREATMENT AND PROGNOSIS

Some studies have indicated that lithium is effective in children, but it is fairly clear that it is not as effective in children as it is in adults. Pediatric lithium doses are, of course, lower than adult doses, but the effective therapeutic range for lithium in the bloodstream when it does work seems to be about the same in children as in adults. (Remember that the therapeutic range in the bloodstream is a measure of lithium concentration. Because children have a smaller total blood volume than adults, a lower dose of lithium for a child will result in the same concentration in the bloodstream.) Getting regular blood tests done is, of course, more challenging with children than with adults, but given the toxicity of lithium, blood-level tests are if anything even more important in children. Several studies used methods that avoid needles and determined lithium levels from saliva rather than from blood, but the results have been disappointing, and so for now these little patients must, unfortunately, have blood tests.

Several studies have indicated that valproate is effective for some young children with bipolar disorder, and some have suggested that it is more effective than lithium in this age range. There is now substantial research supporting the use of atypical antipsychotic medications for pediatric bipolar disorder. These agents appear to be more effective than lithium or anticonvulsant mood stabilizers in young patients. Because of these issues, a combination of medications is commonly required to keep pediatric bipolar-disorder symptoms under control.[5]

How is normal psychological development in children affected by bipolar disorder? Relationships with family members are often strained for these patients, as are relationships with their peers. Their educational development inevitably suffers as well. Clearly, attention to the psychological needs and the special educational requirements of these children is vitally important to minimize the effects of the illness on their psychological development. Thus, perhaps even more than in adults, counseling and therapy must be a high priority when developing treatment plans.

Several tasks lie ahead for those researching bipolar disorder in children. First will be to improve upon the diagnostic process and find out how to better separate bipolar (especially manic) symptoms from other similar diagnostic pictures—especially attention-deficit hyperactivity disorder. Clarifying the relationship between bipolar disorder and ADHD will be a highly instructive area of research for other reasons as well and will surely lead to better understanding of and treatments for both disorders. More research to determine which of the available treatments work best for children and adolescents is also needed, as are long-term follow-up studies to see whether pediatric-onset bipolar disorder looks different from late-adolescent-onset bipolar disorder as the patient grows to adulthood.

--- KEY TAKEAWAYS ---

▶ All forms of bipolar disorder can occur in children and adolescents and by and large show the same clinical picture as in adults.

▶ Although their symptoms can overlap, it is usually possible to differentiate bipolar disorder from ADHD by carefully evaluating for mood symptoms.

▶ Lithium tends not to be as effective in children as it is in adults; however, atypical antipsychotic medications have been shown to be immensely helpful in this age group.

CHAPTER 18

Women with Bipolar Disorder
Special Considerations

Although women are no more likely than men are to suffer from bipolar disorder, the hormonal changes that accompany menstruation and pregnancy affect their course of bipolar disorder and deserve special attention, as do some patterns of symptoms more often experienced by women than by men. In addition, medication use during pregnancy and while breastfeeding requires careful consideration.

SYMPTOM DIFFERENCES IN WOMEN

Of the various differences between the genders in the course of illness and symptoms of bipolar disorder, the greater incidence of rapid cycling in women is the best documented. A review article on bipolar disorder in women looked at ten studies involving several hundred persons with rapid-cycling bipolar disorder and found that 74 percent of patients were women.[1] Thus, the ratio of women to men with rapid-cycling disorder is three to one.

Several reasons have been proposed for this difference. Since thyroid problems have been associated with rapid cycling in bipolar disorder and since women are more likely than men to have certain types of thyroid problems, it was thought that a higher incidence of thyroid disease among women might explain the difference. But when women with rapid-cycling bipolar disorder were tested for thyroid problems, no greater incidence was found. Theories implicating female hormones have also been suggested, but so far they are mostly speculative; no research data exist clearly proving that hormonal differences between men and women explain this difference.

Another theory about the increased incidence of rapid-cycling bipolar disorder in women is related to the finding that women with bipolar disorder have a slightly greater ratio of depressive to manic episodes than men have. Women with bipolar disorder also tend to have more episodes of depression during the course of their illness than men have.[2] This being the case, it may be that women with bipolar disorder are more likely to be treated with antidepressants that can cause them to enter a rapid-cycling phase of the disorder. The types of clinical studies that could prove this theory have yet to be carried out.

The finding that women with bipolar disorder have more depressive episodes than their male counterparts seems to fit with the finding that women are more likely than men to suffer from nonbipolar depression. No one understands this greater tendency of women to suffer from depressive illnesses. Research on the levels of female reproductive hormones in depressed women has generally been unrevealing.

It is now known that there are many differences in brain organization between women and men, differences that have little to do with sex and reproduction. Psychological testing profiles indicate that women are superior to men in their performance on certain tests of language and memory; men perform better on certain specialized tests of three-dimensional visualization. It is thought that there are subtle differences in the way the brains of men and women are "wired" during prenatal development, probably under the influence of hormones in the womb, especially the different levels of testosterone that female and male fetuses are exposed to. The differences between men and women in the incidence and symptom profile of mood disorders may be due to these differences in "wiring." Explaining the significantly higher incidence of serious depression, including bipolar depression, in women is perhaps the most important unanswered question before us in the field of women's mental health.

POSTPARTUM MOOD DISORDERS
AND FAMILY PLANNING

Many clinical studies indicate that women with bipolar disorder are at elevated risk for an episode of illness in the period after giving birth. One review article on bipolar disorder in women put it this way: "There is no other time in the life of any bipolar patient when the risk of an episode is higher than it is for a female bipolar patient in the post-partum period."[3]

The numbers are indeed sobering: studies have shown that between 25 and 30 percent of women with bipolar disorder who become pregnant and deliver will have an episode of depression or mania either during pregnancy or following delivery. Between 80 and 100 percent of women with bipolar disorder who stop taking mood-stabilizer medication during pregnancy will experience relapse soon after discontinuing the medication.[4] Episodes are usually characterized by depressive or mixed symptoms; pure manic symptoms are less common. Thus, many women who experience a "postpartum depression" will turn out to have bipolar disorder, not "unipolar" depression, and the treating physician needs to carefully evaluate any patient who develops serious depression following childbirth for this possibility.

One can speculate on why the period after giving birth is such a high-risk time for women with bipolar disorder: there are the emotional and physical stress of labor and delivery, with the inevitable sleep deprivation; periods of physical pain; and the dramatic changes in the levels of reproductive and stress hormones that attend childbirth. Although the exact reasons remain unknown, it appears that these sorts of environmental issues are not as important as biological factors: younger age and first pregnancy are two, but the most significant appears to be a family history of postpartum mood disorders. In one study, having a relative who had suffered a postpartum episode more than doubled the risk for postpartum relapse in women with bipolar disorder.[5]

Women with bipolar disorder who want to have a child are thus faced with a challenging dilemma. On the one hand, physicians usually recommend that a woman not take any medications during pregnancy, to protect the unborn child from prenatal exposure to pharmaceuticals. On the other hand, it is clear that a woman with bipolar disorder is at high risk for relapse after giving birth and perhaps needs medication late in her pregnancy more than at any other time in her life. Another problem is that several commonly used mood-stabilizing medications have been associated with birth defects.

There are no easy solutions to these problems, but a few facts suggest some ways out. Taking lithium during pregnancy appears to be much safer than originally thought; although there is an increased risk of certain very serious heart malformations in the child, the absolute risk is still low—one to two out of a thousand.[6] Among the anticonvulsants, valproate and carbamazepine have definitely been shown to cause birth defects. Lamotrigine appears to be much safer, as do the atypical antipsychotics.[7]

One fact, however, is clear: simply stopping all medications while trying to get pregnant and for the duration of the pregnancy in order to eliminate all risk to the fetus is *very* risky for the mother. Some women will, of course, be willing to take this risk, and there are many arguments to support this approach. But the first weeks and months—and some say the first few moments—of mother-child contact are essential for mother-child bonding, and this process is disrupted if the mother is depressed or hospitalized with bipolar symptoms. Another perilous scenario is the woman who unknowingly becomes pregnant while taking medication for bipolar disorder and then abruptly stops taking it. This is risky for the child because by the time a woman discovers she is pregnant, the fetus has already been exposed to any medications she is taking for several days to several weeks. Significant organ development has already occurred during this time. I've already mentioned the high risk of relapse in women who stop medication treatment suddenly during pregnancy. *For both of these reasons, I can't stress enough that women with bipolar disorder should plan and prepare for pregnancy so as not to be faced with such difficult choices on short notice.*

Many women with bipolar disorder have healthy babies and remain well in the weeks and months following delivery. Careful planning, conscientious symptom monitoring, and timely resumption of treatment increase the chances of this happening. The woman with bipolar disorder owes it to herself and to her child to think and plan carefully about pregnancy. She should find an obstetrician and a psychiatrist who will support her decision to become pregnant and work closely with her and with each other toward the healthiest possible outcome for both mother and baby.

Is it safe to breastfeed while taking medication? Many medications are secreted in breast milk, including those used to treat bipolar disorder. Careful monitoring for infant exposure to pharmaceuticals by testing breast milk and the baby's blood and urine make it possible for some patients to breastfeed more safely while taking some medications.

PREMENSTRUAL SYNDROMES

There has been intense interest for many years in the mood symptoms that some women experience for several days before the monthly onset of menstruation. Although many women experience some unpleasant physical and psychological symptoms for a few days before their periods, a subgroup of women suffers clinically significant and impairing mood symptoms premenstrually and sometimes mid-cycle as well. Whether the moods of women with bipolar disorder as a group are more likely to sync up with their menstrual cycle is not clear. However, bipolar women who do experience this cycling can have significant and destabilizing mood fluctuations that can make their illness more difficult to control.

It has been shown that women with such monthly mood cycling do not have abnormal reproductive hormone levels. Rather, it appears to be the completely normal but substantial changes of hormonal levels during the menstrual cycle that are responsible for these mood fluctuations. One way to address these symptoms is to take an oral contraceptive. Such medications dampen the normal cycling of hormones and essentially hold hormone levels to what is normally present at the beginning of the menstrual cycle (when the flow begins). To prevent hormonal cycling, the patient takes active medication all the time, skipping the placebo (inactive) pills that are supplied in most contraceptive dispensers. This also means that there is no monthly menstrual flow. Women who notice that menstrually related mood fluctuations consistently cause significant problems for them should consider discussing this approach with their psychiatrist and their gynecologist.

I can't leave the subject of premenstrual mood symptoms without mentioning a study published in the *American Journal of Psychiatry* by several researchers who noticed a significant overlap between premenstrual syndrome (PMS) symptoms and the symptoms of seasonal affective disorder. In both syndromes depressed mood is accompanied by low energy, a tendency to sleep too much rather than too little, and an increase in appetite with carbohydrate craving (as discussed in chapter 15). When the researchers asked patients referred to a PMS clinic whether their PMS was worse during the winter, about two-thirds said that it was. Of the original group, 38 percent met the diagnostic criteria for full-blown seasonal affective disorder. These women, then, had a mood disorder that cycled in at least *two* ways: with the monthly menstrual cycle and with the twelve-month cycle of the seasons.[8] This study shows us once more the intricate and complex relationships between mood and bodily rhythms and cycles and that mood disorders are affected by many different factors in ways we are only beginning to understand.

─────────────── KEY TAKEAWAYS ───────────────

▶ Women with bipolar disorder more frequently have rapid-cycling phases during their illness and have a greater proportion of depressed versus manic/hypomanic episodes.

▶ Family planning is vitally important for women with bipolar disorder because there are complicated issues regarding medications during pregnancy and breastfeeding.

▶ An axiom that cannot be repeated often enough: "There is no other time in the life of any bipolar patient when the risk of an episode is higher than it is for a female bipolar patient in the postpartum period."

▶ Premenstrual worsening of mood symptoms is not uncommon in women with bipolar disorder, and many of them will benefit from taking contraceptive medications to suppress the menstrual cycle.

CHAPTER 19

Alcoholism and Drug Abuse

O f all the statistics associated with bipolar disorder, here is one of the most significant and disturbing: according to one important study, more than 60 percent of persons with bipolar disorder also suffer from alcoholism or drug-abuse problems.[1]

Does having bipolar disorder make individuals more likely to use and abuse drugs and alcohol? Can alcoholism or drug abuse trigger the development of bipolar disorder in someone who is genetically vulnerable? Do bipolar disorder and substance-abuse disorders have a common biochemical or genetic cause? There is evidence to support an answer of yes to all of these questions.

BIPOLAR BINGES

Perhaps the easiest-to-understand model for the observed link between bipolar disorder and alcoholism and drug abuse is the idea that the mood changes of bipolar disorder propel people into situations they would otherwise be able to avoid and cause them to do things they otherwise wouldn't do.

Brad was a forty-two-year-old writer. He had a day job as a copywriter for a small advertising firm, but his creative juices really started flowing late at night when he worked on his "stories." In college Brad won a writing contest and saw his first attempt at writing a short story published in a prestigious national publication. Since then he had published one or two stories a year, sometimes in little literary journals that paid him practically nothing, once in the Atlantic Monthly, *most often in something in between.*

I first met Brad when he was starting to get treatment for alcoholism at the substance-abuse treatment facility affiliated with the hospital where

I worked. A psychiatric consultation was requested because Brad told the staff he was troubled by depression and thought it made his drinking problems worse.

"I know what you're thinking: another alcoholic writer. But I'm not."

"Slow down, Brad," *I said.* "I didn't even know you were a writer until you told me just now." *He was a serious and intense man with dark, deep-set eyes. I had to admit he looked the part of the troubled writer.* "But I'm interested in hearing your ideas about your drinking problem."

"Sorry, I shouldn't jump to conclusions. But people always think of writers as alcoholics. You know, Hemingway, Tennessee Williams, sitting at their typewriters with a glass of Scotch. Well, I don't drink when I write; I drink when I can't write."

This was beginning to sound interesting. "What do you mean?" *I asked.*

Brad drank when he couldn't write because it made him feel better. And it gradually became clear to me that when he couldn't write, it was because he was depressed. "My mind just goes blank for days at a time. I get behind at work, I sleep too much, and I don't even bother turning the computer on at home. I can get the car-wax and potato-chip commercials written at work, but I couldn't be really creative if my life depended on it. This 'what's the use?' feeling comes over me, and I find myself bringing home a fifth of vodka two or three times a week and just sipping the nights away."

"Have you ever used any other drugs? Marijuana? Cocaine?" *I asked.*

"Oh, yes," *Brad said with a deep sigh.* "About three years ago I drained my bank account over a summer—blew it all on cocaine. If I hadn't ended up in the hospital, I might never have stopped."

"What happened?"

"Well, this is really embarrassing. I don't know what got into me, but I got this inspiration to try writing for TV. I had never tried scriptwriting before, but I was sure I could do it. I got an idea for a script about a guy who falls in love with a woman with a cocaine problem. I thought I needed to do some research—you know, where you go to buy the stuff, what those areas of town are like, the people involved."

"Maybe you should have tried the library first."

Brad turned, looking at me intently. At first I thought I had offended him with my little attempt at humor. But I hadn't. "That's just it," *he said.* "That's what I usually* would *have done." He looked away again.* "I'm not a particularly brave person, and certainly not a fool. But I was . . . I don't know quite how to put it . . . uninhibited, confident. I found myself walking down streets at midnight that I would have been nervous walking down in broad daylight. I bought the stuff and had no qualms about using it. And I *was hooked in no time at all. I would get off work, go home, and write until it got dark. Then I'd make a run for the cocaine, kind of cruise around for a while, then come home and snort it. I'd get back to the writing and go at it until the sun came up."*

"When did you sleep?" I asked.

"I didn't, not for days at a time. I didn't need to. I felt energized all the time."

"All the time?"

"Yes, I think cocaine must affect me differently than it does most people. I was feeling high even hours and hours after I had used. Once the high lasted three days."

This was sounding like more than just a drug and alcohol problem. People don't feel high from one dose of cocaine for three days. Something else energized Brad that summer. His mood and behavioral changes had all the hallmarks of hypomania.

"So how did you end up in the hospital?"

"One morning my heart started beating really fast and my chest started to hurt. I left the office and got myself to the emergency room. They wanted to admit me right away, but I wouldn't let them."

"Why not?"

"It didn't seem necessary to me. I thought my heart was fine; I just wanted something for the pain. I know that sounds crazy now, but I think I was a little crazy by then. I don't remember much about what happened next, but they told me I started shouting and fighting. All I know is I got two shots in the butt and didn't wake up until eleven hours later."

Fortunately, Brad's heart was fine, but he was discharged with a prescription for Risperdal to take for a few days for what was called a "cocaine-induced psychosis." His sleep patterns and energy level got back to normal.

"It's funny," he added, "I haven't had even the slightest temptation to use cocaine again. I didn't drink either for the whole next year. But then I found myself slipping into the pit again, and I didn't have the energy to say no anymore. But this time I knew I needed help. I think memories of that cocaine summer made me realize that the drinking might lead to something else again if I didn't get some serious treatment. That's why I checked in here."

I couldn't help asking one more question before telling Brad I thought he probably had bipolar disorder: "Did you finish the script?"

"Yes, I did. It turned out great. I've sent it to a producer, and she's interested. You know, I might even make back the money I spent on my, uh . . . research."

Not all stories like Brad's have such a happy ending. Some persons with bipolar disorder can indeed pull out of substance abuse when their mood episodes come to an end, either spontaneously or with treatment, but for others the substance-abuse problem takes on a life of its own. In the worst-case scenario, the mood disorder and the substance-abuse disorder start feeding on each other, and a vicious cycle of mood symptoms, increased substance abuse, and even more severe mood fluctuations takes over until it's impossible to separate one problem from the other.

Psychiatrists used to talk a great deal about "self-medication" in discussing the relationship between bipolar disorder and substance abuse. The idea was that bipolar patients sometimes started down the road to a full-blown substance-abuse problem by attempting to "treat" their mood symptoms with alcohol or drugs of abuse. Although this certainly occurs in some patients, it doesn't seem to be the most common scenario. While some patients, like Brad, find themselves drinking because it deadens the psychic pain of depression, bipolar patients seem at greater risk for alcohol and drug abuse when they are hypomanic or manic. Brad's cocaine binge is actually the more typical story. The "self-medication" hypothesis might predict that bipolar patients would use stimulants like cocaine to alleviate their depressions. But studies show that, like Brad, bipolar patients are more likely to use cocaine—and to a lesser extent alcohol—to intensify and prolong their hypomanic and manic states.[2]

The link between mania and cocaine abuse has convinced many researchers that it is manic disinhibition and loss of judgment rather than a tendency to "self-medicate" that puts bipolar patients at such high risk for substance abuse.

EFFECT, CAUSE, OR ASSOCIATION?

Another possible relationship between bipolar disorder and substance abuse works in the other direction—that is, alcohol and drug abuse may bring on episodes of abnormal mood in bipolar-disorder patients, perhaps by triggering episodes in persons who are vulnerable to the disorder because of genetic factors. Several studies have shown that bipolar patients who have a substance-abuse disorder have a stormier course to their mood disorder than do patients who do not abuse alcohol or drugs. "Dual-diagnosis" patients, on average, first develop symptoms of their bipolar disorder at a younger age, and in some studies they have been shown to have more frequent hospitalizations. This has been interpreted to indicate that substance abuse may worsen the course of bipolar disorder, perhaps because of some direct effect on the brain caused by repeated use of drugs and alcohol.[3]

Finally, it may be that, like bipolar disorder, vulnerability to addiction has a strong genetic component, and the two problems tend to occur together simply because the genes for both are located close to one another on the chromosomes and tend to be inherited together. I, for one, have seen too many patients like Brad—patients whose bipolar-disorder symptoms and substance abuse seem to trigger and reinforce each other—to believe that these so often tightly intertwined problems are randomly associated.

USE OR ABUSE?

At what point does substance use become "abuse" (table 19.1)? It would be easy for me to launch into a long and complex discussion of diagnostic criteria for substance abuse and chemical dependency, but that probably wouldn't be very helpful. I think the issue is quite clear for individuals with a mood disorder: with the possible exception of occasional alcohol use, I advise persons with a mood disorder to *scrupulously avoid any and all intoxicating substances in any quantity whatsoever*.

All abused substances appear to work by stimulating the "reward" centers of the brain. You have probably heard that laboratory animals will push a lever that delivers an electrical stimulus to certain brain regions rather than another lever that delivers food to their cage, and that they will continue doing so until they're practically dead from hunger. When a similar

---

TABLE 19.1. Signs of alcoholism

Many medical and professional organizations endorse the CAGE questionnaire to identify problem drinking:

1. Have you ever felt you should **C**ut down on your drinking?
2. Have people **A**nnoyed you by criticizing your drinking?
3. Have you ever felt bad or **G**uilty about your drinking?
4. Have you ever had a drink first thing in the morning to steady your nerves or get rid of a hangover (an **E**ye opener)?

One *yes* suggests a possible alcohol problem. More than one *yes* means that an alcohol problem is highly likely.

Source: National Institute on Alcohol Abuse and Alcoholism, *Alcoholism: Getting the Facts*, 1996.

lever device is used to deliver an intravenous dose of alcohol or another drug to laboratory animals, the substances that animals will willingly and persistently self-administer in this way are almost exactly the same ones that humans use to get intoxicated, that we abuse and become addicted to: narcotics, cocaine, and certain stimulants and tranquilizers. Some drugs, like cocaine, affect these centers quickly and powerfully; others, like marijuana, work more slowly, but they all work the same way: by disrupting the normal operation of the brain's "feel-good" circuitry.

Now, you don't need to be a psychiatrist to realize that persons with bipolar disorder already have enough problems with the "feel-good" circuits of the brain and that mucking things up further with "recreational" drugs is a *terrible* idea. There is some evidence to suggest that intoxicating substances actively interfere with the therapeutic effects of the medications used to treat mood disorders. It seems to me that *any* use of intoxicating substances by persons with bipolar disorder is unhealthy and extremely risky and for those reasons amounts to substance abuse.

The question that usually comes next is, can't I even have an occasional glass of wine with dinner? Although I'm hard pressed to forbid my patients ever to drink, it's clear that when it comes to alcohol, less is better. Given the known high risk of bipolar patients for serious substance-abuse problems, the best course is probably no alcohol at all.

A DEADLY COMBINATION

There is one well-established research finding that is much more significant than all the speculation about the nature of the association between bipolar disorder and substance abuse, and even more disturbing than the extremely high rate of substance abuse among people with bipolar disorder. This is the finding that persons who have mood disorders and also abuse alcohol or drugs have a greatly increased risk of suicide. Severe depression complicated by alcoholism or drug abuse has been found to be one of the most frequent diagnostic pictures in study after study of the psychiatric diagnoses of suicide victims. In a 1993 study attempting to make psychiatric diagnoses of suicide victims, clinicians reviewed the medical records and interviewed the relatives of almost fourteen hundred persons who had committed suicide. This study, which found that most of the suicide victims had suffered from a mood disorder, also found that *nearly half* (48 percent) had suffered from alcoholism or drug abuse.[4]

Cannabis: Use at Your Own (Considerable) Risk

Although the research literature on the issue is not extensive, what literature there is indicates that persons with mood disorder should avoid using cannabis.

One of the difficulties with research in this area is that *Cannabis sativa*, the marijuana plant, contains hundreds of psychoactive substances whose effects vary widely. Making things more complicated is the fact that different strains of *C. sativa* can vary greatly in the relative amounts of these different compounds.

The two main psychoactive cannabis compounds (*cannabinoids*) are delta-9-tetrahydrocannabinol (THC) and cannabidiol (CBD). THC is responsible for the cannabis "high" as well as its negative effects, which include anxiety, panic, paranoia, and psychosis, while CBD has antianxiety and other therapeutic effects. Most recreational cannabis has come to consist of higher THC and lower CBD potency, meaning that using cannabis recreationally should be thought of as using THC. This fact likely explains why the preponderance of the research evidence indicates that cannabis has predominantly negative effects on mental health. The cannabis/schizophrenia link has been well established: cannabis doubles the risk of developing schizophrenia and in patients with schizophrenia causes them to have more severe symptoms, higher rates of relapse, longer hospitalizations, and poorer quality of life. Ironically, however, pure CBD preparations are being investigated for their *antipsychotic* effects.

The research on cannabis's effects on mood-disorder patients is less extensive but also strongly indicates that recreational marijuana use is harmful for these individuals. Studies of depression also show increased risk of being diagnosed with major depressive disorder, earlier age of onset, and worse symptom progression. Studies in bipolar patients indicate that cannabis contributes to longer mood episodes, increased mood cycling, lower remission rates, increased suicide risk, and lower recovery.

There are also studies in mood-disorder patients that found no evidence of harm—clearly, more research needs to be done. However, a recent review paper that summarized dozens of studies concluded, "The current literature indicates that there are more harmful consequences compared to benefits associated with long-term cannabis use in bipolar disorder symptomatology and disease progression."*

*D. J. Lowe, J. D. Sasiadek, A. S. Coles, T. P. George, "Cannabis and Mental Illness: A Review," *European Archives of Psychiatry and Clinical Neuroscience* 269, no. 1 (2019): 107-20.

Another point to emphasize here is that when bipolar disorder and a substance-abuse problem coexist, they *both* need treatment. Getting proper treatment for the mood disorder will certainly make the substance-abuse problem easier to treat, but it cannot be assumed that a substance-abuse problem will simply go away when a coexisting mood disorder is treated. An active substance-abuse problem will in fact make the mood disorder difficult to diagnose, let alone treat.

Substance abuse and addiction can best be understood as problem *behaviors*. A certain behavior becomes a problem when the individual engages in it despite negative consequences that are so significant that continuing the behavior is literally self-destructive. A person who continues to drink alcohol or use some other intoxicating substance despite physical, psychological, or social problems that are caused or made worse by it has a substance-abuse problem. Substance abuse is not defined by physical dependence (some substances, such as cocaine, don't even cause physical dependence) or by amount of use. Loss of control and continued use despite negative consequences define substance abuse.

TREATING SUBSTANCE ABUSE AND ADDICTION

The most important prerequisite for the successful treatment of substance abuse, or any problem behavior, is accepting the need to stop the disordered behavior—that is, recognizing that the behavior is causing problems, is out of control, and needs to be given up. This is often the most difficult step. Unless the person overcomes denial ("I don't have a problem; I can stop any time I want to") and accepts his need to change, treatment can't even get started.

One way to conceptualize the process of recognizing this need to change behavior is outlined in the *transtheoretical model*, more commonly called the *stages of change* model, which was initially developed specifically to define the thought patterns and process of behavioral change in smoking cessation.[5] It proposes that individuals who successfully change an unhealthy behavior pass through several stages in the process of change, in a highly predictable way (figure 19.1).

The first phase is called the *pre-contemplative stage*. In this phase, individuals simply don't consider that they may have a problem. They see no reasons for stopping or getting treatment, because they have little or no appreciation of the negative consequences and danger of their behavior.

People with problem behaviors engage in them because doing so benefits them in some way. Drinking alcohol makes you feel good. It is an expected part of many social situations. It decreases anxiety and boosts one's mood a bit, at least initially. In large amounts, it deadens the psychic pain of depression to some extent, at least for a few hours (although we know that alcohol and other intoxicating substances worsen depression when used regularly). During this stage, the individual is continuing the behavior because she judges that its benefits are not outweighed by negative consequences.

The next phase is known as the *contemplative stage*. At this point individuals begin to see that their behavior has at least some negative consequences—to them and their health or to their loved ones. They are beginning to think there might be some advantages to stopping the behavior and may even take some steps to at least investigate what that might entail. They have made no commitment to stop, but they are at least somewhat open to the possibility of stopping. This is one of the most important phases in the cycle, because it is a key place to intervene. People can be stuck here for some time: they may fear the difficulty of stopping, feel uncertain about putting together a plan, or just be "waiting for the right time." This is sometimes as far as a person gets in the process of change, and it can be a torturous time in her life; she now sees the negative results of her actions but is still powerless to stop.

The third phase is known as the *action stage*. Individuals take steps to implement a plan to stop their negative behavior. This is also a crucial stage in the process—if the individual can't tolerate the loss of the behavior's positive effects, he may quickly give up on this plan and move back to the contemplation phase. During the action stage, individuals need support, empathy, and strong encouragement to keep on track and continue in treatment.

If the action individuals take leads to cessation of the behavior, they enter the *maintenance stage*, in which they continue to abstain from negative behaviors and have coping mechanisms and support in place to do so. As with the action phase, individuals may need a great deal of support to remain committed to abstinence. This can be particularly important as their situation improves and the previous negative consequences of the behavior recede. It is easy to see how seductive thoughts like "just one more time" or "I can handle it now" can sneak in.

Psychiatrists and other mental-health professionals are well versed in the available treatment resources in their community for chemical-dependency problems. But perhaps more than most other types of mental-health problems, the treatment of alcohol- and drug-abuse problems requires a wide

The Stages of Behavioral Change

FIGURE 19.1. The stages of change in the transtheoretical model

Illustration by Jenna Macfarlane

The *transtheoretical* model of behavior change proposes that people pass through characteristic and predictable phases on the way to changing a self-defeating behavior, whether it is weight loss, cigarette smoking, alcoholism, or "cutting" behaviors. People make behavioral changes in stages, moving clockwise through the cycle from *pre-contemplative* (not accepting the need to change) to *maintenance* (maintaining the behavioral change). Many slip backward (counterclockwise in the cycle) on their way to recovery, and many suffer a full relapse, moving from maintenance to the pre-contemplative phase and needing to go through the cycle another time, even multiple times, before achieving success.

It's important to emphasize here that whether *others* think that negatives outweigh positives is not important. Only the affected individual's judgment in this matter can lead him to change.

- Pre-contemplation stage:
  - "I don't have a problem"
  - "I can stop any time I want to, but I don't need to or want to."

- Contemplation stage:
  - "Maybe this is a problem, but I'm not ready to change."

- Action Phase:
  - "I have a problem. I definitely need to stop doing this and start developing a plan to do so."

- Maintenance Phase:
  - "I need to be vigilant; it would be so easy to slip up and be right back where I started!"

range of specialized services and support groups. Mental-health professionals will usually refer a patient to a chemical-dependency center or organization for evaluation and treatment of a chemical dependency. Treatment options might include inpatient rehabilitation, outpatient treatment, or a new type of treatment program wherein patients spend the day at the program and return home at night. There are even evening programs that allow people to return to work during the day.

The first step is admitting that there might be a problem. This is often the most difficult step. When in doubt, talking about these concerns with a psychiatrist or therapist is not just important; it can be literally lifesaving.

───────── KEY TAKEAWAYS ─────────

▶ Studies have shown that over half of individuals with bipolar disorder also suffer from addiction.

▶ When they co-occur, *both* the mood disorder and the addiction *must* be treated. Treating the one will not make the other go away.

▶ Intoxicating substances (including cannabis) are best avoided by persons with bipolar disorder.

CHAPTER 20

Borderline Personality Disorder

I n addition to sharing an acronym, *BPD*, bipolar disorder and border-line personality disorder share some other superficial similarities that make it easy to confuse the two. In my experience, misdiagnosing borderline personality disorder (which I'm going to refer to here as BPD) as bipolar disorder is the more frequent error rather than the other way around. BPD is a highly complex disorder, characterized by problems with negative emotions and with emotional regulation and a damaged sense of self, all of which combine to cause relationship problems and put individuals with BPD at much higher risk of self-destructive behaviors such as addiction, eating disorders, self-harming behaviors such as "cutting," and repeated suicidal behaviors.

Primarily, however, individuals with BPD have a great deal of difficulty regulating emotions.

Now, that of course is also a feature of bipolar disorder—but there is a subtle difference in BPD. Whereas persons with bipolar disorder experience periods of abnormal mood in which their mood state bears little or no relationship to what's going on around them, persons with BPD have difficulty modulating what might be called *normal* moods. In BPD, a person's emotional reactions to unpleasant situations come on more quickly, are more intense, and are slower to return to baseline. More importantly, persons with BPD experience these intense reactions all the time, not just during discreet episodes, so much so that their difficulty regulating mood can be thought of as part of the individual's makeup or temperament, which is why the phrase *personality disorder* is part of the terminology for this problem.

Persons with BPD tend to react to situations with negative emotions like anxiety, depression, and anger more readily than others do, to the point where even relatively neutral situations tend to be interpreted negatively and tend to provoke such feelings. It is almost as if these dark moods are the default emotional response to almost any ambiguous situation. As a result, sufferers are battling an ever-present swirl of various painful, uncomfortable emotions. But, compounding their distress, persons with BPD are far less equipped to cope with and modulate these feelings to keep them from taking over. Their emotions change rapidly and unpredictably and easily spiral out of control, leading to extremes of anxiety, sadness, rage, or excitement. They can go from mildly irritated to utterly enraged in a heartbeat, or from feeling merely disappointed to suicidal just as quickly. They cannot talk themselves out of these spirals but tend to "catastrophize"; that is, they immediately imagine the worst-case scenario in every situation and see every problem as disastrous and insolvable. When strong emotions are stirred up, they can even become irrational and show a decline from their usual level of functioning.

Another aspect of BPD is what can be understood as a *damaged sense of self*. Persons with BPD suffer from profound feelings of inadequacy, inferiority, and failure as well as feelings of emptiness and boredom. Now, this damaged sense of self can be seen in many persons who have serious bipolar depression, which has a peculiar way of distorting the way we feel about ourselves that diseases of the body do not. As one of my professors said, "When a person has a toothache, he doesn't start to think that he *is* the toothache." But when a person is seriously depressed, he often starts to attribute his bad feelings to who he "really is" or to something he has done (or not done). Persons who have BPD seem especially prone to this problem, even during times when their depression is not so severe. Recognizing that the way they feel most of the time is different from what they see in those around them, persons with BPD feel like outcasts or outsiders, as if they do not truly belong. Their view of their future is affected too, and they often lack a stable image of who they are or would like to become. Their attitudes, values, goals, and feelings about who they are are often unstable. It's not difficult to see how the combination of chronic negative emotions and a damaged sense of self can lead to a tendency for the person who has BPD to feel helpless, powerless, and at the mercy of forces outside her control.

Lacking the capacity to soothe or comfort themselves when distressed, they need others to help them regulate emotions. This means they require constant reassurance and approval and are often extremely needy or dependent in relationships. They become attached to others quickly and often intensely, developing feelings and expectations of others that are not warranted. This can easily lead to feeling misunderstood, mistreated, or victimized when, inevitably, someone around them proves unwilling or unable to help them in some way. It doesn't take too many of these experiences for them to expect that they will sooner or later be rejected or abandoned by the emotionally significant people in their life. Another aspect of this feature is that, despite their neediness, they are often simultaneously rejecting of others, craving intimacy and caring but tending to rebuff it for fear of being rejected first. The phrase *push-pull relationship* was coined to capture the strained and unstable relationships of persons with the borderline diagnosis, and this leads to interpersonal relationships that are intense and troubled, full of turmoil and conflicts.

The emotional features of the borderline diagnosis make recurrent suicidal behaviors extremely common. Feeling chronically empty and worthless, experiencing extremes of emotions, and being impulsive are a certain recipe for behaviors that can be thought of as the BPD sufferer's dysfunctional attempts to cope: Some individuals with the borderline diagnosis will say that they cut on their body to "keep from feeling numb" or to "just make all of the bad feelings stop." Drug use or binge-eating behaviors often stem from similar motivations.

This dysfunctional coping can take the form of what psychiatrists call *suicidal gestures*. These are attempts at self-harm that are unlikely to cause death but rather seem to be intended to send someone a message. They can usually be better understood as seeking attention and nurturing from others or seeking to demonstrate the depth of the individual's emotional despair.

If it isn't already, I want to make it clear at this point that borderline personality disorder is not easy to diagnose mainly because its symptoms are often shared with many other psychiatric problems (like mood disorders, anxiety disorders, addiction, eating disorders). Only an experienced clinician can make the diagnosis of BPD and then only after getting to know the patient quite well. One of my professors of psychiatry held that it was impossible to make a diagnosis of a personality disorder until after treating the patient for at least six months. That may be a bit of an exaggeration, but it is a good point: even the most experienced therapist cannot make sound judgments about a problem that includes subtleties of personality as well as symptoms that are shared by many other disorders without really getting to know his patient well.

Reading the list of problems that persons with BPD have and the interaction among them, it is probably difficult to imagine that it is a diagnosis with a very good prognosis. But that is indeed the case. An extensive body of literature, much too extensive to review here, has shown that persons with what was once considered a nearly untreatable psychiatric problem do very well with proper treatment. Dialectical behavioral therapy, which is discussed in more detail in chapter 11, has been shown to be especially effective.

Longitudinal research has demonstrated that a substantial proportion of persons diagnosed with BPD recover completely with the right treatment and no longer experience the symptoms or engage in the behaviors associated with the diagnosis.

Features of Borderline Personality Disorder

- *Persistent painful, uncomfortable emotions*
  - Unhappiness, depression or despondency
  - Anxiety
  - Anger and hostility

- *Inability to adequately modulate emotions*
  - Rapid and unpredictable emotional changes
  - Tendency for emotions to spiral out of control, leading to extremes of anxiety, sadness, rage, excitement
  - Inability to soothe or comfort self when distressed, need for assistance to regulate emotions
  - Tendency to "catastrophize," prone to see problems as disastrous and insolvable
  - Quick and intense attachments, unwarranted feelings and expectations of others
  - Fear of rejection or abandonment by those who are emotionally significant
  - Tendency to feel misunderstood, mistreated, or victimized
  - Tendency to become irrational when strong emotions are stirred up and show a decline from usual level of functioning
  - Tendency to act impulsively, without regard for consequences
  - Simultaneously craving intimacy and caring but tending to reject it when offered

- *Unstable, chaotic, and rapidly changing interpersonal relationships*

- *Damaged sense of self*
  - Lack a stable image of who one is or would like to become: attitudes, values, goals, and feelings about self may be unstable and changing
  - Feelings of inadequacy, inferiority, failure
  - Feelings of emptiness and boredom
  - Tendency to feel helpless, powerless, at the mercy of forces outside one's control
  - Feeling like an outcast or outsider, as if one does not truly belong

- Tendency to be overly needy or dependent, requires excessive reassurance or approval

BORDERLINE OR BIPOLAR—OR BOTH?

The problem with diagnosing BPD and differentiating it from bipolar disorder is compounded but the fact that a person can have *both*. There is evidence that persons with BPD are especially likely to also have mood disorders, including bipolar disorder, often bipolar II or a "soft" bipolar disorder. What is the relationship between these two problems?

A group of psychiatrists at Harvard led by Dr. John Gunderson, who has studied the borderline diagnosis for many years and is one of the leading experts in the disorder, attempted to answer this question by following 196 individuals who were carefully diagnosed by experts as having BPD, assessing them for a co-occurring diagnosis of bipolar I or II, and then following them for four years, reevaluating all of them annually to assess whether additional individuals had developed a bipolar disorder. The researchers found that almost one in five patients with a diagnosis of borderline personality either came into the study with bipolar disorder or developed it during the four years they were followed.[1]

This study also found that, as a group, those persons who had BPD and a bipolar disorder had a less than complete recovery in their overall clinical status during the study. That is, they continued to have substantial difficulties in functioning, and they continued to need intensive treatment for their borderline symptoms and behaviors; this was true even if their bipolar disorder was being treated. If this seems counterintuitive, the study authors suggested a possible reason for this finding, warning that "the bipolar diagnosis encourages individuals and their families to have unrealistic expectations about what medications can do" and to make less of a commitment to their treatment for BPD.[2] This is important because intensive psychotherapy, often including both individual therapy as well as family and groups sessions, is part of the hard work of recovery from BPD.

Another way to look at this issue is to see whether persons with a borderline diagnosis benefit from medications that we know help in bipolar disorder. When approached this way, there is solid evidence from research studies that many people who receive the diagnosis of borderline personality do indeed benefit greatly from the medications known to be effective in bipolar disorder. In one of these studies, persons with the borderline diagnosis were given the mood stabilizer lamotrigine and followed for eighteen months.[3] The study was interesting in that it did not look at the effect of the medication on *mood* but rather at its effect on *anger*. It found that volunteers showed a significant decrease in their subjective feelings of anger and aggressive behaviors (toward self or others) and an increase in their ability to control their angry impulses.

So, how can we synthesize these data? On the one hand, it has been proposed that BPD is just another form of bipolar disorder, a proposal that is almost certainly wrong. Nevertheless, there appears to be a connection of some kind between the two diagnoses. It may be that whatever genetic factors put a person at risk for developing BPD also put her at risk of developing bipolar disorder. One of my colleagues at Johns Hopkins, Dr. Dean MacKinnon, has proposed an idea that I admire very much, which is that the symptoms and behaviors that characterize BPD result from an interaction between an individual's biologically determined tendency to experience strong emotions and childhood experiences that are invalidating of those emotions.[4] The idea is that the child's extra-strong emotional reactions are ignored or discounted by their environment, leading the child to feel invalidated, damaged, and "different," leading to the damaged sense of self and dysfunctional behaviors that are seen in BPD.

This exceedingly brief overview of borderline personality disorder only begins to scratch the surface of the complexities of the diagnosis and the poorly understood relationship between BPD and bipolar disorder. You can find more material to explore in the suggested readings in the "Resources" at the end of the book.

KEY TAKEAWAYS

▶ Borderline personality disorder is a severe and complex psychiatric diagnosis that, like bipolar disorder, is characterized by difficulties in mood regulation.

▶ In persons with BPD, intense and negative emotional reactions (depression, anxiety, anger) are the default responses to frustrating experiences, however trivial.

▶ Persons with BPD have a damaged sense of self and chronic feelings of hopelessness, alienation, and emptiness.

▶ These problems often lead them to develop dysfunctional coping behaviors, such as "cutting," addiction, and eating disorders.

▶ Some individuals with BPD suffer from a bipolar disorder as well as BPD and will need treatment for both to do well.

▶ Borderline personality disorder has a very good prognosis, especially with the proper specialized treatment.

CHAPTER 21

Bipolar Disorder
and Creativity

Aristotle said, "No great genius has ever existed without some touch of madness."[1] Most truisms contain a kernel of truth, and that of the "mad genius" seems to as well. Scholars who have studied the lives of highly creative people have discovered that among them there are unexpectedly high numbers of individuals with severe psychiatric illness. Clinicians involved in this work have concluded that bipolar disorder is by far the most common among them. It doesn't require extensive research to come up with a long list of writers, artists, and composers whose biographies indicate that they probably had a mood disorder. Let's take a glimpse into the lives of several of them.

George Gordon, Lord Byron (1788–1824) had periods of fiery expansiveness and hollow despair throughout his life. The recorded observations of his friends and his physicians make a diagnosis of bipolar disorder all but certain in the great English poet. Byron's family history is entirely consistent with this diagnosis—suicide, "madness," and murder can be traced back several generations on both sides of his family tree.

Medical biographers of Vincent van Gogh (1853–1890) have speculated for decades about the illness that drove him to self-mutilation and repeatedly confined him to the Asylum of Saint-Paul at Saint-Rémy. The episodic nature of Van Gogh's illness and the acceleration of its course toward the end of his life are highly suggestive of bipolar disorder. Van Gogh described his dreadful depressions in his letters and was diagnosed with mania by several of his physicians. Van Gogh's family history, like Lord Byron's, seems to confirm the diagnosis of bipolar disorder: Vincent's brother Theo described his own struggles with depression in letters to Vincent, and a third brother, Cor, committed suicide. A person needs only to imagine the brilliant, swirling, sometimes frenzied colors and shapes of Van Gogh's paintings as visual representations of his moods to understand what psychiatric illness best explains the artist's episodes of psychosis (figure 21.1).

**FIGURE 21.1. Vincent van Gogh's painting
of the Maison de Santé Saint-Paul**

The Maison de Santé Saint-Paul is the psychiatric hospital where Van Gogh stayed for a year (1889–1890) recovering from a depressive episode. Saint-Paul's is still an active health care facility for patients with psychiatric illnesses.

Source: Musée d'Orsay, Paris / Scala / Art Resource, NY

The Romantic composer Robert Schumann (1810–1856) wrote of suicide at age eighteen but only a year later reported, "I am so full of music, and so overflowing with melody that I find it simply impossible to write down anything." Schumann suffered his first major episode of psychiatric illness in 1844 at the age of thirty-four, but he had written a description of his depressions several years earlier in a letter to his future wife, Clara: "No one knows the suffering, the sickness, the despair, except those so crushed. In my terrible agitation I went to a doctor and told him everything—how my senses failed me so that I did not know which way to turn in my fright, how I could not be certain of not taking my own life when in this helpless condition." Schumann recovered from this episode to write some of his greatest musical works, including three of his four symphonies, but ten years later he suffered another collapse. In February 1854 Clara recorded, "In the night, not long after we had gone to bed, Robert got up and wrote down a melody which, he said, the angels had sung to him. Then he lay down again and talked deliriously the whole night. When morning came, the angels transformed themselves into devils and sang horrible music, telling him he was a sinner and that they were going to cast him into Hell."[2]

A few weeks later, probably in the grip of an episode of psychotic depression, Schumann ran out of their home and threw himself off a bridge into the icy waters of the Rhine. He was rescued by fishermen and placed in the asylum in Endenich, where he died a year later, possibly of self-starvation. As with van Gogh, biographers have quarreled at times about Schumann's diagnosis, but a glance at the opus numbers of his works grouped by year of composition (figure 21.2) leaves little doubt that he suffered from bipolar disorder. What other illness could better explain these intense fluctuations of productivity, periods of intense creative energy that gave way to psychosis and despair?

The fact that many great artists have suffered from bipolar disorder does not in itself indicate a special link between bipolar disorder and creativity. There have certainly been many other great artists, writers, and composers who as far as we can tell did *not* suffer from major psychiatric illnesses. Johannes Brahms, Schumann's musical protégé, who arguably went on to surpass his mentor's accomplishments as a composer, was as staid and steady a man as ever lived. Brahms ate dinner at the same restaurant in Vienna nearly every day for the last several *decades* of his life, often sitting at the same table and ordering the same items from the menu.

Nevertheless, several researchers who have performed psychobiographical surveys of groups of creative individuals have found that a striking and inordinate number of accomplished artists, writers, and musicians have suffered from bipolar disorder. Most studies have come up with prevalence rates of between 30 and 50 percent—nearly ten times the rate of mood disorders in the general population. Perhaps the most careful of these studies has been done by Kay Redfield Jamison, who examined autobiographical and biographical materials and, when available, the medical records of all major British and Irish poets born between 1705 and 1805. Jamison concluded that over half of these writers suffered from a mood disorder, more than one-third from bipolar disorder. These numbers are so high that one can't help but wonder whether there might be some bias in the research method: Do the more tumultuous biographies of psychiatrically ill artists result in more biographical material being available, thus skewing the results? To avoid such a bias, researchers selected living writers, musicians, and artists on the basis of literary and artistic prizes for further studies, which came up with virtually the same numbers. The prevalence of bipolar disorder is simply much higher in groups of accomplished artists than in the general population (table 21.1).[3]

FIGURE 21.2. The fluctuations of composer Robert Schumann's musical productivity

The severe fluctuations of the German Romantic composer Robert Schumann's musical productivity become strikingly apparent when his musical works (identified here by opus number) are arranged according to the year of their composition. Schumann died in an asylum a little more than a year after his suicide attempt in 1854.

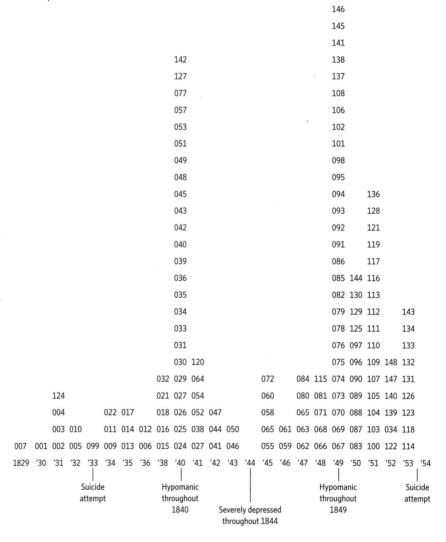

Source: Adapted from Eliot Slater and Alfred Meyer, "Contributions to a Pathology of the Musician Robert Schumann," *Confinia Psychiatrica* 2 (1959): 65–94. Reproduced with the permission of S. Karger, AG, Basel.

TABLE 21.1. Artists, writers, and composers with bipolar disorders

Artists

Paul Gauguin

Vincent van Gogh*

Mark Rothko*

Writers

William Blake

Lord Byron

Ernest Hemingway*

Robert Lowell*

Sylvia Plath*

Anne Sexton*

Virginia Woolf*

Composers

Hector Berlioz

George Frederick Handel

Robert Schumann*

Hugo Wolf*

*Attempted or committed suicide.

How can this striking finding be explained? Emil Kraepelin thought that manic-depressive illness could free a person from the inhibitions that might otherwise stifle creativity: "The volitional excitement which accompanies the disease may . . . set free powers which are otherwise constrained by all kinds of inhibition[s]."[4] Fear of failure, sensitivity to criticism, worry that one has nothing important to contribute—these kinds of inhibitions, of course, vanish during periods of hypomania and mania.

One can argue that the extraordinary mental states experienced by persons with bipolar disorder provide them with rich raw materials for the production of works of great creativity. As I tried to make clear in chapter 1 of this book, the clinical states of mania and major depression often bear little resemblance to normal mood states. They are not simply exaggerations of normal happiness and sadness but rather are normal moods transcended and transformed. Is it any wonder, then, that those who endure them have put such great effort into chronicling and communicating these remarkable experiences? Because of the relapsing and remitting course of the illness, a person who has recovered from mania or major depression can record what it was like. Individuals in the midst of an episode will usually be too disorganized or too lethargic to be productive, but later, when their mood state returns to normal, they can articulate these almost inexpressible feelings and experiences in art, music, and poetry.

It has been suggested that the changes in thinking patterns that occur during the hypomanic and manic states are especially conducive to creative endeavor. When the thinking processes of highly creative individuals (with or without mood disorders) have been studied, it has been found that their thinking tends to be fluid and divergent. Ideas spring from and give rise to other ideas only loosely connected by logic and convention. Unrelated ideas are merged and mingled in novel ways. The loss of logical progression in thinking and a rapid flow of loosely connected ideas are, of course, a fundamental aspect of the hypomanic state.

It has also been suggested that it is not any one mood state, normal or abnormal, that gives rise to the creative powers of these artists, but rather the flux and tensions between the different mood states. Constant changes in mood and temperament give the individual with cyclothymic mood changes a kaleidoscopic view of the world, always changing, always new. Perhaps bipolar disorder stimulates creativity in part because its sufferers experience the world through the emotional prisms of its many and shifting moods, some of them extreme, even violent. As the English poet John Keats observed, "What shocks the virtuous philosopher delights the chameleon poet."[5]

Artists and Entertainers Who Have Disclosed Their Treatment for Bipolar Disorder

- Mariah Carey, singer-songwriter
- Carrie Fisher, writer and actress who portrayed Princess Leia in the Star Wars franchise
- Brian Wilson, singer-songwriter member of the Beach Boys
- Catherine Zeta-Jones, Academy Award–winning actress
- Vivien Leigh, won Academy Awards for Best Actress in *Gone with the Wind* and *A Streetcar Named Desire*; received ECT to treat her illness
- Sinead O'Connor, Irish singer-songwriter
- Jane Pauley, award-winning journalist, currently the anchor of *CBS Sunday Morning*

Individuals with bipolar disorder may be drawn to creative endeavors out of a need to understand and heal themselves through art and the act of creation. The French author and filmmaker Jean Cocteau said, "Art is science made clear."[6] When medicine and psychiatry fail to explain the inner experiences of the disease, when lithium and antidepressants and therapy all flounder and the terrible moods return again and again, people can find ways of understanding and transforming their suffering through poetry, music, and painting.

All these reasons help us to understand why this often-destructive illness can also generate such intense creativity and artistic accomplishment. If creative work requires unique experiences, fluid imagination, confidence in one's abilities, and energetic excitement about the act of creation, bipolar disorder would seem to fit the bill.

But reading the biographies of these bipolar artists reveals the high price they often paid. Bipolar disorder was a mighty but malignant muse for Vincent van Gogh and Ernest Hemingway and Sylvia Plath, all of whom committed suicide. How many more symphonies would Robert Schumann have composed if, like his quiet, steady friend Brahms, he had lived into his sixties?

Perhaps the most intriguing question about the connection between bipolar disorder and creativity is whether the illness was somehow *essential* to the creative powers of these individuals. Van Gogh might have lived to paint many more paintings if he had not suffered from bipolar disorder, but would they have been great paintings? Would he have been a painter at all? Or would he have acquiesced to his father's wishes and contentedly applied himself to becoming a member of the clergy? This is, of course, an unanswerable question when historical figures are involved, but a related question poses a very real dilemma for many individuals with bipolar disorder and their physicians. Does the treatment of bipolar disorder with mood-stabilizing medication suppress creativity and dull the artistic spirit?

Several studies attempting to answer this question were done just after the introduction of lithium as a treatment for bipolar disorder in the 1970s (one of them by Morgans Schou, who, as you may remember from chapter 4, was a pioneer in the use of lithium as a mood stabilizer). Artists and writers were asked whether they thought treatment with lithium had increased, decreased, or had no effect on their productivity. The results are fairly unequivocal and perhaps a little surprising. Over half (57 percent) reported that treatment of their mood disorder with lithium had *increased* their artistic productivity, and another 20 percent thought it had not affected their artistic output. Only one-quarter of these artists and writers believed that lithium had adversely affected their work.[7] Since one of the side effects of lithium in some persons is a dulling of thinking, it is also possible that these individuals were reporting the impact of a medication side effect rather than the impact of mood stabilization. Would artists treated with valproate or carbamazepine have reported the same results?

Over the years a small number of my patients have resisted taking mood stabilizers because they believed that their creative powers would be or actually were adversely affected by these medications. I have usually thought that these individuals were reluctant to take medications for other reasons: unwillingness to accept a diagnosis of bipolar disorder, ambivalence about taking a medication that they feared would "control" them, and other understandable concerns that can usually be resolved with therapy and counseling. People seize upon all kinds of reasons not to take medication; my impression is that this particular plausible-sounding reason is usually a substitute for facing and working through understandably conflicted feelings about taking medication.

The mysterious link between bipolar disorder and creativity, though unexplained by either psychiatrists or philosophers, is real. It poses challenges for patients and dilemmas for clinicians and offers opportunities for researchers. Better understanding of this connection will not only expand our understandings of mood disorders but will perhaps lead us to new insights into the magic of artistry and the creative process.

KEY TAKEAWAYS

▶ There appears to be an intriguing connection between bipolar disorder and creativity. Several studies suggest that highly creative persons suffer from mood disorders at a higher than expected rate compared to the general population.

▶ There is no good evidence that getting treated for bipolar disorder negatively impacts creativity, in fact the opposite may be true.

PART V

Getting Better and Staying Well

There are millions of people living with bipolar disorder today. Many are living healthy, happy, and productive lives, but many others are not. This section of the book is intended to help you maximize your chances of getting into and staying in the first category and staying out of the second.

If you're looking for a simple list of dos and don'ts, I'm afraid you will be disappointed. Instead, in chapter 22, "Living with Bipolar Disorder," I've tried to lay out general principles that underlie the sorts of advice and recommendations that are usually given to patients in the doctor's office or clinic. I hope that after reading this chapter, you'll have a better understanding of why some of the recommendations that you hear from your doctor and therapist are so important.

Chapter 23 offers some principles for dealing with emergencies and highlights the types of emergency situations that patients and their families often fail to prepare for. We're always tempted to put off thinking about and planning for things we hope won't happen. But it is important not to give in to this temptation. I explain here how easy it is to be prepared for emergencies.

Bipolar disorder doesn't affect only the individual with the diagnosis of the illness. Inevitably, family and friends are affected in countless ways, both directly and indirectly. Chapter 24, "The Role of the Family," addresses this aspect of the illness. I talk about what family members can do—and, just as important, what family members cannot and should not try to do—to help their loved one who has bipolar disorder.

CHAPTER 22

Living with Bipolar Disorder

There is no one medication or treatment approach for bipolar disorder that works for everyone. The symptoms of the illness in a specific person are often as unique as the individual, and treatment must be carefully individualized to each patient and his particular symptom pattern. This said, there are some approaches and pieces of advice that I think are always going to be helpful. In fact, the principles I lay out in this chapter are, in my experience, indispensable to staying well and having the best possible control of symptoms.

CONFRONT AND ACCEPT THE ILLNESS

There is no cure for bipolar disorder, only treatment and management. It is a relentless illness whose symptoms inevitably and repeatedly return to torment its sufferers. The only way to keep it at bay is for the patient to be relentless as well—relentless about getting needed treatment and sticking to it. No other piece of advice I can give is as important as this one.

Human beings have an almost unlimited capacity to explain away the obvious. People who don't want to confront serious physical illnesses can ignore and rationalize even the most alarming symptoms: for example, the middle-aged man with a history of high blood pressure who doesn't pay attention to his repeated episodes of chest pain ("Oh, it's just heartburn; must have been something I ate") or the woman who feels a lump in her breast and tells herself, "It's probably just a cyst, I'm sure it will go away." Facing a possibly life-threatening illness is perhaps the most frightening experience we can face. Small wonder that we sometimes put ourselves through some impressive mental gymnastics to avoid the confrontation.

When there are no *physical* signs of illness, no pains or lumps or dizzy spells, it may be all the easier to convince oneself that the symptoms of illness are something else. I don't know how many times I've had a patient ask whether I thought she really needed to continue on a mood stabilizer after a manic episode had resolved: "After all, I was under a lot of stress, and I hadn't slept for weeks. Maybe I just need to take it easy." As we'll see, stress can indeed play a role in precipitating an episode of a mood disorder, *but it's not the cause*. Stress doesn't make people manic or send them into a major depression unless they have bipolar disorder. Neither does drinking too much or sleep deprivation or the loss of a job or the end of a love affair or the hundred other things that you can convince yourself of to explain your symptoms.

People with bipolar disorder can go through years of denial and anger about their illness. I have seen patients repeatedly stop taking medication and drop out of treatment and explain their repeated hospitalizations, shattered relationships, and ruined finances in all sorts of ways: "My wife has it in for me, she put me in the hospital again." "If my boss wouldn't put so much pressure on me, this wouldn't happen." "I think you need to check my thyroid again; I know that's the real problem." Or in its simplest form: "I don't need this medicine, because I'm not crazy."

If you have been diagnosed with bipolar disorder and you have read to this point in the book, you have almost certainly gotten past a great deal of this understandable denial and anger. This is a tremendous accomplishment—it signals a turning point in your recovery. (If you're reading this book to better understand another person with bipolar disorder who hasn't yet made it past denial, chapter 24 is especially for you.) But there's a gap between complete denial and complete ability to confront and accept this illness. Unfortunately, people sometimes try to hold onto the notion that nothing is seriously wrong by refusing to take the problem seriously. It is especially easy and especially problematic to take this view in bipolar disorder.

In bipolar disorder the patient ultimately determines how well *any* treatment is going to work—because it is the *patient* who puts treatment recommendations into action. It is the patient who will determine whether he takes *every* dose of medication, or just 90 percent of the doses, or 50 percent, or even less. The patient will determine whether the blood for her lithium or valproate blood-level test is drawn exactly twelve hours after the last dose or whether she gets to the lab after ten or fifteen hours, throwing the results and the doctor's calculations off by 10 or 20 percent. The patient will determine how many appointments are kept with the doctor and the therapist and how many are missed—and how many are shorter than scheduled because of tardiness. It's so easy to let your guard down, let treatment lapse in little ways, and convince yourself that missing a dose of medication here

Will There Ever Be a *Cure* for Bipolar Disorder?

Until we have a much better understanding of the causes of bipolar disorder, it's hard to imagine what a cure might look like, if by *cure*, one means a one-time intervention that resolves symptoms and eliminates any chance of recurrence. However, at the beginning of the twentieth century, the idea of a cure for cancer seemed an impossible dream, and yet today many forms of cancer are eminently curable. In the past decade, a cure for hepatitis C was found. Gene therapies are under development for various immunological diseases and sickle cell anemia.

Cure becomes a much more difficult thing to imagine when an illness is an essentially developmental problem like schizophrenia appears to be. And one of the daunting problems with developing a cure for bipolar disorder is that there appear to be many "broken" pieces to fix—there are probably dozens of genetic errors that add up, probably in many different combinations, to cause a person to develop the illness.

So the best we can do for now is *control* the symptoms.

Nevertheless, a recent scientific development may lead to dramatic improvements in treatment. This development is a technique by which cells from an adult can be treated to turn them into stem cells that can then be coaxed to develop into neurons and other cells of the nervous system. This breakthrough presents the possibility of taking a few cells from a patient with bipolar disorder, perhaps in a procedure as noninvasive as a "punch" biopsy that your dermatologist may perform to check a suspicious mole, and growing neurons in the lab. Those neurons could then be tested to see exactly what functions have gone awry and to select treatments based upon that information. Such techniques are already in use for cancer treatment and hold great promise for the treatment of other illnesses as well.

Even more exciting is the possibility of using a patient's own stem cells to directly treat the illness. Such interventions to treat neurological diseases like Parkinson's are already in development. Stem cells appear to be able to find their own way to damaged areas of the brain and help rebuild what's been lost in these illnesses. By the time that you read this, a clinical trial under the leadership of Dr. Jair Soares at the UTHealth McGovern Medical School in Houston will be underway involving infusing stem cells into patients with bipolar depression.*

So although we can't speak of a cure just yet, exciting changes in the treatment of bipolar disorder may be just over the horizon.

*Information about this and other clinical trials for bipolar disorder is available at clinicaltrials.gov/.

or there, having that second beer, ignoring a string of sleepless nights, isn't really important. To do so is to turn away from rather than to confront this disease, and often the turning away springs from ambivalence about the need for treatment: *less than complete acceptance of the diagnosis.* To not accept this illness, to not confront it puts treatment success in jeopardy, because in bipolar disorder perhaps more than in any other serious illness, it is the patient who administers the treatment most of the time.

Imagine that a surgeon is evaluating a patient with recurrent abdominal pain. He has done a physical examination and has ordered some lab tests and x-rays. All the evidence points to gall bladder problems, and the surgeon decides that the best treatment among several possibilities is gall bladder removal. Now imagine that the surgeon is in the middle of the operation and suddenly says to the operating room nurse, "You know, this operating room's getting awfully hot, and besides, I'm hungry. I think we'll cancel the operation. I'll give our patient here the antibiotics for another week or so. Maybe we didn't stick with the medication approach long enough after all. But I just don't think I want to go on with this operation right now."

Sound far-fetched? (I certainly hope so!) Well, here's another scenario: A man with bipolar disorder has driven off with the family for their three-week vacation. The family has already traveled fifty miles when the wife says, "Honey, I packed Timmy's asthma medicine, but I didn't see your medication bottle in the cabinet; did you remember to bring your lithium?" The man realizes that he didn't. "Ah . . . sure I did," he tells his wife, and then says to himself, "Three weeks won't make any difference. Besides, I haven't felt depressed or anything in a long time. This is a vacation, after all. And if I get just a little high, it would be OK; I'm sure I could handle it."

Now, what do these scenarios have in common? In both cases, a treatment plan was decided upon, presumably after much consideration and discussion as to the best course of action. In both cases, something comes up that makes continuing with the treatment a bit inconvenient. In both cases, rather than make a rational decision about the best course of action, the person in charge of the treatment uses flimsy logic—accompanied perhaps by a large measure of preexisting ambivalence about the treatment being the correct one in the first place—to justify doing what's easiest. Add in some misinformation—three weeks without lithium *can* make a difference, and nobody can just "handle" evolving mania—and you have a recipe for disaster. No one would go back to a physician who treated him this way, and no one should treat himself this way, either.

Making a commitment to treatment means (1) being active, not passive, in formulating a treatment plan with your providers; (2) taking charge of

Confront and Accept the Illness

- Make the decision that you will do whatever it takes to take control of this illness; otherwise, it *will* take control of you.

- Be *active*, not passive in collaborating with your treatment providers.
  - *Prepare* for your appointments: What is your goal for today's appointment?
  - Write down your observations and any questions ahead of time and bring them to the appointment.
  - Ask your prescriber to give you any changes in treatment plan *in writing*. Don't rely on memory. Hospitals and clinics can usually provide you with an *after-visit summary* with a medication list, blood tests ordered, and so forth. Ask for it!

- Take charge of your treatment—by taking medications as directed, getting blood tests done as ordered, and keeping appointments (and being on time!).

treatment implementation 100 percent of the time; and (3) making the decision that you will do everything possible to take control of this illness rather than be controlled by it.

But can a person be "on guard" all the time? In fact, who would *want* to be? What kind of life is it to be constantly worrying about one's mental health? A terrible one, of course. But worrying all the time is certainly not what I'm suggesting. Rather, accepting and confronting this illness means deciding to do whatever you need to do to be as healthy as you can possibly be. This means sticking with treatment and being frank and open with your treatment professionals. It also means more self-discipline and restraint than you may be used to; it means making some lifestyle changes that I'll call *mood hygiene*.

PRACTICE MOOD HYGIENE

Hygiene is a word that we might not use in medicine as much as we should, and we certainly don't use it as much as we used to. Hygeia was the Greek goddess of health, the daughter—or in some versions of the story, the wife—of Asclepius, the god of medicine. Hygiene, or hygienics, is the science of *the establishment and maintenance of health*—as opposed to the treatment of disease—and has to do with conditions and practices that are conducive to health. The hygienic conditions and practices we think of today usually relate to cleanliness, but the word has a much broader meaning. At the beginning of the twentieth century, institutions such as the Johns Hopkins University School of Hygiene and Public Health (now the Bloomberg School) and the London University School of Hygiene and Tropical Diseases were founded to study methods for *preventing* disease and for promoting and improving the health of whole communities. Predating them both was the Mental Hygiene Association, founded in 1909 by former asylum inmate Clifford Beers (who probably had bipolar disorder). Now called Mental Health America, its purpose is to promote emotional health and well-being and to lobby for better and more readily available treatment for psychiatric illnesses.

So, what do I mean by *mood hygiene*? Simply put, practices and habits that promote good control of mood symptoms. Several areas of research on bipolar disorder show how important preventive measures can be for improving symptom control. Things like stress management and lifestyle regularity make a big difference.

Emil Kraepelin noticed that early in the course of his manic-depressive patients' illnesses, their mood episodes often came on after a stressful event in their lives: "In especial, the attacks begin not infrequently after the illness or death of near relatives. . . . Among other circumstances there are occasionally mentioned quarrels with neighbors or relatives, disputes with lovers . . . excitement about infidelity, financial difficulties. . . . We must regard all alleged injuries as possible sparks for the discharge of individual attacks." Kraepelin was quick to point out that these events were triggers, not causes, and that "the real course of the malady must be sought in permanent internal changes which . . . are innate." Kraepelin noticed, however, that later in the course of the illness, attacks occurred "wholly without external influences," and he proposed that for patients at that stage of the illness, "external influence[s] . . . must not be regarded as a necessary presupposition for the appearance of an attack."[1]

The accuracy of these observations has been borne out in later studies: initial and early mood episodes in patients with bipolar disorder are often related to psychological stressors, but after several episodes, the illness can take on a life of its own, such that later episodes are more likely to arise spontaneously.

An interesting parallel in animals can be demonstrated by repeatedly giving animals small doses of stimulants such as cocaine. Over time, animals become *more* rather than less sensitive to the stimulant, and repeatedly giving the same small dose causes *increasing* amounts of behavioral stimulation in the animal. When these animals' brain cells are closely examined, it is found that a certain gene that had not been active previously was turned on by the repeated stimulant exposure. This same gene can be made to turn on by stressing the animals—by depriving them of water, for example. This work with animals, showing that chemical stimulation as well as stress can bring about long-term changes in behavior—possibly through alterations in gene function—is thought by many experts to be highly relevant to the study of bipolar disorder.[2]

Several direct observations of patients indicate that a similar phenomenon may occur in individuals with bipolar disorder: (1) Patients sometimes show more environmentally triggered mood episodes at first in the course of their illness and more spontaneously occurring episodes later. (2) They sometimes show an acceleration in their illness as they age, with episodes occurring more and more frequently as time goes on. (3) Mood episodes make patients more sensitive to stress and more likely to relapse than they might otherwise be. In a study of fifty-two patients with bipolar disorder followed for two years, those who relapsed during the time of the study were much more likely to have experienced some stressful event. In this group of patients, those with a greater number of prior episodes were *more* sensitive to these stresses: they were more likely to relapse under stress, and they relapsed more quickly.[3]

The converse, however, may be true as well: as time in remission gets longer, people seem to develop a resiliency that helps them stay well. Several years ago, I was leading a seminar for psychiatry residents at Johns Hopkins on the treatment of bipolar disorder with lithium. We were lucky enough to have my colleague Hopkins professor Kay Jamison drop by and join us that afternoon. As we were finishing up, I repeated the maxim that I mentioned earlier in the book to the young doctors, "The second year on lithium is better than the first." Smiling, Dr. Jamison added, "That's right . . . and the *twenty*-second year on lithium is really terrific!" Her point was that longer periods of mood stability confer a kind of resilience on persons with bipolar disorder and lessen the probability that stresses will trigger an episode. Several studies have demonstrated that the treatment and prevention of mood episodes improve the long-term outcome in bipolar disorder. Treatment intervention during the first ten years after diagnosis appears to be especially important; the prevention of manic episodes is vital, too.[4] Working hard to stay well, especially in the first years after diagnosis, makes it easier to stay well over the longer term; put another way, stability begets stability. This means that one of the foundations of mood hygiene needs to be *relapse prevention*. And there should be no doubt in your mind at this point that the most effective relapse-prevention tool is medication.

Persons with bipolar disorder should make peace with the idea of taking medication every day for the foreseeable future. That is an especially hard thing to do in this disease. The symptoms and the need for medication often start when people are in their twenties or even younger, when none of their peers have to bother with medication—when the only people they know who take medication are "old people" and "sick people." It's difficult for a young, physically healthy person who's feeling well to take medication every day.

The idea of taking medication to control one's moods and mental processes is also a daunting one. An early study asked forty-seven persons who were attending a clinic about their attitudes toward taking lithium.[5] Of those who had stopped taking lithium at some point during the course of their treatment, the most frequently given reason was that they were "bothered by the idea of moods being controlled by a medication." On the face of it, this is quite understandable, perhaps even reasonable. Remember, however, that in bipolar disorder the medication allows the patient to be in control of her moods rather than the other way around.

Each individual needs to work out for himself a method for making sure that every single dose of every medication is taken. Pharmacies sell a variety of clever devices to help make this happen. There are pillboxes with built-in clocks and timers, with alarms that can be set to go off when it's time for the next dose. There are boxes that hold a whole week's worth of medication in little compartments, one for every dose, so that the answer to "Did I take my dose this morning?" is always clear and certain: if the little compartment is empty, the dose was taken. Ask your treating physician whether your medication can be taken just once a day, or twice rather than three times a day. Ask about controlled-release forms of medications; several are available, often making it possible to eliminate midday doses, which are inevitably the most difficult ones to fit into a busy life.

The body of evidence showing that medication prevents relapse cannot be argued with; it is simply overwhelming. But there is some evidence that persons who stop medication for bipolar disorder may run more than just the risk of a relapse. There have been several case reports of persons who stopped taking lithium for bipolar disorder, had a relapse, *and then did not respond to lithium when it was restarted*, a phenomenon that has been called *lithium-discontinuation-induced refractoriness*. Out of fifty-four patients who stopped lithium, ten—nearly 20 percent—had a poor response when they restarted it. For these patients, lithium lost some of its effectiveness.[6] The results of this study provide even more proof of the importance of relapse prevention for the long-term course of bipolar disorder. I already mentioned the work showing a better prognosis for persons whose illness is well controlled from the beginning. Lithium-discontinuation-induced refractoriness illustrates the converse of the adage "stability begets stability": *instability begets instability*, at least in some persons.

Next on the list of mood-hygiene practices is *stress and conflict management*. Most of us have little control over when and how stress and conflict come into our lives. But we can learn how to manage stress and conflict better—and here I'll put in another plug for counseling and therapy. This is because I am talking about serious, *vigorous* attention to whatever ongoing sources of serious stress there may be: primary relationship and marital conflicts, job and career problems, and chronic financial or legal problems are good examples. Immediately after diagnosis with bipolar disorder may not be the time to deal with ongoing and chronic problems of these sorts. But several months later, after mood symptoms have been under good control for a while, is a good time for some very serious stocktaking, and professional help is highly recommended.

By *stocktaking* I do not mean some process that can be described in a few paragraphs or distilled into the kinds of "helpful hints" and "dos and don'ts" lists that you might find in a magazine article. Rather, I mean *serious examination and fundamental change*. This may involve changing jobs or even careers, selling a house you can't afford or declaring bankruptcy instead of struggling with an austerity budget, postponing or reconsidering marriage (or divorce), not going back to school. Just as a person who has had a heart attack must do some serious investigation and hard thinking before taking a job as, say, a high-level manager of a big company, the bipolar patient needs to go through the same process before making big decisions. The stress and strain involved in whatever is being considered should be seriously weighed in the decision-making process.

But serious attention to the "big stuff" doesn't mean that the details of everyday life will just take care of themselves. *Structuring your life* is a key aspect of mood hygiene as well. In chapter 15 we reviewed the data and studies on the relationship between sleep and bipolar disorder. Remember that a properly synchronized sleep-wake cycle is important to the regulation of mood and that periods of sleep deprivation precipitate hypomanic and manic symptoms. *Establishing and sticking to a personal schedule* is crucial. This means establishing regular times for going to bed and getting up in the morning—seven days a week, if possible.

> **Mood Hygiene**
>
> - Establish *regular* sleep habits: retire to bed and get up at the same times *every day*.
>
> - Avoid sleep-disrupting habits: cut down on caffeine and avoid electronic tablets, smart phones, and other screens in the late evening.
>
> - Structure and schedule your days: make time for exercise—and relaxation.
>
> - Keep a *mood chart* or use a *mood app* on your smart phone. Search "mood" in your app store to find the one that suits you best.
>
> - Take stock of sources of stress in your life.
>   - Job problems? Relationship problems? Worries about stigma? Therapy, therapy, therapy!
>   - Don't procrastinate: it's a recipe for worry.

Research on sleep shows that many other lifestyle factors contribute to or detract from good sleep. Consider cutting caffeinated beverages out of your diet completely, or at least make a rule for yourself not to drink coffee, tea (including iced tea), or soft drinks containing caffeine after noon. Heavy meals late in the day should be avoided. Regular exercise has been shown to benefit sleep and has many other benefits as well; it helps to stabilize blood pressure, for example, most likely because of the cortisol-lowering effect that it provides. *Schedule* your daily walk and your Monday-Wednesday-Friday swim or visit to the gym. Don't exercise only when you "have the time" or "feel like it." Make it part of your regular schedule, not a luxury.

Don't allow yourself to procrastinate. Putting things off until the last moment invariably increases stress levels. Waiting until the eleventh hour to work on your income tax return and then staying up late tanked up on coffee, searching for receipts and W-2 forms, is not something people with bipolar disorder should let happen to themselves. It's no fun for anybody, but for the bipolar individual, it's downright dangerous. File your taxes early, renew your driver's license early, get your car inspected early—you get the idea. Eliminate procrastination as a way of dealing with things, and you've gone a long way toward eliminating a lot of stress. This advice holds true for putting off dealing with interpersonal problems, too. Smoldering tensions in a relationship; ongoing conflicts with a coworker, a neighbor, or a landlord—these are chronic stresses that will inevitably take their toll on *anyone's* mental health and can exact a higher price on the individual with a mood disorder. Don't put off dealing with these problems, and if you don't know how to approach them, get the professional help you need, whether that means consulting a counselor or a therapist or an attorney.

Alcohol? As I've already said, *the less, the better*.

As I explained in a previous chapter, the stress hormone cortisol has a direct injurious effect on neurons in the hippocampus, an area of the brain that is at the center of mood control. Psychological stress, sleep deprivation, lack of exercise, alcohol and drugs, and even an unhealthy diet are all environmental factors that have been shown to raise cortisol levels in the blood. Whatever you can do to keep cortisol levels down is going to make it easier for your medication to work to keep you well.

Some people find it helpful to keep a record of their moods, a *mood chart*. This can be a journal or diary if you're so inclined, but simpler and less time-consuming techniques can work just as well. If you need to keep an appointment calendar anyway, it's a simple matter to make a notation of your mood every day using a numerical scale. Clinicians commonly ask patients to rate their mood on a 1 to 10 scale, with 1 being the most depressed they've ever felt, 10 the best mood they've ever had, and 5 a normal, neutral, everyday mood. If 1 to 10 seems too confining, use a scale of 1 to 100. It's important to rate your mood at the same time every day to control for diurnal mood variations. Simply record your mood ratings every day by jotting down a number in your appointment book, recording it in your computer time-management program, or marking it on a calendar you keep on your bedside table. One of the first things I ask my patients to do when we're having trouble with persistent mood cycling is to keep a more detailed mood chart that also captures changes in their sleep pattern, menstrual cycle, levels of anxiety, and medication changes.

A quick internet search is all it takes to find any number of blank mood charts you can easily print out. You will also find several websites that allow you to set up an account and track your symptoms online, and mood-tracker apps for smart phones are available, too. Keeping this kind of record will provide you and your clinical team with invaluable information that can help show what medications are or are not working, determine whether there is a premenstrual or seasonal component to mood changes, and, of course, detect evolving depressive or hypomanic episodes early.

All of this is much easier said than done for persons with bipolar disorder. Regularizing your life in these ways may seem quite foreign and strange, not to mention boring. If throughout your life you've learned to wait for the good moods to get things done and just put off thinking about things during the inevitable return of the bad ones, such planning and regularity won't come easily. But a growing body of research supports the notion that external regulators like regular sleep and activity schedules help with mood stability.

BUILD YOUR SUPPORT SYSTEM

Everyone should have a team of supporters and well-wishers to help them get through difficult times. Persons with bipolar disorder are no exception. All the advice I've given you so far will be much easier to put into practice if you've got a team behind you.

The most important members of the team are likely to be your family and friends. A trusted family member or friend can be extremely helpful by acting as an objective observer of mood changes. One problem that persons with bipolar disorder all struggle with at one time or another is difficulty figuring out which mood changes are normal and which are not. I have seen patients go from one extreme to another in this regard. They may explain away severe and obviously pathological mood changes as "normal ups and downs" while they are in denial about the illness. Then they may overreact and worry that every low mood after a disappointment, every enthusiasm over a new project or relationship means that their medication isn't working. The physician and the therapist can help with this, of course, but someone who is concerned and caring and closer to home can be an invaluable ally in this regard. An astute friend or family member who knows how to communicate observations in a caring, nonprovocative way upon noticing sustained changes in mood is one of the best supports you can have. You may need to give the person you choose permission to be blunt with you. The best person for this task might not be someone who lives in the same house with you; that person may be too close to the situation to be objective. Look around you and choose carefully.

This topic leads to the question, to whom should you disclose your diagnosis? Two good rules are that the disclosure should be made only to those who *need to know* and only to those who *can help and want to help*. The "need to know" category includes, of course, the family doctor, all treating physicians, and any health professional who might be in a position to prescribe medication—even dentists, for example. If you have an attorney or accountant who handles your affairs on an ongoing basis, that person probably needs to know, too.

With employers, things get a bit trickier. If you are asked to disclose conditions you are being treated for as part of receiving medical insurance or other benefits, then you need to disclose your diagnosis. Failure to do so can result in benefits being denied at a later date and claims for reimbursement of treatment costs not being paid. Disclosure up front can avoid a lot of problems down the line, whether this means sharing facts about diagnosis with a new employer or with the current employer at the time of diagnosis. Letting an employer know that shift changes, frequent long business trips, and late hours are things you will not be able to take on because of a medical condition is not only a reasonable request but also a workplace right protected by the Americans with Disabilities Act. I routinely write letters for my patients who are nurses or others who work night shifts, requesting that they not be assigned shift work—and reminding them that the ADA requires them to provide "reasonable accommodations" to employees to keep them healthy. Your provider will be able to supply documentation to support such a request, too. Basing the employer-employee relationship on openness and honesty is always good policy. (The same is true for all other relationships, of course.)

Although employers are legally prohibited from discriminating against individuals with medical problems in hiring and firing decisions, they can make life difficult for employees they want to get rid of. "Choose your battles" would seem to be good advice here. If you sense hostility at your workplace toward persons receiving psychiatric treatment, you might be doing yourself a favor to look for a different employer rather than for an employment-law attorney.

As for peers and coworkers, the "helping" criterion would seem to be the applicable one, and careful consideration is necessary here. If you find that you're telling coworkers about your diagnosis to get sympathy, to get special consideration, or to get out of unpleasant assignments, you're headed for trouble. There's no better way to breed resentment and conflict on the job. You don't want to develop a reputation as one of those people who use some factor beyond their control to get coworkers to cover for them in various ways. That's not building a support system; it's manipulation, and it will make things worse, not better.

I cannot speak too highly of *support groups* for persons with mood disorders. Under the auspices of several national support organizations, hundreds of groups provide support to thousands of individuals with bipolar disorder. (See "Resources" at the end of this book for information on these organizations.) Support groups organized by and for individuals with mood disorders and their families not only provide peer support but also are sources of accurate information about the resources available in a particular community.

The Americans with Disabilities Act (ADA)

The initial Americans with Disabilities Act to prohibit discrimination on the basis of disability was introduced to Congress in 1988 and was signed into law by President George H. W. Bush on July 26, 1990. The ADA provides a wide range of protections for persons with physical and mental disabilities and includes protections for individuals with conditions that are episodic or currently in remission if the condition would be impairing if active. Obviously, by this definition, bipolar disorder is a disability.

The ADA specifies strict limitations on what employers can ask job applicants or employees about disabilities and in most cases prohibits requiring a prospective employee to undergo a medical examination or provide medical records as a condition of being hired. It specifies that all medical information be kept confidential and separate from other employee records.

An important protection for persons with bipolar disorder is the requirement that employers provide *reasonable accommodations* to employees with a disability, including accommodations in work assignments and scheduling changes. This last accommodation is the one that I frequently need to encourage my patients to take advantage of. You've read about how important it is for persons with bipolar disorder to avoid sleep deprivation and establish regular sleep habits. Night shifts, on-call nights, and swing shifts are risky for persons with bipolar disorder; don't hesitate or be embarrassed to ask your prescriber to write a letter asking for this accommodation for you from your employer.

If you request a reasonable accommodation and your employer refuses, he is breaking the law. If you believe your rights under the ADA are being violated, *do* call a lawyer!

I sometimes hear a patient say that he doesn't want to attend a support group because he "doesn't want to sit and listen to other people's problems." Certainly, sitting through an hour of whining is no fun and probably not helpful, but that's not what a support group should be (if the one you find yourself in is, think about looking for another group). A good support group brings together individuals who share a common problem and want to learn from each other about coping with it better. It's one thing to ask your doctor about the side effects of a medication that you're contemplating starting, but talking to someone who is actually taking it for the same problem you have provides a different and valuable perspective. Within a support group, you may have an opportunity to ask other persons with bipolar disorder how *they* told their boss or their children about their diagnosis, what *they* do to remember a complicated medication schedule, and a thousand other questions.

Another advantage of attending a support group is the reassurance you'll get when you meet other persons with bipolar disorder who are doing well and leading healthy, happy, and productive lives. Don't be surprised, however, if these folks seem to be in the minority in your group. It's not that doing well is a rare outcome, not at all. Rather, many persons simply "outgrow" support groups as they do better and better. You can think of these folks as having gotten what they needed from a support group and having moved on.

DON'T BE A "BIPOLAR VICTIM"

Individuals with any incurable but treatable medical problem must learn how to walk the fine line between not taking their illness seriously enough and taking it *too* seriously. We psychiatrists see the consequences of not taking bipolar disorder seriously enough every day in our offices and clinics—and, more often than not, in hospitals and emergency rooms. Individuals who stop taking medication, who won't get the treatment they need for a substance-abuse problem, who ignore ongoing environmental stresses and interpersonal problems until they are overwhelmed by them—these individuals are truly victims of bipolar disorder who abdicate to the whims and erratic rhythms of their illness rather than do what they can to control their symptoms. But there's another kind of victim as well: the person who worries about her symptoms and illness all the time, who avoids challenges and withdraws from work and the community into a world of medications, blood tests, doctor's visits, and support-group meetings. I think most people with bipolar disorder spend some time on both sides of this fine line as they sort out the impact of the illness on their view of themselves and figure out how to integrate what they need to do about the illness into their lifestyle. Neither extreme is healthy, and it takes time, good advice, and hard work to find the proper balance.

Perhaps the biggest obstacle to finding this balance is *stigma*. Sociologist Erving Goffman explained the grisly origins of that word in the introduction to his 1963 book on the subject, *Stigma: Notes on the Management of Spoiled Identity*: "The Greeks, who were apparently strong on visual aids, originated the term *stigma* to refer to bodily signs designed to expose something unusual and bad about the moral status of the signifier. The signs were cut or burnt into the body and advertised that the bearer was . . . a blemished person, ritually polluted, to be avoided, especially in public places." Goffman originally became interested in the issues of stigma, prejudice, and discrimination against physically handicapped individuals who had some immediately visible sign of being different: persons who were blind or disfigured or who had had a limb amputated. He soon came to realize, however, that the same issues were relevant, but became much more complicated, when there was no outward sign of the stigmatized condition, as in "the blemishes of individual character . . . mental disorder, imprisonment, addiction."[7]

Fortunately, psychiatric conditions such as bipolar disorder are not often considered "blemishes of individual character" anymore, but they are stigmatized just the same. Persons with psychiatric conditions are too often regarded as untreatable and thus unpredictable and dangerous, or at the least unreliable and incompetent. Too many films and television programs still ridicule or demonize individuals with psychiatric illnesses, and words like *crazy* and *insane* are generalized terms of contempt that you can hear in any schoolyard during recess. People with bipolar disorder have usually incorporated these prejudiced and negative views into their own way of thinking from a young age—a process psychologists refer to as the *internalization* of stigma. Therefore, when they are diagnosed with bipolar disorder, they have to deal not only with the prejudices and unfair biases others may have toward them but also with their *own* internalized negative ideas and feelings about persons with a psychiatric illness. People can react to this in opposite ways, either not accepting the diagnosis and remaining in denial about it, or giving in to their negative thinking and feelings and becoming "a bipolar" rather than "a person who has bipolar illness," telling everyone and anyone about their illness and using it as an excuse to avoid responsibilities and challenges. In either case, the individual has become a victim of the illness.

How can you avoid becoming a victim? You've taken a big step by reading this book. Accurate information about what bipolar disorder is and is not provides an excellent defense against prejudiced thinking and bad decisions based on misinformation. A close second to getting accurate information is getting the support, feedback, and advice—and the opportunity to ask questions and just vent your fears and frustrations—that counseling, therapy, and support groups provide. No one needs to confront this problem and sort through all the conflicting emotions and feelings alone—and no one should.

--------------- KEY TAKEAWAYS ---------------

▶ Your mental-health team will prescribe your treatment, but *you* are in charge of implementing it.

▶ Practice *mood hygiene*. Avoiding sleep deprivation is perhaps the most important component of these healthy habits.

▶ Know you rights under the Americans with Disabilities Act.

▶ Get the support you need to do the best job that you can in taking care of yourself. Join the Depression and Bipolar Support Alliance, NAMI, Mental Health America, or another of the organizations listed in the "Resources" section of this book—better yet, volunteer and be a "stigma buster"!

CHAPTER 23

Planning for Emergencies

The decisions we are forced to make in a crisis are frequently not the decisions we would have made under other circumstances. When an emergency arises for which we are unprepared, we usually have to improvise a response as we go along. In this chapter I identify several potential emergencies that may face the individual with bipolar disorder and his family and discuss how to prepare for and deal with them. One of the best ways to prepare for an emergency is to have a crisis plan ready beforehand.

Because we have such effective treatments available for bipolar disorder, we sometimes forget that it is a potentially lethal illness. And when you are dealing with a disease that can become life threatening, the last thing you want is an improvised response to an emergency situation.

People usually enjoy making plans—vacation plans, wedding plans, retirement plans. Planning for a psychiatric emergency is much less enjoyable but, unfortunately, much more important. Unlike vacation plans, these are plans that no one would be disappointed about not getting to use. But if you do need them, odds are you'll be very glad you made them.

I could sense the frustration in Lisa's voice as I listened to her speaking into the emergency room phone. She was a psychiatric nurse and we were both at the ER.

"I hear you, Mrs. Washington, but the magistrate won't approve a petition for involuntary treatment just because your husband isn't taking his medication. I need more information before we can—"

Suddenly she stopped and put the phone down. "I can't believe it; she hung up on me." Lisa looked down at her notepad, then turned to me. "Does the name Jesse Washington mean anything to you? That was his wife. She wanted someone to come out to their house and bring him in to the emergency room. She said he's very depressed."

"The name doesn't ring any bells with me," I replied. "Let's try the

computer to see if he's ever had any treatment here before. Then we can try calling her back." As Lisa stepped over to the emergency room's computer terminal, I glanced at my watch. "Lisa, I'm going to go grab some lunch. You know how to reach me."

Twenty minutes later, a text from Lisa arrived, a message to call the emergency room.

"Frank, this is Lisa. Mr. and Mrs. Washington are here in the ER. Well, that's not exactly true. Mrs. Washington is here, but Mr. Washington won't get out of the car. Do you think you could come down?"

I hadn't done any parking-lot therapy for a while, and as I walked past the Authorized Personnel Only Please sign that marked the door to the emergency department, I wondered who and what would be waiting for me. At the nursing station, I asked the secretary where the psychiatric nurse was. I had no sooner asked the question than Lisa walked in. "I went out and persuaded him to come in. They're in room 5. He's not doing too well; I think he'll need to be admitted. I'll call the unit and see if we have any beds."

"Has he been here before?" I asked.

"The last time he was here was about ten years ago, so he only has a paper chart and it's in off-site storage. We might get it in 48 hours, but . . ." She turned the computer screen so I could see it. "The only thing we have in the electronic record is that he was admitted to the mood-disorders unit for eleven days and the discharge diagnosis was bipolar disorder, manic episode."

"Well, that's some help. Let's go see them."

As soon as I opened the door to the interview room, I could see that (as usual) Lisa had sized up the situation pretty accurately. Mr. and Mrs. Washington looked to be in their early fifties. He was sitting in a corner, staring at the floor, and he looked as if he hadn't shaved in about a week. Mrs. Washington was sitting next to him but got up as I entered the room. "I practically had to carry him to get him into the car to come here," she said. "I've been desperate. He hasn't eaten anything in four days. We've only been married for a year, and I didn't realize—I mean, I didn't know how bad. . . . I called his psychiatrist's office, but they said she wasn't practicing anymore."

It took a while to get Mrs. Washington calmed down and even longer to get the whole story. Mr. Washington was obviously in the grip of serious depression and was barely able to talk, let alone give any kind of history of his problems.

Mrs. Washington showed me an empty bottle of lithium capsules with a "filled" date three months old and "no refills" clearly indicated. I recognized the name of the prescribing psychiatrist as a colleague who had retired about six months before. I knew for a fact that she had sent letters announcing her retirement almost a year before she quit her practice group.

I was getting the more recent history from the patient's wife when I heard a knock on the door. Lisa peeked in. "Dr. Mondimore, can I see you for a moment?"

"Excuse me," I said and stepped outside. Lisa was holding the "preferred-provider" and HMO list that was posted on the ER bulletin board. "His insurance doesn't cover him here. If he needs to be admitted, he'll have to go to Harris Memorial."

"Great," I grumbled. "He definitely needs to be in the hospital, but his wife had a terrible time getting him here. I don't think we should let her transport him. Can you have the secretary call the hospital transportation people?"

Lisa frowned. "Our transportation won't take patients to a hospital outside our system. We'll need to call an ambulance."

"That will cost these folks several hundred dollars. We can't use our people for a three-mile ride?" Lisa gave me her very best "I don't make the rules, I just follow them" look and said nothing. I took a deep breath and prepared to go tell the Washingtons that it would probably be several more hours before Jesse would be in the hospital.

Mr. Washington appeared to be operating under the assumption that his bipolar disorder had gone away for good (mistake number 1). So when the letter came from the office of his psychiatrist announcing her retirement, he put off making arrangements to establish care with a new one (mistake number 2). When the emergency came along, he had no treating physician familiar with his situation. He and his wife had obviously not had a very detailed discussion about bipolar disorder, about what she should do if symptoms flared up, leaving Jesse unable to make good decisions about treatment (mistake number 3). Mrs. Washington was not familiar with the law and the procedures in their community regarding involuntary commitment of persons with psychiatric illness (mistake number 4). And last but not least, the Washingtons were unfamiliar with the requirements of their medical insurance plan and went to a hospital where their insurance would not approve hospitalization (mistake number 5).

How long would it have taken to prevent all these mistakes? An hour or two? Maybe three? Obviously, this would have been time well spent. Let's review some of the things it is important to know about in planning for this type of emergency.

KNOW WHOM TO CALL FOR HELP

I've always thought that the people who can handle almost anything are those who know when they need help and whom to call for it. Persons with bipolar disorder owe it to themselves to be under the care of a psychiatrist who is familiar with their symptoms and the course of their illness. That means establishing yourself with a new physician when you move to a new community or if any other factor, such as the retirement of your psychiatrist, leaves you "uncovered." Changes in insurance plans sometimes force a change in psychiatrists. Don't put off making an appointment to get established as a new patient. Because administrative hassles and delays can prolong the time it takes for records to be transferred from one office to another, ask your providers for a copy of your records or a letter of introduction that you can take to your new doctor at the first appointment.

Don't hesitate to ask the psychiatrist how her practice is covered after hours. And how easy is it to get a routine office appointment? Are appointment slots set aside so that urgent appointments can be set up within a day or two? Every psychiatrist or mental-health clinic should have some means of seeing patients within twenty-four hours in cases of true emergency. One that does not is one to steer clear of.

Be sure you know how to contact the psychiatrist or his office at any time of the day or night and what arrangements are in place to handle emergencies. Does the psychiatrist see his own emergencies, or does everyone in the practice take emergency on-call duty on a rotating basis? The on-call system, though not ideal, is often the standard in a practice; it means that you may well not see your regular doctor in an acute emergency. Are you prepared for such an arrangement in order to be under the care of a psychiatrist who comes highly recommended?

What hospitals does your prescriber or her practice have a relationship with? Does she admit to the hospital you prefer? To the hospital where your insurance covers inpatient psychiatric treatment?

If the answers to these questions are not satisfactory, consider your options. Ask your family doctor, family members, friends, or members of your support group for recommendations. Call the local chapter of the National Mental Health Association, the Depression and Bipolar Support Alliance, or some other advocacy group for a referral. (These groups are listed in "Resources" at the end of this book.) Sometimes your options are limited by medical insurance coverage—which brings us to another important aspect of being prepared.

INSURANCE ISSUES

Be familiar with the details of your medical insurance coverage for psychiatric illness. Although the situation is changing, many plans treat psychiatric illnesses differently from nonpsychiatric illnesses. For example, they may have different and stricter limits on hospitalization coverage, the number of outpatient visits they will pay for, and the percentage or amounts that patients must pay out of pocket (copayments) for certain services. Do you have a lifetime cap on psychiatric services? There might be a limit on days of hospitalization or on the number of outpatient visits per year, or there might be a dollar-amount limit to coverage. Are you limited to certain hospitals or practice groups or covered at a lower rate if you don't go to certain hospitals or psychiatrists? If your insurance company denies coverage for a hospitalization or for several days of hospitalization, what are the procedures by which you can appeal the decision?

Remember that a visit to an emergency department is often also considered a hospital service when it comes to insurance coverage, and a visit to the ED of a hospital outside your network may cost thousands of dollars and not be covered at all.

Hospital stays of all types have become shorter, and psychiatric hospitalization is no exception. Hospitalization is now reserved almost exclusively for life-threatening emergencies, and patients are discharged as soon as possible. Patients are no longer hospitalized in a psychiatric unit or a psychiatric hospital for weeks or months. Does your psychiatrist have access to a psychiatric day program? These services go by several different names including *partial hospitalization* and *intensive outpatient treatment*, but they are all alternatives to traditional hospital treatment that provide hospital-like monitoring and treatment during the day but allow patients to return home in the evening to spend the night. It is a useful treatment option for bipolar disorder because it offers a way to provide daily monitoring of mood symptoms and treatment response without the disruption to personal and family life that staying in a hospital causes. Some insurers cover day programs—even insist on it—but others do not.

Nearly all insurers have some form of *utilization review* for their policyholders. Most contract this role to a *managed care organization* (MCO) that supervises or manages how much medical care you receive. The utilization review is accomplished in a variety of ways, some of which may be visible to you, some not. The main purpose is to minimize your use of the more expensive types of medical care, usually meaning hospitalization and treatment by specialists. In an HMO, you may have to be referred by a primary physician to any specialists—including psychiatrists—in order to be covered. Lab tests may be covered only if your primary physician approves them (this can make it inconvenient to get the blood tests needed to monitor therapy with lithium and some other psychiatric drugs). If you are admitted to a hospital, your doctor is likely be called every few days by someone from the MCO asking why you still need to be there. If the reviewer (usually a nurse) thinks you should be discharged, he will tell your doctor (and you) that coverage will be denied after a certain date and that you will be financially responsible for any additional inpatient treatment. (A variety of appeals procedures usually kick in at this point if your doctor disagrees.) Managed care, which was once usually limited to inpatient treatment, is now applied to outpatient treatment as well, and psychiatrists are being asked to fill out forms specifying a treatment plan and requesting a certain number of office visits.

If the insurance plan includes coverage for pharmacy charges, you may not have a choice of brands of medication but will need to take a generic equivalent instead of the exact medication your psychiatrist prescribes. Some plans cover only certain drugs in a broadly defined class of medications, thus limiting the doctor's prescribing options. Your insurance company may allow you to receive only thirty days of medication at a time or may impose such a limit unless you use a mail-order pharmacy. Your doctor may need to justify prescriptions and ask permission to prescribe a higher dose of a medication than usual or to use a medication off label to treat you. Taking your prescription to the pharmacy is often only the first step in getting your medication; if a *preauthorization* is needed, there will be a series of phone calls and faxes back and forth between the pharmacy, doctor's office, and benefits manager, a process that often takes several days. If some sort of appeals process is necessary, it can take weeks. All of this means that you should scrupulously avoid waiting until the last minute to call for a refill.

Even then, some medications simply will not be covered under any circumstances. I once wrote a letter to a pharmacy benefits manager for permission to prescribe a medication off label to treat a patient. I included a dozen or so research articles supporting the request. We were denied because there had been no "large placebo-controlled clinical trial" testing the particular situation that this patient was in. This was an impossibly high standard to set: if a particular clinical situation doesn't arise very often, no one will invest in a multimillion-dollar clinical trial to test it.

Managed-care methods save millions upon millions of health care dollars. Some people argue that as a result more people have access to better medical care because the system is more efficient and effective. Others argue that *managed care* is an oxymoron. But the fact is that managed-care methods are used in all types of insurance coverage now. Your type of medical insurance will almost certainly determine which hospital you can be admitted to, and it may determine which doctor you can see. Your insurance company will probably supervise the length of your hospitalizations and possibly control the number of office visits you can have, which medications can be prescribed for you, and likely what doses can be prescribed. Therefore, you should closely scrutinize all aspects of your insurance coverage for psychiatric illness, both your existing policy and any new policies that you may have to choose from because of life changes. Don't be beguiled

---

The Broken American Health Care System

I wrote this having just watched the 2020 Democratic candidates for the presidency debate one another on television. That evening, the debate was dominated by the candidates' differing ideas for and disagreements about the American health care system.

It's a sad fact that, as of this writing, Americans pay far more for health care than the citizens of any developed country, but for these many billions of dollars, they get less care and have worse outcomes. By any measure of health care quality,* from life expectancy (ranking #31, worse than Costa Rica and Slovenia), to infant mortality (#38), to deaths during childbirth (#46), the United States lags far behind countries like Japan, Great Britain, Canada, and Germany.

Why do we pay so much for so little?

One reason is that for a vast swath of the US population, access to health care is controlled by for-profit companies. The 2014 compensation package for the CEO of UnitedHealth Group, one of the largest health insurers in the country, was more than $66 million. The company's profit 2017 was $163 billion—that is more than one hundred times the total budget of the National Institute of Mental Health. You read that correctly. In 2017, $163 billion was siphoned out of the American health care system and put in the pockets of shareholders; diverting just 1 percent of those profits could operate dozens of free mental health clinics or double the amount of research NIMH could fund.

Be aware, stay informed, and vote like your life depends on it—because it does.

*World Bank data, 2015, datacatalog.worldbank.org.

by the smiling faces on glossy brochures from insurance companies when it comes to picking a plan. Ask colleagues and coworkers and persons in your support group about their experiences with different plans and companies. Don't put yourself in the position of getting an emergency room surprise.

SAFETY ISSUES AND HOSPITALIZATION

The most dangerous emergency situation for persons with bipolar disorder, and one that frequently leads to hospitalization, is the development of suicidal thoughts and behaviors. In studies from the 1940s, suicide rates of 30 and even 60 percent were reported in groups of bipolar patients. Thankfully, the availability of modern treatments for bipolar disorder has greatly changed these grim numbers. Nevertheless, the rate of suicide deaths in persons with bipolar disorder has been estimated to be at least fifteen times higher than that seen in the general population.[1] It may seem obvious to say that the most effective way of minimizing the risk of suicide in bipolar disorder is relapse prevention. But if I had said "*relapse* prevention is *suicide* prevention" in the previous chapter, you might have thought I was just being dramatic. Do not *ever* lose sight of the fact that bipolar disorder is a potentially fatal disease: relapse prevention *is* suicide prevention.

Individuals with bipolar disorder should not have firearms in the home. There are numerous scientific studies showing that this increases the chances of a violent death occurring in that home, either by suicide or by homicide.[2] Where an illness whose symptoms can include suicidal depression and heightened irritability with loss of inhibitions is concerned, there is never, *ever*, any justification whatsoever for having a firearm of any type in the home. Period.

The emergence of self-destructive thoughts and impulses is frightening both to the patient and to those around her. The tremendous stigma and disgrace that have been associated with suicide for centuries still make people reluctant to discuss these thoughts when they occur. That context and notions such as "only crazy people kill themselves" complicate what is really a much simpler clinical issue: suicidal thinking is a serious symptom of this illness, which must be evaluated quickly by a professional and managed swiftly and effectively. Patients can be intensely ashamed of suicidal thoughts and believe that the development of self-destructive impulses is a kind of failure. Of course it is not a failing in any way; it is a symptom of an illness. It is important to understand the development of suicidal feelings in a bipolar patient as a dangerous symptom of serious illness, as dangerous as the onset of chest pains in a heart patient. When they occur, it's not a time to wonder about what they mean. *It's time to call for help.* And like chest pains in a heart patient, suicidal feelings in a mood-disorder patient are often a reason for hospitalization.

Psychiatric hospitalization can be experienced as a terrible failure. Again, the clinical perspective tells us otherwise. Although we have become much better at treating bipolar disorder, our treatment methods are by no means perfect. Sometimes, despite everyone's best efforts, relapses occur and serious symptoms like suicidal feelings emerge and require hospitalization. Such an occurrence is not time for self-blame or questions like "What did I do wrong?" Rather, it's time for healing.

Remember that the word we often used in the past for psychiatric hospitals was *asylum*, a term defined as "a place offering protection and safety."[3] Individuals whose will has been temporarily seized by this terrible illness and who are on the verge of terrible and desperate action deserve a place of protection and safety. No apologies are *ever* necessary, no reproach ever justified.

One more reminder: bipolar disorder can raise issues of personal safety. These issues need to be anticipated, discussed, planned for, and promptly addressed if and when they arise. Because family members are often a crucial part of dealing with these emergencies, I'll discuss their role further in the next chapter.

KEY TAKEAWAYS

▶ Have an emergency plan. Decisions made in crisis mode are usually not the best ones.

▶ Thoroughly research insurance plans before signing up.

▶ Consider executing a mental-health power of attorney.

▶ Do *NOT* have firearms in the home.

CHAPTER 24

The Role of the Family

The challenges of living with bipolar disorder are not limited to those who have the disease. Family and friends face these challenges as well. It's intensely painful to see a loved one suffer from the desperate bleakness of major depression, and just as painful and frightening to see him in the frenzied grip of mania. As in any illness, the role of the family includes support, understanding, and encouragement of the person who is ill. The first step in being able to provide this kind of support is understanding some important facts about the illness.

RECOGNIZING SYMPTOMS

Never forget that the person with bipolar disorder does not have control of her mood state. Those of us who do not suffer from a mood disorder sometimes expect mood-disorder patients to be able to exert the same control over their emotions and behavior that we ourselves are able to. When we sense that we are letting our emotions get the better of us and want to subdue them, we tell ourselves things like "Snap out of it," "Get hold of yourself," "Try to pull yourself out of it." We are taught that self-control is a sign of maturity and self-discipline. We are indoctrinated to think of people who don't control their emotions very well as being immature, lazy, self-indulgent, or foolish. But you can only exert self-control if the control mechanisms are working properly, and in people with mood disorders, they are not.

People with mood disorders cannot "snap out of it," much as they would like to (and it's important to remember that they want *desperately* to be able to). Telling a depressed person things like "Pull yourself out of it" is cruel and may reinforce the feelings of worthlessness, guilt, and failure already present as symptoms of the illness. Telling a manic person, "Slow down and get hold of yourself" is simply wishful thinking; that person is like a tractor trailer careening down a mountain highway with no brakes.

So the first challenge facing family and friends is to change the way they look at behaviors that might be symptoms of the illness—behaviors like not wanting to get out of bed, being irritable and short tempered, being "hyper" and reckless or overly critical and pessimistic. Our first reaction to these sorts of behaviors and attitudes is to regard them as laziness, meanness, or immaturity and to be critical of them. In a person with bipolar disorder, criticism almost always makes things worse: it reinforces the depressed patient's feelings of worthlessness and failure, and it alienates and angers the hypomanic or manic patient.

This is a hard lesson to learn. Don't always take behaviors and statements at face value. Learn to ask yourself, "Could this be a symptom?" before you react. Little children frequently say "I hate you" when they are angry at their parents, but good parents know that it's just the anger of the moment talking; this is not the child's true feeling. Manic patients will say "I hate you" too, and it's the illness talking, an illness that has hijacked the patient's emotions. The depressed patient will say, "It's hopeless; I don't want your help." Again, it's the illness and not your loved one rejecting your concern.

I'm now going to make things really difficult by warning against the other extreme: interpreting *every* strong emotion in a person with a mood disorder as a symptom. This other extreme is just as important to guard against. I have seen many couples in which one partner has a bipolar disorder and the healthy partner wields the diagnosis as a weapon to emotionally subdue the other. (Come to think of it, that doesn't sound very "healthy," does it?)

"Vicky's medication needs an adjustment. I'm sure of it."

Vicky stared down at the floor angrily as Peter went on. "She won't give up on this crazy idea about going back to college." I winced a little at Peter's use of the word crazy, *a word that can make a person with a psychiatric illness feel like they've just been slapped in the face. I made a mental note to bring it to his attention later, but to do so now might make it look as if I was "taking sides."*

"Peter," I said, "I'd like to hear from Vicky about this. She's been doing well for over two years now; I think it may be time to have a serious discussion about her idea."

Vicky looked up. "I was six months away from graduating from Bryn Mawr when I got sick the first time. I've called State, St. James College, and Everett, and I could get my degree with only a year of study at any of them."

Vicky was in her midthirties, an intense, vibrant woman who I suspected was probably brilliant as well. Peter had been transferred to town by his company a month after Vicky had gotten out of the hospital following a nearly lethal suicide attempt. It had taken three hospitalizations for her to be properly diagnosed as having bipolar disorder—after nearly ten years of roller-coaster moods. She had been treated for a depressive disorder, for a personality disorder, even for schizophrenia before she started on valproate and had a big turnaround. She had done so well, in fact, that I had seen her only half a dozen times over the past two years. About half the time her husband came along to her appointments. Every couple of months I noticed a book review she had written in the local newspaper, and on one visit she mentioned working on a biography of Mary Todd Lincoln. Going back to college seemed well within her capabilities.

Peter sighed, then went on. "It makes me really nervous to see her up late at night looking at college entrance requirements over the internet. And we've gotten dozens of college catalogs through the mail that she's called or written for. I'm afraid she's getting manic, and I just can't go through that again."

Vicky's eyes flashed, and she drew in her breath, then slowly released it. "Peter's not used to me being this confident and energized about anything. We've only been married for four years, and for nearly two of those I was more or less depressed. This is me, not mania." Her voice became just the slightest bit louder. "But he's treating me like a child, an incompetent." She looked over at her husband. "A lunatic, right? I'm finally getting back to my *goals and career after ten years, and what did you call it? 'Crazy'?"*

Now it was Peter's turn to look angry. "You see, Doctor? Do you see what I mean, how angry she gets? She's not usually like this. Before we came here today, she—"

"Oh, God, stop it." Vicky said quietly, through clenched teeth. Tears were flowing now.

"OK, you two, let's cool down for a moment," I said. I could sense that this was a continuation of a power struggle between Peter and Vicky that had probably been going on for weeks, maybe even months. But I also had the sense that Vicky was assessing herself accurately and that Peter was overreacting. Vicky was not being carried away by her feelings—not at the moment, at least; if anything, she was showing a lot of restraint. Peter was *treating her like a child.*

"Vicky," I said, "perhaps Peter doesn't understand your reasons for wanting to go back to college."

"I admit it might seem like a waste of time," she said. "But that degree means a lot to me. I was devastated when I had to withdraw from college.

I felt like a complete failure. Maybe I just need to prove to myself that I can do it. That I'm not . . ." She hesitated before spitting it out: "Not crazy."

Peter was calmer, too. "It's not that we can't afford it," he said. "I just worry that it will be too much for her, that she'll get sick again. And she gets so angry when we talk about it; she seems obsessed with this idea. That's not normal, is it?"

"I don't think trying to decide how much obsessiveness is normal or abnormal is going to help us here, Peter," I said. "It seems to me that the problem is that Vicky is investing a lot of time and emotional energy in a project that you don't think is worthwhile."

"That's right," Peter said decisively.

"But I think it's worthwhile," Vicky said. "Just because I have a psychiatric illness doesn't invalidate me as a person. It doesn't mean I need someone to make all my decisions for me."

"Honey, I'm just trying to help you, to protect you—"

Vicky snapped back, "I don't want to be protected, I want to have a real life."

"Wait a minute, wait a minute," I said. "I think we were getting somewhere. Let's go back to Vicky's reasons for wanting to go back to school."

This struggle between Peter and Vicky illustrates a common problem that can come up in families in which an individual has been diagnosed with a bipolar illness. It's possible to jump to the conclusion that everything the ill person does that might be foolish or risky is a symptom of illness, even to the point of hauling the person into the psychiatrist's office for a "medication adjustment" every time he disagrees with his spouse, partner, or parents. As with Peter and Vicky, a vicious cycle can take over: some bold idea or enthusiasm, or even plain old foolishness or stubbornness, is labeled as "getting manic," and feelings of anger and resentment are stirred up in the person with the diagnosis. When these angry feelings are expressed, they seem to confirm the family's suspicion that the person is "getting sick again," so more criticism ensues, followed by more anger, and so on. "He's getting sick again" sometimes becomes a self-fulfilling prophecy: so much anger and emotional stress are generated that a relapse *does* occur, because the person with the illness stops taking the medication that controls his symptoms out of frustration and anger and shame: "Why bother staying well, if I'm *always* treated as if I were sick?"

So how does one walk this fine line between not taking every feeling and behavior at face value in a person with bipolar disorder, on the one hand,

and not invalidating real feelings by calling them symptoms, on the other? I think communication is the key: honest and open communication. Ask the person with the illness about her moods; make observations about behaviors; express concerns in a caring, supportive way. Go along with your family member to doctors' appointments, and share your observations and concerns during the visit in the family member's presence. Above all, do not call the therapist or psychiatrist and say, "I don't want my [husband, wife, son, daughter] to know that I called you, but I think it's important to tell you that . . ." There's nothing more infuriating or demeaning than to have someone reporting on you behind your back.

But it's also possible to err on the side of not being involved enough in treatment for fear of being a "tattletale," assuming that the clinicians will notice the same things you've noticed about changes in moods or behaviors. One of the most valuable ways a family member can help is to provide a clear, undistorted view of the situation to the clinical team treating the illness. In my experience, family members are frequently the first to pick up on subtle changes in behaviors and attitudes that signal the beginning of a relapse. I don't know how many times I have seen patients in the clinic or even in the emergency room who reassured me that they were feeling fine; their behavior and mood seemed normal, so I sent them on their way with a note in the chart that they were doing well. Then I received a panicked phone call from a spouse or other relative a few hours later: "Didn't he tell you that he's lost ten pounds?" ". . . that she hasn't slept in three nights?" ". . . that he got fired from his job?" Contrary to popular belief, psychiatrists cannot read minds! Become involved with treatment, and communicate your concerns openly, sincerely, and supportively—almost anything that might otherwise seem intrusive can be forgiven.

Remember that your goal is to have your family member trust you when she feels most vulnerable and fragile. She is already dealing with feelings of deep shame, failure, and loss of control related to having a psychiatric illness. Be supportive, and yes, be constructively critical when criticism is warranted. But above all, be open, honest, and sincere.

INVOLUNTARY TREATMENT AND OTHER LEGAL ISSUES

In every community there are laws and procedures to safeguard individuals who are unable to care for themselves. Laws that allow the removal of children from the care of parents who are abusing them are the most obvious example. Another set of laws allows individuals to be treated for psychiatric illnesses against their will in certain circumstances. One of the most difficult things a person might be called on to do for a family member with bipolar disorder is to initiate involuntary treatment or commitment. But given the power of this illness (especially bipolar I) to cloud judgment and create dangerous situations, there is sometimes no choice but to force the treatment issue in this way. It is always a last resort, but it can literally be lifesaving.

Commitment laws are usually state laws and so vary from one state to another; in addition to these state-by-state variations, local procedures can vary from community to community. Therefore, I can't provide a step-by-step procedure here, only general principles. But in my experience, it's not the procedures that confuse people; it's the general principles, so I think a brief discussion is worthwhile.

Laws and legal procedures governing the provision of psychiatric treatment—or any kind of medical treatment, for that matter—against a person's stated wishes are based on the knowledge that an individual whose judgment is clouded by the symptoms of an illness often does not make the same decisions about treatment that he would make otherwise. The delirious motor-vehicle-accident victim who has suffered massive blood loss may moan, "I want to go home," as she loses consciousness on the stretcher, but the ER team will ignore such a statement and proceed to do what they have to do to save the person's life. It is presumed that if the person were alert and thinking clearly and understood the implications of "going home," she would not make such a request. Similar principles underlie psychiatric commitment laws: treatment is given to persons against their will if clouded judgment prevents them from making good decisions about their treatment. Depressed individuals may be so hopeless that they believe treatment has no chance of helping. Thinking processes in mania can be so disorganized and scattered that seeking out and cooperating with treatment is not possible. In either case there are mechanisms to get needed treatment for persons whose psychiatric symptoms blind them to the need for it.

Fortunately, these laws also have safeguards built in to prevent confinement in a psychiatric hospital for the wrong reasons. Decades ago it was easy to invoke commitment law; it often required only the signature of a relative or family physician to hospitalize a person for weeks or months—even years. People were hospitalized for all kinds of bogus reasons, and serious abuses of individual rights occurred. Laws became much stricter in the 1960s and 1970s to prevent such abuses. The main change was the addition of *dangerousness* as a commitment criterion. Unless an individual's behavior endangers himself—usually meaning suicidal behavior—or others, the person cannot be committed for involuntary psychiatric treatment.

Requests or petitions for involuntary commitment do not necessarily mean that the person who is alleged to be psychiatrically ill will be hospitalized. Friends and relatives cannot admit a patient to a hospital; only a doctor can. The family's request for involuntary commitment usually will allow the patient to be transported to an emergency room, where a physician will make a decision about hospitalization. The patient may be released if she does not meet legal criteria.

Involuntary commitment is a legal procedure in which an individual is confined against his will and temporarily loses some rights of self-determination. For this reason, the law and the courts take involuntary psychiatric treatment seriously, and many safeguards against abuses are built into the procedures. The person requesting the involuntary commitment must usually appear in person at the local courthouse or police station to give information and, in some jurisdictions, make a sworn statement before a judge or magistrate. Family or friends will be asked for specific and detailed information about the behaviors they have observed. This is often frustrating for those trying to get help for their loved one. They may think that it's uncaring for them to be asked such a lot of questions or that their judgment or motives are being questioned. It's important to remember that in the days when individuals could be confined to psychiatric hospitals simply because a relative or doctor "thought it was best" for them, there were significant abuses of civil rights. When there is serious attention on the part of the issuing magistrate or judge to documenting the facts and questioning the need for involuntary treatment, it means that the system is working.

There is a judicial review (a "commitment hearing") at some point (usually a few days after admission to a hospital), wherein a judge or hearing officer determines whether the commitment procedure was done properly and legally. Although this is a legal proceeding, it is not a big courtroom scene. Usually a conference room in the hospital is used, only a few people are present, and the proceedings are kept confidential (they are not a matter of public record). The patient is allowed legal representation; in fact, an attorney will be appointed to represent the patient if she cannot afford to hire one.

Involuntary commitment for psychiatric treatment does not usually affect a person's other legal rights. Wills or other legal instruments he has executed are not invalidated, and patients do not become legally "incompetent" in other areas. Hospitalization and treatment are the only issues that are addressed in commitment hearings.

Occasionally individuals with severe, poorly controlled bipolar disorder and their families make legal arrangements to safeguard the individuals' financial assets in case another severe episode of the illness comes upon them. This can involve actually having a legally appointed guardian who might control access to bank accounts, prevent the sale of property or other assets, and so forth. Although rarely necessary, this is a valuable option that can go a long way toward preventing financial ruin caused by manic spending sprees. A document called a *power of attorney* can convey certain specific responsibilities and powers—and not others—and does not constitute guardianship. Careful consideration and consultation with an attorney are, of course, necessary so that legally binding documents with safeguards appropriate to the situation can be drafted.

I am aware that the topic of this section of the chapter is a frightening one, especially to persons with bipolar disorder, to whom it might seem that liberty and the right of self-determination can be taken away all too easily. At the risk of sounding glib, however, I want to reassure you that involuntary commitment of an individual is *not* a quick and easy procedure. On the contrary, in my experience most people are surprised at how difficult it is to invoke these laws, how many safeguards are built into the procedures, and how seriously the strict interpretation of the laws is taken by everyone involved. The laws covering involuntary commitment have been carefully written in the interest of helping, not simply confining, people with severe psychiatric illnesses. In my experience they are effective at doing just that.

MORE ON SAFETY

Never forget that bipolar disorder can occasionally precipitate truly dangerous behavior. Kay Jamison wrote of the "dark, fierce and damaging energy" of mania and the even darker specter of suicidal violence that haunts those with serious depression.[1] Violence is often a difficult subject to deal with because the idea is deeply embedded in us from an early age that violence is primitive and uncivilized and represents a kind of failure or breakdown in character. Of course we recognize that the person in the grip of psychiatric illness is not violent because of some personal failing, and perhaps because of this there is sometimes a hesitation to admit the need for a proper response to a situation that is getting out of control: when there is some threat of violence, toward either self or others.

I've already talked a bit about suicidal thinking, and it bears repeating that people with bipolar disorder are at much higher risk for suicidal behavior than is the general population. Although family members cannot and should not be expected to take the place of psychiatric professionals in evaluating suicide risk, it is important to have some familiarity with the issue. Again, patients who are starting to have suicidal thoughts are often intensely ashamed of them. They will often hint about "feeling desperate," about "not being able to go on," but they may not verbalize actual self-destructive thoughts. It's important not to ignore these statements but rather to clarify them. Don't be afraid to ask, "Are you having thoughts of hurting yourself?" People are usually relieved to be able to talk about these feelings and get them out into the open where they can be dealt with. But they may need permission and support to do so.

Remember that the period of recovery from a depressive episode can be a time of especially high risk for suicidal behavior. People who have been immobilized by depression sometimes develop a higher risk for hurting themselves as they begin to get better and their energy level and ability to act improve. Patients having mixed symptoms—depressed mood and agitated, restless, hyperactive behavior—may also be at higher risk for self-harm. In fact, there is some evidence that mixed or dysphoric mania is the most dangerous mood state in this regard.[2]

Another factor that increases the risk of suicide is substance abuse, especially alcohol abuse. Alcohol not only worsens a person's mood, but it lowers inhibitions. People will do things when they are drunk that they wouldn't do otherwise. Increased use of alcohol increases the risk of suicidal behaviors and is definitely a worrisome development that needs to be confronted and acted upon.

The development of serious suicidal risk calls for action. Have an emergency plan, and be prepared to use it. Don't hesitate to invoke involuntary commitment procedures if you are really worried and the patient is disputing the need for evaluation.

A less frequent but nevertheless real risk of violence is the violence toward others that can occur in mania. Friends and family members should not hesitate to call for help if they feel imminently threatened.

Many communities have teams of mental-health professionals who have specialized training in de-escalating persons with psychiatric problems who have become agitated. In some communities, these crisis intervention teams are part of the local police department and the team consists of specially trained police officers who are accompanied by a clinical social worker or other mental-health professional.

In 1992, the police department of the City of Houston established an entire division specializing in mental-health issues. Houston trains not only patrol officers but also 911 dispatchers and jail personnel to recognize and appropriately respond to situations involving persons with mental illness.

In an ideal world, a 911 call for help with an imminently violent person with bipolar disorder would result in a rapid response from a team of various professionals accustomed to dealing with psychiatrically ill individuals, trained in crisis intervention and safe physical restraint techniques, and familiar with psychiatric emergency services in the community who can transport the patient quickly and safely to the appropriate health care facility so that she can receive proper treatment. Unfortunately, we do not live in an ideal world and many communities do not provide this level of services. Tragedies have resulted when inadequately trained police officers overreacted in confrontations with aggressively agitated psychiatric patients. Such tragedies highlight the importance of being familiar with the full range of available emergency services in your community and developing emergency plans with your or your loved one's treatment team.

GETTING SUPPORT

It's important for family members to recognize their own need for support, encouragement, and understanding in dealing with this illness. Mental-health professionals go home every day and leave their work of dealing with psychiatric illnesses behind, an option that family members often do not have. It can be exhausting to live with a hypomanic person and frustrating to deal with a seriously depressed person day after day. The changes and unpredictability of the moods of someone with bipolar disorder intrude into home life and can be the source of severe stress in relationships, straining them to the breaking point.

Perhaps the most difficult challenge is that posed by a family member with bipolar disorder who is resistant to obtaining treatment. The most astonishing learning experience that medical students and interns have is with their first patient who repeatedly refuses to continue with a treatment that will keep him well and out of the hospital. I remember as a resident reading the chart of a bipolar patient who had been admitted to the hospital dozens of times after stopping lithium. "Why on earth," I wondered, "would a person make such a foolish decision again and again?" I remember thinking that taking three capsules of lithium a day seemed a trivial inconvenience compared with spending what added up to several years of this patient's life in a psychiatric hospital. I've since learned that making

The Depression and Bipolar Support Alliance

www.dbsalliance.org

Mission Statement: "DBSA provides hope, help, support, and education to improve the lives of people who have mood disorders."

The DBSA has extensive online resources for patients and families and sponsors nearly six hundred support groups throughout the country and abroad. Online support groups are available as well.

peace with the illness and with the idea of staying in treatment is much more difficult than healthy people realize (see chapter 20). But the harder lesson is that there is no way anyone can *force* a person to take responsibility for her treatment. Unless the patient makes the commitment to do so, no amount of love and support, sympathy and understanding, cajoling or even threatening can make someone take this step. Even family members who understand this at some level may feel guilty, inadequate, and angry at times dealing with this situation. These are completely normal feelings. Family members should not be ashamed of experiencing frustration and anger but rather get help with these emotions.

Even when the patient does take responsibility and is trying to stay well, relapses can occur. Family members might then wonder what *they* did wrong. Did I put too much pressure on him? Could I have been more supportive? Why didn't I notice the symptoms coming on sooner and get her to the doctor? A hundred questions, a thousand *if onlys*, another round of guilt, frustration, and anger.

On the other side of this issue is another set of questions: How much understanding and support for the bipolar person might be too much? What is protective, and what is overprotective? Should you call your loved one's boss with excuses regarding why he isn't at work? Should you pay off credit card debts from hypomanic spending sprees caused by dropping out of treatment? What actions constitute helping a sick person, and what actions are helping a person to be sick? These are thorny, complex questions that have no easy answers.

For all these reasons, it's vital that family members go along with the patient to support groups—and go to support groups themselves even if the patient will not go—and consider getting counseling or therapy for themselves to deal with the stresses caused by this illness. Comprehensive programs for the treatment of persons with bipolar disorder are increasingly emphasizing family involvement.

Like many other chronic illnesses, bipolar disorder afflicts one but affects many in the family. It's important that *all* those affected get the help, support, and encouragement they need.

———————————— KEY TAKEAWAYS ————————————

▶ Family members should familiarize themselves with the signs of a developing mood episode. That being said, persons with bipolar disorder are allowed to have normal feelings.

▶ Become familiar with involuntary treatment procedures and community resources in your area and have an emergency plan at the ready, especially if the diagnosis is bipolar I disorder and there is a history of suicidal behaviors.

▶ Family members need support, too!

PART VI

Summing Up and Looking Ahead

A short final chapter looks into the future at some of the exciting possibilities that we hope will help us to better understand bipolar disorder, to better diagnose and treat it, and, yes, perhaps one day to *cure* this illness.

CHAPTER 25

Putting It All Together and Looking to the Future

We are making enormous progress in the field of psychiatry. The diagnosis of bipolar disorder and other psychiatric illnesses is becoming more accurate all the time. The available treatments for these illnesses are more effective, and there are more of them. But these advances have come about largely through trial and error, not through a better scientific understanding of the causes of the diseases. This situation is changing, however. Thousands of scientists in two different disciplines are conducting research that will eventually lead to a fuller understanding of psychiatric illnesses and to new and more effective treatment approaches.

The first of these is the field of *neuroscience*, the study of the biology and chemistry of the brain and nervous system. At the beginning of the twentieth century, the physical and psychiatric examination of patients with brain disorders and the microscopic study of brain tissue obtained from them after death were the only available methods to investigate the diseases of the brain. Animal experiments complemented these studies, but this work resulted in only the vaguest outline of the organization of brain function. The location of brain areas important for speech, movement, vision, and so forth were discovered, but psychiatric illnesses remained so mysterious that ideas having nothing to do with biology, theories such as psychoanalysis, were the only ones that seemed to offer any hope of understanding these problems.

By the end of the century, however, breakthrough followed upon breakthrough, mostly in the field of the chemistry of brain functioning, as neurotransmitters were discovered, more powerful electron microscopes allowed the visualization of synapses and other cellular structures, and sophisticated chemical probes allowed scientists to work out the mechanisms by which neurons grow and communicate with each other. Understanding continues to accumulate concerning the fine details of how neurons develop and link to and communicate with each other through complex networks, and how brain cells and their networks adapt and change in the living organism in response to experience.

Now, new technologies for brain imaging permit scientists to see the brain at work in living persons for the first time. These imaging techniques can trace changes in blood flow within the brain, locate areas that are hyper- or hypoactive, and detect abnormally high or low levels of brain chemicals such as serotonin and dopamine. This information is revealing how the interplay of activity between different brain areas is important in the regulation of mood, and it is making it possible to identify the responsible circuitry. With these new techniques, we can see how the brain of a person with a mood disorder functions differently from that of a person who does not have the disorder. Perhaps an even greater benefit will result because we can see the changes that occur in the brain when a person receives treatment and is beginning to feel well again. Transcranial magnetic stimulation and deep brain stimulation for the treatment of mood disorders came about because of advances in neuroscience. One can argue that these new brain-stimulation techniques are a direct result of neuroscience research; they represent the very first psychiatric treatments that were developed based on science and research rather than stumbled upon accidentally.

The second of these innovative scientific disciplines is the field of *genetics*. Here again, it is the development of new biochemical methods and molecular probes that has made this new research possible. With the announcement that the Human Genome Project had mapped all of the genetic material in the human chromosomes, a new era in the understanding of genetics began. The discovery of new genes is announced every day, and it is only a matter of time before the genetic mechanisms of mood disorders are unraveled. But this is only one of the goals of work in this field. Just as important is understanding the epigenetic mechanisms by which genes turn on and off and other mechanisms that regulate the expression and work of the instructions encoded in the DNA molecule.

The first genetic approach to pay off in changing treatment is likely to be *pharmacogenomics*, the field within genetics that investigates genetic factors associated with responses to particular pharmaceuticals rather than with risk of disease. The promise of pharmacogenomics is that therapeutic agents can be rationally selected based on a person's genetic profile rather than the trial-and-error process patients must now endure. In the not-too-distant future, a blood test will show whether lithium or valproate or lamotrigine or some as yet undiscovered drug will be the best treatment for a particular individual with bipolar disorder. A blood test may be able to identify the bipolar patients who can safely take an antidepressant.

As the genetic basis of mood disorders is discovered, it may turn out that our classification system for them is all wrong and a whole new diagnostic system will be needed for psychiatric illnesses, perhaps one based on the genes that are involved in individual patients. Instead of "bipolar disorder II," we may be diagnosing patients with something like "DISC I disorder," a diagnostic label derived from the name of a gene.[1]

The two fields of neuroscience and psychiatric genetics are closing in on the causes and mechanisms of mood disorders from different directions. As these two enterprises advance, they will begin to inform each other—that is, advances in one field will lead to advances in the other. The discovery that a gene for a particular protein is linked to a mood disorder will tell neuroscientists that that protein is important in the regulation of mood. The discovery of an enzyme in neurons that is important in neuroplasticity, the process of neuronal retuning that appears to go awry in mood disorders, will tell geneticists to focus on the gene for that enzyme in their association studies. Little by little, the whole picture will become increasingly clear.

Skin cells from a simple biopsy can be transformed into stem cells or even neurons that can be cultured in the laboratory and tested for responses to particular drugs. It will be a while yet before this technique is widely available for individual patients, but when it is, it will represent the ultimate in personalized medicine and take much of the guesswork out of treatment.

As our understanding of the biology of mood disorders improves, we get closer to better diagnostic methods and safer and more effective treatments. The number of new medications continues to grow, and many more new pharmaceuticals are "in the pipeline," some of them based on clues about the biological causes of these illnesses. The era of finding new medications essentially by accident is coming to a close; researchers are already designing treatments more effectively and more rationally. More sophisticated use of nonpharmaceutical treatments such as transcranial magnetic stimulation may make it possible to use lower doses of medications or may help medications work more quickly.

As we take the step from isolating genes to determining the function of those genes, there is the possibility of *gene therapy*: repairing the code in the DNA that causes mood disorders. The obstacles to be overcome before we can look for this type of cure can only be called monumental, even daunting. Stem-cell infusions are being used to treat a variety of neurological illnesses. As scientists are learn more and more about the neurological basis of bipolar disorder, a cure might be possible.

As the mechanisms of illness development become known and the genetic vulnerabilities are identified, another exciting possibility emerges: *prevention*. Genetic data and a better understanding of what triggers the illness may allow the development of programs aimed at preventing the development of illness in individuals known to be at higher risk for a particular disorder.

So, there is much reason to expect great strides in our ability to diagnose and effectively treat bipolar disorder. But we have *already* made great strides—individuals with bipolar disorder must not let denial or fear stand in the way of taking advantage of the excellent treatments that are now available. Ignorance is no excuse, either. Support organizations provide up-to-date information about bipolar disorder through newsletters, brochures, websites, and most importantly, in the support groups they sponsor (see the list of resources that follows this chapter). With the ever-growing online resources now available, anyone with access to a computer can, with the click of a mouse, get the very latest information on new pharmaceuticals and other treatments.

Like many other serious illnesses, bipolar disorder can be life threatening. Unlike some other potentially lethal conditions, however, it has a unique capacity to rob individuals of their spirit, to take over their humanity. And yet some of its sufferers have taken inspiration from their struggle with this illness to produce music and art and literature that have inspired and exhilarated the world.

People with bipolar disorder frequently ask me, "Will I have to take medication for the rest of my life?" I always tell them that no one knows the answer to that question because no one knows exactly what the treatment of mood disorders might be in the future. Pediatricians practicing in the 1930s probably could not have imagined that vaccines would one day practically eliminate diphtheria, polio, measles, and other childhood diseases, the common, frequently crippling, and sometimes fatal illnesses they diagnosed so frequently in their patients but were so helpless to treat. The astonishing developments in neuroscience and genetics hold just this much promise for people afflicted with mood disorders. There is every reason to expect that the time is not too far off when treatments for bipolar disorder will be more effective than *we* can now imagine.

Resources

SUGGESTED READING

Cheney, Terry. *Manic: A Memoir*. New York: William Morrow, 2009.
This is not an easy read. Words like *brutal* and *unflinching* capture the author's no-holds-barred descriptions of the terrifying journey that she traveled with her illness before achieving acceptance and the cautious but persistent optimism and steely determination that now sustain her. Not for the faint of heart but truly inspirational.

Jamison, Kay Redfield. *Touched with Fire: Manic-Depressive Illness and the Artistic Temperament*. New York: Free Press, 1993.
A thorough survey of creative individuals who suffered from bipolar disorder, and an excellent discussion of the connections between creativity and mood disorders.

Jamison, Kay Redfield. *An Unquiet Mind: A Memoir of Moods and Madness*. New York: Vintage Books, 1996.
A powerful and moving narrative written with grace and wit by an international expert on the illness who suffers from it herself. This treasure of a book contains some of the most engrossing and vivid descriptions of the experience of bipolar disorder ever written. A must-read for anyone touched by bipolar disorder.

Jahren, Hope. *Lab Girl*. New York: Alfred A. Knopf, 2016.
Who knew trees were so amazing? Written by a brilliant, award-winning scientist who happens to suffer from bipolar disorder. Not your typical bipolar memoir, more here on the struggles of being a woman in science and the author's deep knowledge of the lives of trees, which she relates with infectious enthusiasm. Professor Jahren's brief discussions of her very severe bouts of illness are little more than side notes—as they should be.

Kraepelin, Emil. *Manic-Depressive Insanity and Paranoia*. Trans. R. M. Barclay, ed. G. M. Robertson. 1921; reprint, New York: Arno Press, 1976.
Many college and university libraries have a copy of this book and digital versions are readily available online. Arguably the very first textbook on the illness ever written, it is definitely worth reading.

Miklowitz, David. *The Bipolar Disorder Survival Guide: What You and Your Family Need to Know*. 3rd ed. New York: Guilford Press, 2019.
This book emphasizes the patient's role in managing bipolar disorder symptoms, in simple and easy-to-understand terms. A good introduction.

Mondimore, Francis Mark, and Patrick Kelly. *Adolescent Depression: A Guide for Parents*. 2nd ed. Baltimore: Johns Hopkins University Press, 2015.
OK, I'm biased in favor of this one. But if you're looking for a book that focuses on the diagnosis and treatment of mood disorders (including bipolar disorder) in young people coping with them, I think this is the one to buy. "I heartily recommend this book to parents and relatives of adolescents who have or may have mood disorders. It . . . helps parents to understand the complexities of the problem [and] is optimistic of the likelihood of improvement with correct diagnosis and treatment." Marcia Slomowitz, MD, *Journal of Clinical Psychiatry*.

Mondimore, Francis Mark, and Patrick Kelly. *Borderline Personality Disorder, New Reasons for Hope*. Baltimore: Johns Hopkins University Press, 2011.
"This exceptionally well-written book explains the many complexities of borderline personality disorder and dismantles much of the confusion surrounding the disorder. The authors are to be commended for a book that serves everyone in the BPD community: patients, family members, and professionals alike." Perry D. Hoffman, PhD, President, National Education Alliance for Borderline Personality Disorder.

Noonan, Susan J. *Take Control of Your Depression: What You Can Do to Feel Better Now*. Baltimore: Johns Hopkins University Press, 2018
This slim volume is packed with truly helpful advice about managing the symptoms of depression, informed by the author's own struggle with a depressive illness as well as her expertise as a physician and background in public health. Dr. Noonan doesn't just offer suggestions but lays out exercises and lifestyle recommendations that are concise and eminently practical. All are presented simply, compassionately, and in small, realistic steps that recognize how difficult it is for a depressed person to get things done.

Rosenthal, Norman E. *Winter Blues: Seasonal Affective Disorder, What It Is and How to Overcome It*. New York: Guilford Press, 1993.
A comprehensive and highly readable discussion of seasonal affective disorder.

Sapolsky, Robert M. *Why Zebras Don't Get Ulcers*. New York: Holt, 2004.
A very accessible overview of the biology of stress, the impact stress has on physical and mental health, and what you can do about it.

Styron, William. *Darkness Visible: A Memoir of Madness*. New York: Random House, 1990.
I recommend this book to medical students as one of the best accounts of the symptoms of depression available. A good book for family members to read to better understand the experience of serious depression.

SUPPORT AND ADVOCACY ORGANIZATIONS

All of the following organizations provide information and resources, and some offer referrals to support groups as well as to clinicians in your community who are skilled in treating mood disorders. Contact them all and become a member of each! In addition to the direct services they provide to consumers, they are active in combating the stigmatization of psychiatric illnesses, in lobbying for better medical insurance coverage for psychiatric disorders, and in supporting research.

Depression and Bipolar Support Alliance (DBSA)
55 E Jackson Blvd, Suite 490
Chicago, IL 60604
800-826-3632
www.dbsalliance.org

National Alliance for the Mentally Ill (NAMI)
3803 N. Fairfax Drive, Suite 100
Arlington, VA 22203
703-524-7600
www.nami.org

**Mental Health America
(formerly, the National Mental Health Association)**
500 Montgomery Street, Suite 820
Alexandria, VA 22314
800-969-6642
www.mentalheathamerica.org

INTERNET RESOURCES

All of the support and advocacy groups listed in the previous section have websites, and the astonishing range of resources on the internet continues to grow. Remember, however, that inaccurate information, bias, and just plain nonsense can also be found on the internet. It is important to consider information sources very carefully.

Here are some excellent resources:

International Society for Bipolar Disorders
www.isbd.org
For scientists and clinicians specializing in bipolar disorders, the site also lists the latest research articles on bipolar disorder research from around the world.

Medscape
www.medscape.com
This is primarily a news site for medical professionals, but it also has a "patient information" section with many useful articles and links to other resources.

National Network of Depression Centers
www.nndc.org
The NNDC is a research consortium made up of leading academic medical centers but the NNDC website also contains informative articles on new research written for general audiences. Check in often to read about the very latest breakthroughs.

PubMed
www.ncbi.nlm.nih.gov/entrez/query.fcgi
Free access to the most comprehensive medical database in the world, maintained by the US National Library of Medicine. Anyone can use PubMed to search through fifteen million scientific journal citations on any medical topic. The vast majority of the citations include an abstract (short summary) of the article, and your local public library can often help you obtain a copy of the complete text.

WebMD
www.webmd.com
One of the best sources of information on just about any medical problem. Organized into "Condition Centers," including centers for bipolar disorder and depression, that pull together many resources for common illnesses.

Notes

Preface

1. Kathleen Merikangas, Robert Jin, Jian-Ping He, Ronald C. Kessler, Sing Lee, Nancy A. Sampson, Maria Carmen Viana, Laura Helena Andrade, Chiyi Hu, Elie G. Karam, Maria Ladea, Maria Elena Medina Mora, Mark Oakley Browne, Yutaka Ono, Jose Posada-Villa, Rajesh Sagar, and Zahari Zarkov, "Prevalence and Correlates of Bipolar Spectrum Disorder in the World Mental Health Survey Initiative," *Archives of General Psychiatry* 68, no. 3 (2011): 241–51.
2. For a discussion of the diagnosis of bipolar disorder in these historical personalities, see Kay Redfield Jamison, *Touched with Fire: Manic-Depressive Illness and the Artistic Temperament* (New York: Free Press, 1993).
3. WebMD, "Famous People with Bipolar Disorder," 2019, www.webmd.com/bipolar-disorder/ss/slideshow-celebrities-bipolar-disorder.
4. "National Survey of NDMDA Members Finds Long Delay in Diagnosis of Manic-Depressive Illness," in News and Notes, *Hospital and Community Psychiatry* 44, no. 8 (1993): 800–801.
5. J. Dagani, G. Signorini, O. Nielssen, M. Bani, A. Pastore, G. Girolamo, and M. Large, "Meta-analysis of the Interval between the Onset and Management of Bipolar Disorder," *Canadian Journal of Psychiatry / Revue Canadienne de Psychiatrie* 62, no. 4 (2017): 247–58.
6. F. K. Goodwin, B. Fireman , G. E. Simon, E. M Hunkeler, J. Lee, and D. Revicki, "Suicide Risk in Bipolar Disorder during Treatment with Lithium and Divalproex," *Journal of the American Medical Association* 290 (2003): 1467–73.
7. L. Tondo, M. Pompili, A. Forte, and R. J. Baldessarini, "Suicide Attempts in Bipolar Disorders: Comprehensive Review of 101 Reports," *Acta Psychiatrica Scandinavia* 133 (2016): 174–86.

Chapter 1. Normal and Abnormal Mood

1. *Webster's Third New International Dictionary, Unabridged*, s.v. "mood," unabridged.merriam-webster.com.
2. Although I have made these clinical vignettes as realistic as possible by using symptom details culled from many patients, they are fictitious and do not portray any person, living or dead.
3. The word *mania* has ancient origins, deriving from the Greek word *mainesthai*, which means simply "to be insane." Early English physicians sometimes used the word *madness* to describe the syndrome of disorganized hyperactivity that we now call mania. But during the eighteenth and nineteenth centuries, European physicians writing about mental disorders increasingly employed *mania* (in French *la manie* and in German *die Manie*) to describe the elevated or irritable mood states of bipolar disorder. When Emil Kraepelin used *manic-depressive insanity* in his groundbreaking work on bipolar disorder, the term *mania* for the excited phase of the disorder became firmly established.
4. Henry J. Berkley, *A Treatise on Mental Diseases* (1900; reprint, New York: Arno Press, 1980), 143.
5. Kay Redfield Jamison, *An Unquiet Mind: A Memoir of Moods and Madness* (New York: Vintage Books, 1996), 36.

6. Frederick K. Goodwin and Kay Redfield Jamison, *Manic-Depressive Illness* (New York: Oxford University Press, 1990), 23.

7. Quoted in Goodwin and Jamison, *Manic-Depressive Illness*, 26–27.

8. Emil Kraepelin, *Manic-Depressive Insanity and Paranoia*, trans. R. M. Barclay, ed. G. M. Robertson (1921; reprint, New York: Arno Press, 1976), 31. This is a translation of volumes 3 and 4 of the 8th edition (1913) of Kraepelin's textbook *Psychiatrie*, which originally appeared in 1896.

9. Goodwin and Jamison, *Manic-Depressive Illness*, 29.

10. Kraepelin, *Manic-Depressive Insanity*, 31.

11. For a discussion of the concept of motivated behaviors in psychiatry, see Paul McHugh and Philip Slavney, *The Perspectives of Psychiatry* (Baltimore: Johns Hopkins University Press, 1998), 151–238.

12. Kraepelin, *Manic-Depressive Insanity*, 62.

13. Kraepelin, *Manic-Depressive Insanity*, 56, 64.

14. J. D. Campbell, *Manic-Depressive Disease: Clinical and Psychiatric Significance* (Philadelphia: J. D. Lippincott, 1953), 159–60, quoted in Goodwin and Jamison, *Manic-Depressive Illness*, 24.

15. Jamison, *Unquiet Mind*, 83.

16. Kraepelin, *Manic-Depressive Insanity*, 70.

17. Berkley, *Treatise on Mental Diseases*, 160.

18. Quoted in Edward Hare, "The Two Manias: Study of the Evolution of the Modern Concept of Mania," *British Journal of Psychiatry* 138 (1981): 89–99.

19. Norman Endler, *Holiday of Darkness: A Psychologist's Personal Journey out of His Depression* (New York: John Wiley and Sons, 1982), 4.

20. Endler, *Holiday of Darkness*, 86.

21. William Styron, *Darkness Visible: A Memoir of Madness* (New York: Random House, 1990), 19.

22. Endler, *Holiday of Darkness*, 48–49.

23. Styron, *Darkness Visible*, 17.

24. Endler, *Holiday of Darkness*, 29.

25. Kraepelin, *Manic-Depressive Insanity*, 75.

26. F. Scott Fitzgerald, *The Crackup* (New York: New Directions, 1956), 75.

27. Styron, *Darkness Visible*, 17.

28. Endler, *Holiday of Darkness*, 54.

29. Styron, *Darkness Visible*, 43–44.

30. Endler, *Holiday of Darkness*, 54.

31. Kraepelin, *Manic-Depressive Insanity*, 84.

32. Kraepelin, *Manic-Depressive Insanity*, 89.

33. Styron, *Darkness Visible*, 58.

34. Kraepelin, *Manic-Depressive Insanity*, 97.

35. Jamison, *Unquiet Mind*, 45.

36. Kraepelin, *Manic-Depressive Insanity*, 104.

37. Kraepelin, *Manic-Depressive Insanity*, 99.

Chapter 2. The Categories of Bipolar Disorder

1. Kathleen Merikangas, Robert Jin, Jian-Ping He, Ronald C. Kessler, Sing Lee, Nancy A. Sampson, Maria Carmen Viana, Laura Helena Andrade, Chiyi Hu, Elie G. Karam, Maria Ladea, Maria Elena Medina Mora, Mark Oakley Browne, Yutaka Ono, Jose Posada-Villa, Rajesh Sagar, and Zahari Zarkov, "Prevalence and

Correlates of Bipolar Spectrum Disorder in the World Mental Health Survey Initiative," *Archives of General Psychiatry* 68, no. 3 (2011): 241–51.

2. The diagnostic classifications used when these older studies were done have changed. In most cases, patients with "manic-depressive illness" in these studies had full-blown manic episodes and severe depressions and thus would today probably be diagnosed with bipolar I. Nevertheless, cases that would today be diagnosed differently (as bipolar II, for example) may have been mixed in. Thus, the findings and statistics must be interpreted with some caution.

3. Thomas A. C. Rennie, "Prognosis in Manic-Depressive Psychosis," *American Journal of Psychiatry* 98 (1942): 801–14, quoted in Frederick K. Goodwin and Kay Redfield Jamison, *Manic-Depressive Illness* (New York: Oxford University Press, 1990), 133.

4. Emil Kraepelin, *Manic-Depressive Insanity and Paranoia*, trans. R. M. Barclay, ed. G. M. Robertson (1921; reprint, New York: Arno Press, 1976), 136.

5. Kraepelin, *Manic-Depressive Insanity*, 3, 137.

6. G. Winokur, P. Clayton, and T. Reich, *Manic-Depressive Illness* (St. Louis: C. V. Mosby, 1969), quoted in Goodwin and Jamison, *Manic-Depressive Illness*, 141.

7. Athansio Koukopoulas, Daniela Reginaldi, Giampolo Minnai, Gino Serre, Luca Pani, and Neil Johnson, "The Long-Term Prophylaxis of Affective Disorders," in *Depression and Mania: From Neurobiology to Treatment*, ed. G. Gessa, W. Fratta, L. Pina, and G. Serre (New York: Raven Press, 1995), 127–47.

8. P. Grof, "Sixty Years of Lithium Responders," *Neuropsychobiology* 62, no. 1 (2010): 8–16.

9. Lewis L. Judd, Hagop S. Akiskal, Pamela J. Schettler, Jean Endicott, Jack Maser, David A. Solomon, Andrew C. Leon, John A. Rice, and Martin B. Keller, "The Long-Term Natural History of the Weekly Symptomatic Status of Bipolar I Disorder," *Archives of General Psychiatry* 59, no. 6 (2002): 530–37.

10. A. Cochran, M. McInnis, and D. Forger, "Data-Driven Classification of Bipolar I Disorder from Longitudinal Course of Mood," *Translational Psychiatry* 6, no. 10 (2016): 1–7.

11. William Coryell, Nancy Andreasen, Jean Endicott, and Martin Keller, "The Significance of Past Mania or Hypomania in the Course and Outcome of Major Depression," *American Journal of Psychiatry* 144 (1987): 309–15.

12. Merikangas et al., "Prevalence and Correlates."

13. J. H. Baek, D. Y. Park, J. Choi, J. S. Kim, J. S. Choi, K. Ha, J. S. Kwon, and K. S. Hong, "Differences between Bipolar I and Bipolar II Disorders in Clinical Features, Comorbidity and Family History," *Journal of Affective Disorders* 131 (2011): 59–67.

14. Baek et al., "Differences between Bipolar I and Bipolar II."

15. Baek et al., "Differences between Bipolar I and Bipolar II."

16. Kraepelin, *Manic-Depressive Insanity*, 131.

17. Anna R. Van Meter, Eric A. Youngstrom, and Robert L. Findling, "Cyclothymic Disorder: A Critical Review," *Clinical Psychology Review* 32, no. 4 (2012): 229–43.

18. G. Perugi, E. Hantouche, G. Vannucchi, and O. Pinto, "Cyclothymia Reloaded: A Reappraisal of the Most Misconceived Affective Disorder," *Journal of Affective Disorders* 183 (2015): 119–33.

19. Kraepelin, *Manic-Depressive Insanity*, 132.

20. H. Akiskal, E. Hantouche, and J. F. Allilaire, "Bipolar II with and without Cyclothymic Temperament: 'Dark' and 'Sunny' Expressions of Soft Bipolarity," *Journal of Affective Disorders* 73, no. 1 (2003): 49–57.

21. H. Akiskal, M. K. Khani, and A. Scott- Strauss, "Cyclothymic Temperamental Disorders," *Psychiatric Clinics of North America* 2 (1979): 527–54, quoted in Frederick K. Goodwin and Kay Redfield Jamison, *Manic-Depressive Illness* (New York: Oxford University Press, 1990), 54.

22. Anna Van Meter, Eric A. Youngstrom, Christine Demeter, and Robert L. Findling, "Examining the Validity of Cyclothymic Disorder in a Youth Sample: Replication and Extension," *Journal of Abnormal Child Psychology* 41, no. 3 (2013): 367–78.

23. Kraepelin, *Manic-Depressive Insanity*, 2.

24. Hagop Akiskal and Gopinath Mallya, "Criteria for 'Soft' Bipolar Spectrum: Treatment Implications," *Psychopharmacology Bulletin* 23, no. 1 (1987): 68–73.

Chapter 3. Bipolar Disorder and the *DSM-5*

1. Alfred Kinsey, Wardell Pomeroy, and Clyde Martin, *Sexual Behavior in the Human Male* (Philadelphia: W. B. Saunders, 1948), 678, 639.

Chapter 4. The Mood Disease

1. Quoted in Stanley W. Jackson, *Melancholia and Depression, from Hippocratic Times to Modern Times* (New Haven, CT: Yale University Press, 1986), 251 ("peevish," "complain[ed]," and "At the height"); and in Frederick K. Goodwin and Kay Redfield Jamison, *Manic-Depressive Illness* (New York: Oxford University Press, 1990), 58 ("In my opinion").

2. Quoted in Jackson, *Melancholia and Depression*, 253–54.

3. Quoted in Jackson, *Melancholia and Depression*, 257.

4. See Jackson, *Melancholia and Depression*, 262–63.

5. Emil Kraepelin, *Manic-Depressive Insanity and Paranoia*, trans. R. M. Barclay, ed. G. M. Robertson (1921; reprint, New York: Arno Press, 1976), 1.

6. See David Healy, *Mania: A Short History of Bipolar Disorder* (Baltimore: Johns Hopkins University Press, 2008).

7. John F. J. Cade, "Lithium Salts in the Treatment of Psychotic Excitement," *Medical Journal of Australia* 36 (1949): 349–52.

8. For a superb account of this shameful story, see Götz Aly, Peter Chroust, and Christian Pross, *Cleansing the Fatherland: Nazi Medicine and Racial Hygiene* (Baltimore: Johns Hopkins University Press, 1994).

9. Ronald R. Fieve, *Moodswing: The Third Revolution in Psychiatry* (New York: Bantam Books, 1975), 3.

10. M. Schou, N. Juel-Nielsen, E. Strömgren, and H. Voldby, "The Treatment of Manic Psychoses by the Administration of Lithium Salts," *Journal of Neurology, Neurosurgery, and Psychiatry* 17 (1954): 250–60.

11. Roland Kuhn, "The Treatment of Depressive States with G 22355 (Imipramine Hydrochloride)," *American Journal of Psychiatry* 115 (1958): 461.

12. M. Schou, N. Juel-Nelson, E. Strömgren and H. Voldby, "The Treatment of Manic Psychoses with the Administration of Lithium Salts," *Journal of Neurology, Neurosurgery and Psychiatry* 17 (1954): 256.

Chapter 5. Mood-Stabilizing Medications

1. Anastase Georgotas and Samuel Gershon, "Historical Perspectives and Current Highlights on Lithium Treatment in Manic-Depressive Illness," *Journal of Clinical Psychopharmacology* 1, no. 1 (1981): 27–31.

2. Paul Baalstrup and Morgans Schou, "Lithium as a Prophylactic Agent: Its Effect against Recurrent Depressions and Manic-Depressive Psychosis," *Archives of General Psychiatry* 16, no. 2 (1967): 162–72.

3. B. Blackwell and M. Shephard, "Prophylactic Lithium: Another Therapeutic Myth?" *Lancet* 1 (1968): 968–71.

4. P. Baalstrup, J. Poulsen, M. Schou, K. Thomsen, and A. Amdisen, "Prophylactic Lithium: Double-Blind Discontinuation in Manic and Recurrent-Depressive Disorders," *Lancet* 2 (1970): 326–30.

5. American Psychiatric Association, "Practice Guidelines for the Treatment of Bipolar Disorder," *American Journal of Psychiatry* 151, suppl. (1994): 6.

6. To be more precise, the therapeutic index is the ratio of the largest dose producing no toxic symptoms to the smallest dose routinely producing the desired therapeutic effects.

7. Alan Gelenberg, John Kane, Martin Keller, Phillip Lavori, Jerrold Rosenbaum, Karyl Cole, and Janet Lavelle, "Comparison of Standard and Low Levels of Lithium for Maintenance Treatment of Bipolar Disorder," *New England Journal of Medicine* 321, no. 22 (1989): 1489–93.

8. Morgans Schou, "Forty Years of Lithium Treatment," *Archives of General Psychiatry* 54 (1997): 9–13.

9. Schou, "Forty Years of Lithium Treatment," 11.

10. R. J. Knebel, N. Rosenlicht, and L. Collins, "Lithium Carbonate Maintenance Therapy in a Hemodialysis Patient with End-Stage Renal Disease," *American Journal of Psychiatry* 167, no. 11 (2010): 1409–10.

11. For an excellent review, see T. J. Raedler and K. Wiedermann, "Lithium-Induced Nephropathies," *Psychopharmacology Bulletin* 40, no. 2 (2007): 134–49.

12. American Psychiatric Association, "Practice Guidelines for the Treatment of Bipolar Disorder," 7.

13. Frederick K. Goodwin and Kay Redfield Jamison, *Manic-Depressive Illness* (New York: Oxford University Press, 1990), 707.

14. Jonathan Sporn and Gary Sachs, "The Anticonvulsant Lamotrigine in Treatment-Resistant Manic-Depressive Illness," *Journal of Clinical Psychopharmacology* 17, no. 3 (1997): 185–89.

15. Joseph R. Calabrese, S. Hossein Fatemi, and Mark J. Woyshville, "Antidepressant Effects of Lamotrigine in Rapid Cycling Bipolar Disorder," *American Journal of Psychiatry* 153, no. 9 (1996): 1236.

16. C. L. Bowden, J. R. Calabrese, G. Sachs, L. N. Yatham, S. A. Asghar, M. Hompland, P. Montgomery, N. Earl, T. M. Smoot, and J. DeVeaugh-Geiss (Lamictal 606 Study Group), "A Placebo-Controlled 18-Month Trial of Lamotrigine and Lithium Maintenance Treatment in Recently Manic or Hypomanic Patients with Bipolar I Disorder," *Archives of General Psychiatry* 60, no. 4 (2003): 392; J. R. Calabrese, C. L. Bowden, G. Sachs, L. N. Yatham, K. Behnke, O. P. Mehtonen, P. Montgomery, J. Ascher, W. Paska, N. Earl, and J. DeVeaugh-Geiss (Lamictal 605 Study Group), "A Placebo-Controlled 18-Month Trial of Lamotrigine and Lithium Maintenance Treatment in Recently Depressed Patients with Bipolar I Disorder," *Journal of Clinical Psychiatry* 64, no. 9 (2003): 1013–24.

17. T. Terao, A. Ishida, T. Kimura, M. Yarita, and T. Hara, "Preventive Effects of Lamotrigine in Bipolar II Versus Bipolar I Disorder," *Journal of Clinical Psychiatry* 78, no. 8 (2017): e1000–e1005.

18. J. R. Calabrese, J. R. Sullivan, C. L. Bowden, T. Suppes, J. F. Goldberg, G. S. Sachs, M. D. Shelton, F. K. Goodwin, M. A. Frye, and V. Kusumakar, "Rash in Multicenter Trials of Lamotrigine in Mood Disorders: Clinical Relevance and Management," *Journal of Clinical Psychiatry* 63, no. 11 (2002): 1012–19.

19. J. C. Ballenger and R. M. Post, "Carbamazepine in Manic-Depressive Illness: A New Treatment," *American Journal of Psychiatry* 137, no. 7 (1980): 782–90.

20. B. Lerer, M. Moore, E. Meyendorff, S. R. Cho, and S. Gershon, "Carbamazepine versus Lithium in Mania: A Double-Blind Study," *Journal of Clinical Psychiatry* 48, no. 3 (1987): 89–93.

21. Robert Post, Thomas Uhde, James Ballenger, and Kathleen Squillace, "Prophylactic Efficacy of Carbamazepine in Manic-Depressive Illness," *American Journal of Psychiatry* 140, no. 12 (1983): 1602–4.

22. R. H. Weisler, A. H. Kalali, and T. A. Ketter, "A Multicenter, Randomized, Double-Blind, Placebo-Controlled Trial of Extended-Release Carbamazepine Capsules as Monotherapy for Bipolar Disorder Patients with Manic or Mixed Episodes," *Journal of Clinical Psychiatry* 65, no. 4 (2004): 478–84.

23. F. Centorrino, M. J. Albert, J. M. Berry, J. P. Kelleher, V. Fellman, G. Line, A. E. Koukopoulos, J. E. Kidwell, K. V. Fogarty, and R. J. Baldessarini, "Oxcarbazepine: Clinical Experience with Hospitalized Psychiatric Patients," *Bipolar Disorders* 5, no. 5 (2003): 370–74.

24. See Charles Bowden and Susan McElroy, "History of the Development of Valproate for the Treatment of Bipolar Disorder," *Journal of Clinical Psychiatry* 56, suppl. 3 (1995): 3–5.

25. Charles L. Bowden, "Predictors of Response to Divalproex and Lithium," *Journal of Clinical Psychiatry* 56, suppl. 3 (1995): 25–29.

26. D. J. Muzina, K. Gao, D. E. Kemp, S. Khalife, S. J. Ganocy, P. K. Chan, M. B. Seranno, C. M. Conroy, and J. R. Calabrese, "Acute Efficacy of Divalproex Sodium versus Placebo in Mood-Stabilizer-Naïve Bipolar I or Bipolar II Depression: A Double-Blind, Randomized, Placebo Controlled Trial," *Journal of Clinical Psychiatry* 72, no. 6 (2011): 813–19; C. L. Bowden, J. R. Calabrese, S. L. McElroy, L. Gyulai, A. Wassef, H. G. Pope, J. C. Chou, P. E. Keck, L. J. Rhodes, A. C. Swann, R. M. Hirshfeld, and P. J. Wozniak, "A Randomized, Placebo-Controlled 12-Month Trial of Divalproex and Lithium in the Treatment of Outpatients with Bipolar I Disorder: Divalproex Maintenance Study Group," *Archives of General Psychiatry* 57, no. 5 (2000): 481–89.

27. K. A. Macritchie, J. R. Geddes, J. Scott, D. R. Haslam, and G. M. Goodwin, "Valproic Acid, Valproate, and Divalproex in the Maintenance Phase of Bipolar Disorder," *Cochrane Database of Systematic Reviews* 3 (2001): Art. No. CD003196.

28. American Psychiatric Association, "Practice Guidelines for the Treatment of Bipolar Disorder," 10.

29. See Frederick Jacobsen, "Low-Dose Valproate: A New Treatment for Cyclothymia, Mild Rapid-Cycling Disorders, and Premenstrual Syndrome," *Journal of Clinical Psychiatry* 54, no. 6 (1993): 229–34. Also J. A. Delito, "The Effect of Valproate on Bipolar Spectrum Temperamental Disorders," *Journal of Clinical Psychiatry* 54, no. 8 (1993): 300–304.

30. Gary Sachs, "Bipolar Mood Disorder: Practical Strategies for Acute and Maintenance Phase Treatment," *Journal of Clinical Psychopharmacology* 16, no. 2, suppl. 1 (1996): 32S–47S.

31. Joseph F. Goldberg, Katherine E. Burdick, and Carrie J. Endick, "Preliminary Randomized, Double-Blind, Placebo-Controlled Trial of Pramipexole Added to Mood Stabilizers for Treatment-Resistant Bipolar Depression," *American Journal of Psychiatry* 161, no. 3 (2004): 564–66.

32. Michael Berk, David Copolov, Olivia Dean, Kristy Lu, Sue Jeavons, Ian Schapkaitz, Murray Anderson-Hunt, and Ashley Bush, "N-Acetyl Cysteine for Depressive Symptoms in Bipolar Disorder—A Double-Blind Randomized Placebo-Controlled

Trial," *Biological Psychiatry* 64, no. 6 (2008): 468–75; M. Berk, O. Dean, S. Cotton, C. Gama, F. Kapczinski, B. Fernandes, K. Kohlmann, S. Jeavons, K. Hewett, C. Allwang, H. Cobb, A. Bush, I. Schapkaitz, S. Dodd, and G. Malhi, "The Efficacy of N-Acetylcysteine as an Adjunctive Treatment in Bipolar Depression: An Open Label Trial," *Journal of Affective Disorders* 135, nos. 1–3 (2011): 389–94.

Chapter 6. Antipsychotic Medications

1. In a study of 11,555 patients treated with clozapine, 73 developed agranulocytosis (of whom 2 died of the infectious complications of the condition). Jose Alvir, Jeffrey Lieberman, Allan Safferman, Jeffrey Schwimmer, and John Schaaf, "Clozapine-Induced Agranulocytosis: Incidence and Risk Factors in the United States," *New England Journal of Medicine* 329 (1993): 162–67.
2. Joseph Calabrese, Susan Kimmel, Mark Woyshville, Daniel Rapport, Carl Faust, Paul Thompson, and Herbert Meltzer, "Clozapine for Treatment-Refractory Mania," *American Journal of Psychiatry* 153, no. 6 (1996): 759–64.
3. Carlos Zarate Jr., Mauricio Tohen, Michael Banov, Michelle Weiss, and Jonathan Cole, "Is Clozapine a Mood Stabilizer?" *Journal of Clinical Psychiatry* 56, no. 3 (1995): 108–12.
4. G. Parker and G. Malhi, "Are the Atypical Antipsychotic Drugs Antidepressants?" *Journal of Clinical Psychopharmacology* 59, no. 3 (2002): 94–95.
5. T. Baptista, N. M. Kin, S. Beaulieu, and E. A. de Baptista, "Obesity and Related Metabolic Abnormalities during Antipsychotic Drug Administration: Mechanisms, Management, and Research Perspectives," *Pharmacopsychiatry* 35, no. 6 (2002): 205–19.
6. W. Ray, C. Chung, K. Murray, K. Hall, and C. Stein, "Atypical Antipsychotic Drugs and the Risk of Sudden Cardiac Death," *New England Journal of Medicine*, 360 (2009) 225–35.

Chapter 7. Antidepressant Medications

1. H. S. Lee, D. H. Song, C. H. Kim, and H. K. Choi, "An Open Clinical Trial of Fluoxetine in the Treatment of Premature Ejaculation," *Journal of Clinical Psychopharmacology* 16, no. 5 (1996): 379–82.
2. G. S. Sachs, A. A. Nierenberg, J. R. Calabrese, L. B. Marangell, S. R. Wisniewski, L. Gyulai, E. S. Friedman, C. L. Bowden, M. D. Fossey, M. J. Ostacher, T. A. Ketter, J. Patel, P. Hauser, D. Rappaport, and J. M. Martinez, "Effectiveness of Adjunctive Antidepressant Treatment for Bipolar Depression," *New England Journal of Medicine* 356, no. 17 (2007): 1711–22.

Chapter 8. New (and Old) Medications and Pipeline Drugs

1. A. G. Szmulewicz, F. Angriman , C. Samamé, A. Ferraris, D. Vigo, and S. A. Strejilevich, "Dopaminergic Agents in the Treatment of Bipolar Depression: A Systematic Review and Meta-analysis," *Acta Psychiatrica Scandinavia* 135 (2017): 527–38.
2. A. Tundo, R. de Filippis, and F. De Crescenzo, "Pramipexole in the Treatment of Unipolar and Bipolar Depression: A Systematic Review and Meta-analysis," *Acta Psychiatrica Scandinavia* 140, no. 2 (2019): 116–25.
3. B. Dell'Osso and T. A. Ketter, "Assessing Efficacy/Effectiveness and Safety/ Tolerability Profiles of Adjunctive Pramipexole in Bipolar Depression: Acute

versus Long-Term Data," *International Clinical Psychopharmacology* 28, no. 6 (2013): 297–304.

4. S. Meltzer-Brody, H. Colquhoun, R. Riesenberg, C. Epperson, K. Deligiannidis, D. Rubinow, H. Li, A. J. Sankoh, C. Clemson, A. Schacterle, J. Jonas, and S. Kanes, "Brexanolone Injection in Post-partum Depression: Two Multicentre, Double-Blind, Randomised, Placebo-Controlled, Phase 3 Trials," *Lancet* 392, no. 10152 (2018): 1058–70.

5. E. Brown, J. Park, C. E. Marx, L. S. Hynan, C. Gardner, D. Davila, A. Nakamura, P. Sunderajan, A. Lo, and T. Holmes, "A Randomized, Double-Blind, Placebo-Controlled Trial of Pregnenolone for Bipolar Depression," *Neuropsychopharmacology* 39, no. 12 (2014): 2867–73.

6. Sage Therapeutics, Inc., Sage Therapeutics Announces Second Quarter 2018 Financial Results and Highlights Pipeline and Business Progress, press release, 2018, investor.sagerx.com/news-releases/news-release-details/sage-therapeutics-announces-second-quarter-2018-financial.

7. M. G. Carta, K. M. Bhat, and A. Preti, "GABAergic Neuroactive Steroids: A New Frontier in Bipolar Disorders?" *Behavioral and Brain Functions* 8 (2012): 61.

Chapter 9: More Medications, Hormones, and Dietary Supplements

1. For a discussion of these drugs to treat anxiety in bipolar disorder, see P. E. Keck, J. R. Strawn, and S. L. McElroy, "Pharmacologic Treatment Considerations in Co-occurring Bipolar and Anxiety Disorder," *Journal of Clinical Psychiatry* 67, suppl. 1 (2006): 8–15.

2. Keck, Strawn, and McElroy, "Pharmacologic Treatment Considerations."

3. Y. Dündar, A. Boland, J. Strobl, S. Dodd, A. Haycox, A. Bagust, J. Bogg, R. Dickson, and T. Walley, "Newer Hypnotic Drugs for the Short-Term Management of Insomnia: A Systematic Review and Economic Evaluation," *Health Technology Assessment* 8, no. 24 (2004): iii–x.

4. Z. Xie, F. Chen, W. A. Li, X. Geng, C. Li, X. Meng, Y. Feng, W. Liu, and F. Yu, "A Review of Sleep Disorders and Melatonin," *Neurological Research* 39, no. 6 (2017) 559–65.

5. F. Auld, F. L. Maschauer, I. Morrison, D. J. Skene, and R. L. Riha, "Evidence for the Efficacy of Melatonin in the Treatment of Primary Adult Sleep Disorders," *Sleep Medicine Reviews* 34 (2017): 10–22.

6. A. Kuriyama, M. Honda, and Y. Hayashino, "Ramelteon for the Treatment of Insomnia in Adults: A Systematic Review and Meta-analysis," *Sleep Medicine* 15, no. 4 (2014): 385–92.

7. M. S. Bauer, P. C. Whybrow, and A. Winokur, "Rapid Cycling Bipolar Affective Disorder I: Association with Grade I Hypothyroidism," *Archives of General Psychiatry* 47, no. 5 (1990): 427–32.

8. H. A. Oomen, A. J. Schipperijn, and H. A. Drexhage, "The Prevalence of Affective Disorder and in Particular of a Rapid Cycling of Bipolar Disorder in Patients with Abnormal Thyroid Function Tests," *Clinical Endocrinology* 45, no. 2 (1996): 215–23.

9. D. P. Cole, M. E. Thase, A. G. Mallinger, J. C. Soares, J. F. Luther, D. J. Kupfer, and E. Frank, "Slower Treatment Response in Bipolar Depression Predicted by Lower Pre-treatment Thyroid Function," *American Journal of Psychiatry* 159, no. 1 (2002): 116–21.

10. There have been controversies as to whether all thyroid hormone preparations made by different manufacturers are equivalent and interchangeable.

Lawrence K. Altman, "Caution Urged over Switch in Thyroid Drug," *New York Times*, April 17, 1997. The problem can be avoided by ensuring that you take the same preparation of levothyroxine, whether brand name or generic, all the time and also by getting your thyroid hormone levels tested regularly.

11. J. Sarris, D. Mischoulon, and I. Schweitzer, "Omega-3 for Bipolar Disorder: Meta-analysis of Use in Mania and Bipolar Depression," *Journal of Clinical Psychiatry* 73, no. 1 (2012): 81–86.

12. M. Berk, D. Copoloc, O. Dean, K. Lu, S. Jeavons, I. Schapkaitz, M. Anderson-Hunt, and A. Bush, "N-Acetyl Cysteine for Depressive Symptoms in Bipolar Disorder— a Double-Blind Randomized Placebo-Controlled Trial," *Biological Psychiatry* 64, no. 6 (2008): 468–75; M. Berk, O. Dean, S. Cotton, C. Gama, F. Kapczinski, B. Fernandes, K. Kohlmann, S. Jeavons, K. Hewerr, C. Allwang, K. Cobb, A. Bush, I. Schapkaitz, S. Dodd, and G. Malhi, "The Efficacy of N-Acetylcysteine as an Adjunctive Treatment in Bipolar Depression: An Open Label Trial," *Journal of Affective Disorders* 135, nos. 1–3 (2011): 389–94.

13. K. Linde, G. Ramirez, C. D. Mulrow, A. Pauls, and W. Weidenhammer, "St. John's Wort for Depression—An Overview and Meta-analysis of Randomised Clinical Trials," *British Medical Journal* 313, no. 7052 (1996): 253–58.

14. R. C. Shelton, M. B. Keller, A. Gelenberg, D. L. Dunner, R. Hirschfeld, M. E. Thase, J. Russell, R. B. Lydiard, P. Crits-Christoph, R. Gallop, L. Todd, D. Hellerstein, P. Goodnick, G. Keitner, S. M. Stahl, and U. Halbreich, "Effectiveness of St. John's Wort in Major Depression: A Randomized Controlled Trial," *Journal of the American Medical Association* 285, no. 15 (2001): 1978–86.

15. A. J. Gelenberg, R. C. Shelton, P. Crits-Christoph, M. B. Keller, D. L. Dunner, R. M. Hirschfeld, M. E. Thase, J. M. Russell, R. B. Lydiard, R. J. Gallop, L. Todd, D. J. Hellerstein, P. J. Goodnick, G. I. Keitner, S. M. Stahl, U. Halbreich, and H. S. Hopkins, "The Effectiveness of St. John's Wort in Major Depressive Disorder: A Naturalistic Phase 2 Follow-Up in Which Nonresponders Were Provided Alternate Medication," *Journal of Clinical Psychiatry* 65, no. 8 (2004): 1114–19.

16. E. Moses and A. Mallinger, "St. John's Wort: Three Cases of Possible Mania Induction," *Journal of Clinical Psychopharmacology* 20, no. 1 (2000): 115–17.

Chapter 10. Brain-Stimulation Treatments

1. M. Valance, "The Experience of Electro-Convulsive Therapy by a Practising Psychiatrist," *British Journal of Psychiatry* 111 (1965): 365–67.

2. Larry Squire, Pamela Slater, and Patricia Miller, "Retrograde Amnesia and Bilateral Electroconvulsive Therapy, Long Term Follow-Up," *Archives of General Psychiatry* 38 (1981): 89–95.

3. Larry R. Squire and Pamela C. Slater, "Electroconvulsive Therapy and Complaints of Memory Dysfunction: A Prospective Three-Year Follow-Up Study," *British Journal of Psychiatry* 142 (1983): 1–8.

4. E. Anderson and I. Reti, "ECT in Pregnancy: A Review of the Literature from 1941 to 2007," *Psychosomatic Medicine* 71, no. 2 (2009): 235–42.

5. Frederick K. Goodwin and Kay Redfield Jamison, *Manic-Depressive Illness*, 2nd ed. (New York: Oxford University Press, 2007), 782.

6. Sukdeb Mukherjee, Harold Sackeim, and David Schnur, "Electroconvulsive Therapy of Acute Manic Episodes: A Review of Fifty Years' Experience," *American Journal of Psychiatry* 151 (1994): 169–76.

7. S. Mukherjee, H. Sackeim, and C. Lee, "Unilateral ECT in the Treatment of Manic Episodes," *Convulsive Therapy* 4 (1988): 74–80.

8. Much of the work comparing the effectiveness of ECT with that of medication compares it with lithium. As studies comparing it with newer agents (such as the anticonvulsants) are done, statements about ECT's superiority to medical treatments for mania may need to be revised. However, given that the new mood stabilizers are perhaps *less* effective than lithium for depression, ECT's claims as a more predictably effective treatment for bipolar depression remain unchallenged.

9. See Mark S. George, Eric Wasserman, and Robert Post, "Transcranial Magnetic Stimulation: A Neuropsychiatric Tool for the Twenty-First Century," *Journal of Neuropsychiatry and Clinical Neurosciences* 8 (1996): 373–82.

10. Mark George, Eric Wasserman, Tim Kimbrell, John Little, Wendol Williams, Aimee Danielson, Benjamin Greenberg, Mark Hallett, and Robert Post, "Mood Improvement following Daily Left Prefrontal Repetitive Transcranial Magnetic Stimulation in Patients with Depression: A Placebo Controlled Crossover Trial," *American Journal of Psychiatry* 154 (1997): 1752–56.

11. A. Pascual-Leone, B. Rubio, F. Pallardo, and M. D. Catala, "Beneficial Effect of Rapid-Rate Transcranial Magnetic Stimulation of the Left Dorsolateral Prefrontal Cortex in Drug-Resistant Depression," *Lancet* 348 (1996): 233–37; and Charles Epstein, Gary Figiel, William McDonald, Jody Amazon-Leece, and Linda Figiel, "Rapid Rate Transcranial Magnetic Stimulation in Young and Middle-Aged Refractory Depressed Patients," *Psychiatric Annals* 28 (1998): 36–39.

12. J. Mutz, D. R. Edgcumbe, A. R. Brunoni, and C. H. Y. Fu, "Efficacy and Acceptability of Non-invasive Brain Stimulation for the Treatment of Adult Unipolar and Bipolar Depression: A Systematic Review and Meta-analysis of Randomised Sham-Controlled Trials," *Neuroscience and Biobehavioral Reviews* 92 (2018): 291–303.

13. B. Marangell, A. J. Rush, M. S. George, H. A. Sackeim, C. R. Johnson, M. M. Husain, Z. Nahas, and S. H. Lisanby, "Vagus Nerve Stimulation (VNS) for Major Depressive Episodes: One Year Outcomes," *Biological Psychiatry* 51, no. 4 (2002): 280–87.

14. S. T. Aaronson, P. Sears, F. Ruvuna, M. Bunker, C. R. Conway, D. D. Dougherty, F. W. Reimherr, T. L. Schwartz, and J. M. Zajecka, "A 5-Year Observational Study of Patients with Treatment-Resistant Depression Treated with Vagus Nerve Stimulation or Treatment as Usual: Comparison of Response, Remission, and Suicidality," *American Journal of Psychiatry* 174, no. 7 (2017): 640–48.

15. C. K. Loo, M. M. Husain, W. M. McDonald, S. Aaronson, J. P. O'Reardon, A. Alonzo, C. S. Weickert, D. M. Martin, S. M. McClintock, A. Mohan, and S. H. Lisanby, "International Randomized-Controlled Trial of Transcranial Direct Current Stimulation in Depression," *Brain Stimulation* 11 (2018): 125–33.

16. Loo et al., "International Randomized-Controlled Trial of Transcranial Direct Current Stimulation in Depression."

Chapter 11. Counseling and Psychotherapy

1. S. A. Soo, Z. W. Zhang, S. J. Khong, J. E. W. Low, V. S. Thambyrajah, S. Alhabsyi, Q. Chew, M. Y. Sum, R. S. McIntyre, and K. Sim, "Randomized Controlled Trials of Psychoeducation Modalities in the Management of Bipolar Disorder: A Systematic Review," *Journal of Clinical Psychiatry* 79, no. 3 (2018): ii.

2. Jan Scott, "Psychotherapy for Bipolar Disorder," *British Journal of Psychiatry* 167 (1995): 581–88.

3. Nick Kanas, "Group Psychotherapy with Bipolar Patients: A Review and Synthesis," *International Journal of Group Psychotherapy* 43 (1993): 321–33.

4. L. E. Pollack, "Content Analysis of Groups for Inpatients with Bipolar Disorder," *Applied Nursing Research* 6 (1993): 19–27.

5. D. Miklowitz, J. Price, E. Holmes, J. Rendell, S. Bell, K. Budge, J. Christensen, J. Wallace, J. Simon, N. Armstrong, L. McPeake, G. Goodwin, and J. Geddes, "Facilitated Integrated Mood Management for Adults with Bipolar Disorder," *Bipolar Disorder* 14, no. 2 (2012): 185–97.

6. See Donald Meichenbaum and Roy Cameron, "Cognitive-Behavior Therapy," in *Contemporary Behavior Therapy: Conceptional and Empirical Foundations*, ed. G. Terence Wilson and Cyril M. Franks (New York: Guilford Press, 1982), 310–37.

7. T. R. Goldstein, R. K. Fersch-Podrat, M. Rivera, D. A. Axelson, J. Merranko, H. Yu, D. A. Brent, and B. Birmaher, "Dialectical Behavior Therapy for Adolescents with Bipolar Disorder: Results from a Pilot Randomized Trial," *Journal of Child and Adolescent Psychopharmacology* 25 (2015): 140–49.

8. V. L. Ives-Deliperi, F. Howells, D. J. Stein, E. M. Meintjes, and N. Horn, "The Effects of Mindfulness-Based Cognitive Therapy in Patients with Bipolar Disorder: A Controlled Functional MRI Investigation," *Journal of Affective Disorders* 150 (2013): 1152–57.

9. D. J. Miklowitz, D. A. Axelson, B. Birmaher, E. L. George, D. O. Taylor, C. D. Schneck, C. A. Beresford, L. M. Dickinson, W. E. Craighead, and D. A. Brent, "Family-Focused Treatment for Adolescents with Bipolar Disorder: Results of a 2-Year Randomized Trial," *Archives of General Psychiatry* 65 (2008): 1053–61.

10. Kay Redfield Jamison, *An Unquiet Mind: A Memoir of Moods and Madness* (New York: Vintage Books, 1996), 88–89.

11. Soo et al., "Randomized Controlled Trials of Psychoeducation Modalities."

Chapter 12. Treatment Approaches in Bipolar Disorder

1. The word *empirical* is derived from the Greek word *empeirikos*, which means "a doctor relying on experience alone."

2. T. Suppes, A. C. Swann, E. B. Dennehy, E. D. Habermacher, M. Mason, M. L. Crismon, M. G. Toprac, J. Rush, S. P. Shon, and K. Z. Altshuler, "The Texas Medication Algorithm Project: Development and Feasibility Testing of a Treatment Algorithm for Patients with Bipolar Disorder," *Journal of Clinical Psychiatry* 62 (2001): 439–47.

3. C. Bowden, R. Perlis, M. Thase, T. Ketter, M. Ostacher, J. Calabrese, N. Reilly-Harrington, J. Gonzaliz, V. Singh, A. Neirenberg, and G. Sachs, "Aims and Results of the NIMH Systematic Treatment Enhancement Program for Bipolar Disorder (STEP-BD)," *CNS Neuroscience and Therapeutics* 18, no. 3 (2012): 243–49.

Chapter 14. More Bipolar Biology

1. Robert Sapolsky, *Why Zebras Don't Get Ulcers*, 3rd ed. (New York: Holt Paperbacks, 2004), 7.

2. C. J. Morales-Medina, F. Sanchez, G. Flores, Y. Dumont, and R. Quirion, "Morphological Reorganization after Repeated Corticosterone Administration in the Hippocampus, Nucleus Accumbens, and Amygdala," *Journal of Chemical Neuroanatomy* 38, no. 4 (2009): 266–72.

3. M. Pompili, G. Serafini, M. Innamorati, G. Serra, A. Forte, D. Lester, G. Ducci, P. Girardi, and R. Tatarelli, "White Matter Hyperintensities, Suicide Risk and Late-Onset Affective Disorders: An Overview of the Current Literature," *La Clinica Terapeutica* 161, no. 6 (2010): 555–63.

4. M. J. Kempton, Z. Salvador, M. R. Munafò, J. R. Geddes, A. Simmons, S. Frangou, and S. C. Williams, "Structural Neuroimaging Studies in Major Depressive Disorder: Meta-analysis and Comparison with Bipolar Disorder," *Archives of General Psychiatry* 68 (2011): 675–90.

Chapter 15. The Science of Cycles

1. A. J. Lewy, H. A. Kern, N. E. Rosenthal, and T. A. Wehr, "Bright Artificial Light Treatment of a Manic-Depressive Patient with a Seasonal Mood Cycle," *American Journal of Psychiatry* 139 (1982): 1496–98.
2. Emil Kraepelin, *Manic-Depressive Insanity and Paranoia*, trans. R. M. Barclay, ed. G. M. Robertson (1921; reprint, New York: Arno Press, 1976), 139.
3. Norman E. Rosenthal, *Winter Blues: Seasonal Affective Disorder, What It Is and How to Overcome It* (New York: Guilford Press, 1993), 6.
4. Rosenthal, *Winter Blues*, 9.
5. Diane Boivin, Charles Czeisler, Derk-Jan Dijk, Jeanne Duffy, Simon Folkard, David Minors, Peter Totterdell, and James Waterhouse, "Complex Interaction of the Sleep-Wake Cycle and Circadian Phase Modulates Mood in Healthy Subjects," *Archives of General Psychiatry* 54 (1997): 145–52.
6. Michael Terman, Leora Amira, Jiuan Terman, and Donald Ross, "Predictors of Response and Non-response to Light Treatment for Winter Depression," *American Journal of Psychiatry* 153 (1996): 1423–29.
7. Alan O. Kogan and Patricia Guilford, "Side Effects of Short-Term 10,000-Lux Light Therapy," *American Journal of Psychiatry* 155 (1998): 293–94.
8. For an extensive discussion of circadian rhythms and bipolar disorder, see Frederick K. Goodwin and Kay Redfield Jamison, *Manic-Depressive Illness*, 2nd ed. (New York: Oxford University Press, 2007), chapter 16, "Sleep and Circadian Rhythms," 659–88.
9. F. Benedetti, B. Barbini, A. Lucca, E. Campori, C. Colombo, and E. Smeraldi, "Sleep Deprivation Hastens the Antidepressant Action of Fluoxetine," *European Archives of Psychiatry and Clinical Neuroscience* 247 (1997): 100–103.
10. T. Wehr, D. Sack, and N. Rosenthal, "Sleep Reduction as a Final Common Pathway in the Genesis of Mania," *American Journal of Psychiatry* 144 (1987): 201–4.

Chapter 16. The Genetics of Bipolar Disorder

1. Emil Kraepelin, *Manic-Depressive Insanity and Paranoia*, trans. R. M. Barclay, ed. G. M. Robertson (1921; reprint, New York: Arno Press, 1976), 165.
2. M. Ikeda, T. Saito, K. Kondo, and N. Iwata, "Genome-Wide Association Studies of Bipolar Disorder: A Systematic Review of Recent Findings and Their Clinical Implications," *Psychiatry and Clinical Neurosciences* 72, no. 2 (2018): 52–63.
3. M. DelBello and B. Geller, "Review of Studies of Child and Adolescent Offspring of Bipolar Parents," *Bipolar Disorder* 3 (2001): 325–34.

Chapter 17. Bipolar Disorder in Children and Adolescents

1. B. Birmaher, "Bipolar Disorder in Children and Adolescents," *Child and Adolescent Mental Health* 18, no. 3 (2013): 140–48.
2. Barbara Geller, Kai Sun, Betsy Zimerman, Joan Luby, Jeanne Frazier, and Marlene Williams, "Complex and Rapid-Cycling in Bipolar Children and Adolescents: A Preliminary Study," *Journal of Affective Disorders* 34 (1995): 259–68.

3. M. Strober and G. Carlson, "Bipolar Illness in Adolescents with Major Depression: Clinical, Genetic, and Psychopharmacologic Predictors in a Three- to Four-Year Prospective Follow-Up Investigation," *Archives of General Psychiatry* 39, no. 5 (1982): 549–55.

4. S. V. Faraone, J. Biederman, D. Mennin, J. Wozniak, and T. Spencer, "Attention-Deficit Hyperactivity Disorder with Bipolar Disorder: A Familial Subtype?" *Journal of the American Academy of Child and Adolescent Psychiatry* 36, no. 10 (1997): 1378–87.

5. B. Goldstein, B. Birmaher, G. A. Carlson, M. P. DelBello, R. L. Findling, M. Fristad, R. A Kowatch, D. J. Miklowitz, F. G. Nery, G. Perez-Algorta, A. Van Meter, C. P. Zeni, C. U. Correll, H. W. Kim, J. Wozniak, K. D. Chang, M. Hillegers, and E. A. Youngstrom, "The International Society for Bipolar Disorders Task Force Report on Pediatric Bipolar Disorder: Knowledge to Date and Directions for Future Research," *Bipolar Disorders* 19, no. 7 (2017): 524–43.

Chapter 18. Women with Bipolar Disorder

1. Ellen Leibenluft, "Women with Bipolar Illness: Clinical and Research Issues," *American Journal of Psychiatry* 153 (1996): 163–73.

2. Leibenluft, "Women with Bipolar Illness," 164.

3. K. Yonkers, S. Vigod, and L. Ross, "Diagnosis, Pathophysiology, and Management of Mood Disorders in Pregnant and Postpartum Women," *Obstetrics and Gynecology* 117, no. 4 (2011): 961–77.

4. Yonkers, Vigod, and Ross, "Diagnosis, Pathophysiology, and Management of Mood Disorders in Pregnant and Postpartum Women," 961.

5. J. Payne, D. MacKinnon, F. Mondimore, M. McGinnis, B. Schweitzer, R. Zamoiski, F. McMahon, J. Nurnberger, J. Rice, W. Scheftner, W. Coryell, W. Berrittini, J. Kelsoe, W. Byerley, E. Gershon, J. DePaulo, and J. Potash, "Familial Aggregation of Postpartum Mood Symptoms in Bipolar Disorder Pedigrees," *Bipolar Disorder* 10, no. 1 (2008): 38–44.

6. K. Yonkers, K. Wisner, Z. Stowe, E. Leibenluft, L. Cohen, L. Miller, R. Manber, A. Viguera, and T. Suppes, "Management of Bipolar Disorder during Pregnancy and the Postpartum Period," *American Journal of Psychiatry* 60, no. 1 (2004): 608–20.

7. J. Moore and P. Aggarwal, "Lamotrigine Use in Pregnancy," *Expert Opinions in Pharmacotherapy* 13, no. 8 (2012): 1213–16; A. Einarson and R. Boskovic, "Use and Safety of Antipsychotic Drugs during Pregnancy," *Journal of Psychiatric Practice* 15, no. 3 (2009): 183–92.

8. Douglas Maskall, Raymond Lam, Shala Misri, Lakshmi Yatham, and Athanasios Zis, "Seasonality of Symptoms in Women with Late Luteal Phase Dysphoric Disorder," *American Journal of Psychiatry* 154 (1997): 1436–41.

Chapter 19. Alcoholism and Drug Abuse

1. D. A. Reger, M. E. Farm, and D. S. Rae, "Comorbidity of Mental Disorders with Alcohol and Other Drug Abuse: Results from the Epidemiologic Catchment Area Study," *Journal of the American Medical Association* 264 (1990): 2511–18.

2. Results quoted in Kathleen Brady and Susan Sonne, "The Relationship between Substance Abuse and Bipolar Disorder," *Journal of Clinical Psychiatry* 56, suppl. 3 (1995): 19–24.

3. Susan Sonne, Kathleen Brady, and W. Alexander Morton, "Substance Abuse and Bipolar Affective Disorder," *Journal of Nervous and Mental Disease* 182 (1994): 349–52.

4. Markus Henriksson, Hillevi Aro, Mauri Marttunnen, Martti Heikkinen, Erkki Isometsä, Kimmo Kuoppasalmi, and Jouko Lönnqvist, "Mental Disorders and Comorbidity in Suicide," *American Journal of Psychiatry* 150 (1993): 935–40.

5. J. Prochaska and W. Velicer, "The Transtheoretical Model of Health Behavior Change," *American Journal of Health Promotion* 12, no. 1 (1997): 38–48.

Chapter 20. Borderline Personality Disorder

1. J. G. Gunderson, I. Weinberg, M. T. Daversa, K. D. Kueppenbender, M. C. Zanarini, M. T. Shea, A. E. Skodol, C. A. Sanislow, S. Yen, L. C. Morey, C. M. Grilo, T. H. McGlashan, R. L. Stout, and I. Dyc, "Descriptive and Longitudinal Observations on the Relationship of Borderline Personality Disorder and Bipolar Disorder," *American Journal of Psychiatry* 163, no. 7 (2006): 1173–78.

2. Gunderson et al., "Descriptive and Longitudinal Observations on the Relationship of Borderline Personality Disorder and Bipolar Disorder," 1177.

3. P. Leiberich, M. K. Nickel, K. Tritt, and F. Pedrosa Gil, "Lamotrigine Treatment of Aggression in Female Borderline Patients, Part II: An 18-Month Follow-Up." *Journal of Psychopharmacology* 22, no. 7 (2008): 805–8.

4. D. F. MacKinnon and R. Pies, "Affective Instability as Rapid Cycling: Theoretical and Clinical Implications for Borderline Personality and Bipolar Spectrum Disorders," *Bipolar Disorders* 8, no. 1 (2006): 1–14.

Chapter 21. Bipolar Disorder and Creativity

1. Aristotle, attributed by Seneca in *Moral Essays*, "De tranquillitate animi" ["On Tranquility of Mind"], sec. 17, subsec. 10, quoted in *The Columbia Dictionary of Quotations* (New York: Columbia University Press, 1993; CD ROM ed., 1994).

2. Quoted in Kay Redfield Jamison, *Touched with Fire: Manic-Depressive Illness and the Artistic Temperament* (New York: Free Press, 1993), 203–5.

3. These studies are described and cited in Jamison, *Touched with Fire*.

4. Emil Kraepelin, *Manic-Depressive Insanity and Paranoia*, trans. R. M. Barclay, ed. G. M. Robertson (1921; reprint, New York: Arno Press, 1976), 17.

5. Quoted in Jamison, *Touched with Fire*, 126.

6. Jean Cocteau, "Le coq et l'arlequin," in *Le rappel à l'ordre* (1926), quoted in *Columbia Dictionary of Quotations*, CD ROM ed.

7. These studies are cited and described in Frederick K. Goodwin and Kay Redfield Jamison, *Manic-Depressive Illness*, 2nd ed. (New York: Oxford University Press, 2007), 379–410.

Chapter 22. Living with Bipolar Disorder

1. Emil Kraepelin, *Manic-Depressive Insanity and Paranoia*, trans. R. M. Barclay, ed. G. M. Robertson (1921; reprint, New York: Arno Press, 1976), 179–81.

2. For a complete discussion of these animal models, see Robert Post, "Transduction of Psychosocial Stress into the Neurobiology of Recurrent Affective Disorder," *American Journal of Psychiatry* 149 (1992): 999–1010.

3. Constance Hammen and Michael Gitlin, "Stress Reactivity in Bipolar Patients and Its Relation to Prior History of Disorder," *American Journal of Psychiatry* 154 (1997): 856–57.

4. T. Treuer and M. Tohen, "Predicting the Course and Outcome of Bipolar Disorder: A Review," *European Psychiatry* 25 (2010): 328–33.

5. K. R. Jamison, R. H. Gerner, and F. K. Goodwin, "Patient and Physician Attitudes toward Lithium: Relationship to Compliance," *Archives of General Psychiatry* 36 (1979): 866–69.

6. Mario Maj, Raffaele Pirozzi, and Lorenza Magliano, "Non-response to Re-instituted Lithium Prophylaxis in Previously Responsive Bipolar Patients: Prevalence and Predictors," *American Journal of Psychiatry* 152 (1995): 1810–11. A similar study concluded that "the efficacy of lithium did not differ significantly" when it was started a second time in patients who had stopped it. But almost 13 percent of these patients needed *another* medication added to the restarted lithium to achieve remission. (This seems to me to indicate that the lithium was *not* as effective the second time around.) See Leonardo Tondo, Ross Baldessarini, Gianfranco Floris, and Nereida Rudas, "Effectiveness of Restarting Lithium Treatment after Its Discontinuation in Bipolar I and Bipolar II Patients," *American Journal of Psychiatry* 154 (1997): 548–50.

7. Erving Goffman, *Stigma: Notes on the Management of Spoiled Identity* (Englewood Cliffs, NJ: Prentice-Hall, 1963), 1, 2.

Chapter 23. Planning for Emergencies

1. E. C. Harris and B. Barraclough, "Suicide as an Outcome for Mental Disorders: A Meta-analysis," *British Journal of Psychiatry* 170 (1997): 205–28.

2. See, for example, J. E. Bailey, A. L. Kellerman, G. W. Somes, J. G. Banton, F. Rivara, and N. Rushforth, "Risk Factors for Violent Death of Women in the Home," *Archives of Internal Medicine* 157 (1997): 777–82.

3. *American Heritage Dictionary of the English Language*, 3rd ed. (New York: Houghton Mifflin, 1992).

Chapter 24. The Role of the Family

1. Kay Redfield Jamison, *An Unquiet Mind: A Memoir of Moods and Madness* (New York: Vintage Books, 1996), 120.

2. Stephen Strakowski, Susan McElroy, Paul Keck, and Scott West, "Suicidality among Patients with Mixed and Manic Bipolar Disorder," *American Journal of Psychiatry* 153 (1996): 674–76.

Chapter 25. Putting It All Together and Looking to the Future

1. DISC I is the name of a gene discovered in 1970 that is now known to code for a protein important for the development of neurons. Among other things, this protein is essential for the growth of axons and dendrites, the fibers that connect one neuron to others in the nervous system. An abnormal variation (mutation) of the gene was first identified in a family whose members had an unusually high risk of mental illness. Almost half of the family members with the mutation had schizophrenia, bipolar disorder, major depression, or another psychiatric problem. The acronym comes from *disrupted in schizophrenia* because schizophrenia was the most common illness in affected family members. Subsequent research has indicated that DISC I may be important in bipolar disorder as well.

Index

INDEX **331**